Introduction to Clinical Allied Healthcare

Second Edition

by Debra Garber, RN, BSN, MICN, EMT-P

Clinical Allied Healthcare Series

Kay Cox-Stevens, RN, MA
Series Editor

Career Publishing Inc.
Orange, CA

Series Editor and Executive Director: Kay Cox-Stevens
Senior Editor and Project Coordinator: Valerie L. Harris
Assistant Editors: Laura Mertens and Joani Saari
Illustrators: Alan J. Borie and Valerie L. Harris
   Additional Graphics obtained from the LifeART™ Collections from Techpool Studios, Inc., Cleveland, OH.
Photographs: Pages 2-13, 2-14 (top), 2-17 (bottom), 3-3, 3-5 (bottom), 4-3, 5-5, 5-8, 5-12, 7-6 through 7-10, 8-3,
   9-6, 9-14, 9-24, 9-28, 10-35, 10-38, 11-7, 11-10, 11-11, 17-6, 17-10, 18-26 courtesy K. St. Clair Garber,
   EMS Options Unlimited, Zephyr Cove, Nevada. Printed with permission.
   Additional photographs courtesy Gazelle Technologies, Inc. and PhotoDisc, Inc. Used under license.
Cover Design: Harris Graphics
Cover Photographs: (L) & (R) Courtesy K. St. Clair Garber, EMS Options Unlimited, Zephyr Cove, Nevada.
   Printed with permission.
   (Center) Courtesy Gazelle Technologies, Inc. Used under license.

This publication is designed to provide accurate and authoritative information in regard to the subject
matter covered. It is sold with the understanding that the publisher is not engaged in rendering legal,
medical or other professional service. If legal advice or other expert assistance is required, the service
of a competent professional person should be sought.

Disclaimer: Information has been obtained by Career Publishing Inc., from sources believed to be
reliable. However, because of the possibility of human or mechanical error by our sources, Career
Publishing Inc., does not guarantee the accuracy, adequacy, or completeness of any information and is
not responsible for any errors or omissions or the results obtained from the use of such information. The
publisher and editors shall not be held liable in any degree for any loss or injury by any such omission,
error, misprinting or ambiguity. If you have questions regarding the content of this publication, the
editorial staff is available to provide information and assistance.

ISBN 0-89262-551-1
Library of Congress Catalog Card Number 98-070063

PRINTED AND BOUND IN THE UNITED STATES OF AMERICA

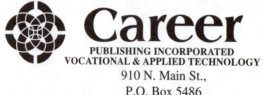

Career
PUBLISHING INCORPORATED
VOCATIONAL & APPLIED TECHNOLOGY
910 N. Main St.,
P.O. Box 5486
Orange, CA 92863-5486

National/Canada
1 (800) 854-4014
Includes Canada, Alaska,
and Hawaii

FAX 1-714-532-0180

10 9 8 7 6 5 4 3 2

Dedication

Once again, I dedicate this text to my loving husband, Kenneth, who is an exemplary role model for showing sincere compassion as well as caring for people who are ill and injured. I love you with all my heart!

This second edition is also dedicated to the loving memory of Daddy.

iv

Contents

Acknowledgements xiv

Welcome to the Student! xv

Introduction xvii

Contributors xviii

Editor's Note xix

Chapter One
Introduction to Healthcare Facilities 1-1
    Objectives 1-1
    Key Terms 1-2
    A Brief History of Healthcare Facilities 1-2
    Types of Healthcare Facilities 1-4
    Nonprofit Organizations 1-6
    Explore Your Options 1-7
    Chapter Summary 1-7
    Student Enrichment Activities 1-9

Chapter Two
The Acute Care Hospital 2-1
    Objectives 2-1
    Key Terms 2-2
    Understanding the Organizational Structure 2-2
    Types of Acute Care Hospitals 2-3
    Hospital Departments 2-5
    Administration 2-6
    Support Services 2-6
    Diagnostic Services 2-9
    Therapeutic Services 2-11
    Nursing Services 2-12
    The Hospital Environment 2-19
    Chapter Summary 2-20
    Student Enrichment Activities 2-21

Chapter Three
Hospital Employees and Medical Staff 3-1
 Objectives 3-1
 Key Terms 3-2
 Career Opportunities in Healthcare 3-2
 Assistants 3-2
 Nurses 3-3
 Health Unit Coordinators 3-5
 Doctors 3-5
 Areas of Specialty 3-7
 Chapter Summary 3-15
 Student Enrichment Activities 3-17

Chapter Four
The Allied Health Worker, the Law, and Professional Ethics 4-1
 Objectives 4-1
 Key Terms 4-2
 Patient Trust 4-2
 Scope of Practice 4-3
 Ethics 4-4
 The Patient's Bill of Rights 4-4
 Contractual Relationships 4-6
 Intentional Torts 4-8
 Consent 4-10
 Advance Directives 4-10
 Confidentiality 4-11
 AIDS and Patient Confidentiality 4-11
 Legal Terms 4-13
 National Student Health Organizations 4-14
 Chapter Summary 4-15
 Student Enrichment Activities 4-17

Chapter Five
Understanding the Patient as a Person 5-1
 Objectives 5-1
 Key Terms 5-2
 The Challenge: Understanding Your Patient 5-2
 From Infancy to Geriatrics 5-2
 Infancy 5-4
 Early Childhood 5-5
 Late Childhood 5-6
 Adolescence 5-8
 Early Adulthood 5-10
 Middle Adulthood 5-11

Late Adulthood 5-12
Stress and the Patient 5-13
Death and Dying 5-15
Chapter Summary 5-18
Student Enrichment Activities 5-19

Chapter Six
Communication Skills **6-1**
Objectives 6-1
Key Terms 6-2
The Need for Effective Communication 6-2
Senders and Receivers 6-2
Verbal and Non-Verbal Communication 6-3
Transmitting the Intended Message 6-4
Receiving the Message 6-5
Human Needs 6-8
Meeting Those Needs 6-11
Defense Mechanisms 6-12
Communication Devices 6-13
Chapter Summary 6-19
Student Enrichment Activities 6-21

Chapter Seven
The Safe Workplace **7-1**
Objectives 7-1
Key Terms 7-2
Safety at Work 7-2
Proper Body Mechanics 7-2
The Anatomy of a Healthy Back 7-3
Back Tips for Everyone 7-4
Needle Sticks 7-7
Patient Safety 7-7
Transfers 7-8
Preventing Injuries With Siderails 7-11
Preventing Falls 7-12
Patients Who Smoke 7-13
Cardiopulmonary Resuscitation (CPR) 7-14
Equipment and Safety 7-14
Electric Shock 7-15
Avoiding Chemical Injuries 7-16
Fire Safety 7-18
Chapter Summary 7-21
Student Enrichment Activities 7-23

Chapter Eight
Disasters: Preparedness, Hazards, and Prevention 8-1
   Objectives 8-1
   Key Terms 8-2
   Expecting the Unexpected 8-2
   Disaster Triage 8-2
   Disaster Preparedness 8-4
   Occupational Safety and Hazards 8-6
   Other Hazards and Potential Disasters 8-7
   Safety = Accident Prevention 8-9
   Chapter Summary 8-10
   Student Enrichment Activities 8-11

Chapter Nine
Infection Control 9-1
   Objectives 9-1
   Key Terms 9-2
   Invisible Enemies 9-2
   Centers for Disease Control and Prevention 9-3
   The Infection Control Department 9-3
   How the Infection Cycle Starts 9-4
   How to Interrupt the Infection Cycle 9-6
   Microorganisms and Disease 9-8
   Medical and Surgical Asepsis 9-10
   Handwashing—The Key to Medical Asepsis 9-11
   Disinfection 9-13
   Sterilization 9-14
   Sterile Technique 9-15
   Disposable Supplies and Infection Control 9-19
   Avoiding Contaminated Sharps 9-19
   The Risks—Hepatitis and AIDS 9-21
   Keeping Pathogens in Their Place With Isolation 9-24
   Standard and Transmission-based Precautions 9-25
   Chapter Summary 9-29
   Student Enrichment Activities 9-31

Chapter Ten
Fundamental Skills 10-1
   Objectives 10-1
   Key Terms 10-2
   The Importance of Skillfulness 10-2
   Vital Signs 10-2
   Homeostasis and Methods of Heat Loss 10-3
   Oral and Rectal Temperatures 10-3

Axillary and Tympanic Temperatures 10-14
The Pulse 10-19
Respiration 10-25
Blood Pressure 10-31
Continuous Monitoring of Blood Pressure Automatically 10-38
Weight and Height 10-41
Chapter Summary 10-45
Student Enrichment Activities 10-47

Chapter Eleven
Fundamental Patient Care Equipment 11-1
Objectives 11-1
Key Terms 11-2
The Importance of Proper Equipment
    Identification and Operation 11-2
Beds and Gurneys 11-3
Traction Devices 11-5
Ambulation Equipment 11-5
Respiratory Devices 11-7
Intravenous Therapy 11-8
Excretory Equipment 11-9
The Patient Lift 11-10
The Crash Cart 11-11
Special Patient Care Items 11-11
The Patient Care Unit 11-12
Chapter Summary 11-15
Student Enrichment Activities 11-17

Chapter Twelve
Introduction to Medical Terminology 12-1
Objectives 12-1
Key Terms 12-2
The Importance of Accurate Terminology 12-2
Determining the Meaning 12-2
The Word Elements 12-4
Abbreviations for Use in Documentation 12-14
Symbols 12-21
Chapter Summary 12-21
Student Enrichment Activities 12-23

Chapter Thirteen
An Introduction to the Human Body 13-1
   Objectives 13-1
   Key Terms 13-2
   Understanding Human Body Function 13-2
   Cells: The Basis of Life 13-2
   Tissues 13-5
   Body Planes and Directional Terms 13-7
   The Body Cavities 13-9
   Chapter Summary 13-10
   Student Enrichment Activities 13-11

Chapter Fourteen
Support, Movement, and Protection:
The Skeletal, Muscular, and Integumentary Systems 14-1
   Objectives 14-1
   Key Terms 14-2
   The Systems That Shape Our Bodies 14-2
   The Skeletal System and Joints 14-2
   Disorders of the Skeletal System 14-5
   Diagnostic Tests for the Skeletal System 14-5
   Joints: Articulation and Movement 14-6
   Diseases and Injuries of the Joints 14-6
   Diagnostic Tests for Joints 14-8
   The Muscular System 14-8
   Muscular Diseases 14-13
   Diagnostic Tests for the Muscular System 14-13
   The Integumentary System 14-14
   Skin Diseases and Disorders 14-17
   Diagnostic Tests for the Skin 14-18
   Chapter Summary 14-18
   Student Enrichment Activities 14-19

Chapter Fifteen
Transporting and Transmitting:
The Circulatory, Lymphatic, and Nervous Systems 15-1
   Objectives 15-1
   Key Terms 15-2
   The Body's Transportation Systems 15-2
   The Circulatory System 15-2
   Blood Vessels 15-3
   Blood and Blood Cells 15-4
   The Pump of Life 15-6
   The Circulatory Path 15-8

Conditions of the Circulatory System 15-10
Diagnostic Tests for the Circulatory System 15-11
The Lymphatic System 15-12
Conditions of the Lymphatic System 15-14
Diagnostic Tests for the Lymphatic System 15-14
The Nervous System 15-14
The Central Nervous System 15-16
The Peripheral Nervous System 15-18
Nervous System Conditions 15-20
Diagnostic Tests for the Nervous System 15-21
Chapter Summary 15-21
Student Enrichment Activities 15-23

Chapter Sixteen
 Excretion: The Respiratory, Digestive, and Urinary Systems 16-1
Objectives 16-1
Key Terms 16-2
Excretion: The Body's Disposal Systems 16-2
The Respiratory System 16-2
The Breathing Process 16-5
Conditions of the Lung and Associated Structures 16-6
Diagnostic Tests for the Respiratory System 16-7
The Digestive System 16-8
Diagnostic Tests for the Alimentary Canal 16-12
The Accessory Organs 16-13
Diagnostic Tests for the Accessory Organs 16-15
The Urinary System 16-16
Conditions Affecting the Urinary System 16-19
Diagnostic Tests for the Urinary System 16-20
Chapter Summary 16-21
Student Enrichment Activities 16-23

Chapter Seventeen
 The Specialties: The Sensory, Endocrine, and Reproductive Systems ... 17-1
Objectives 17-1
Key Terms 17-2
The Special Systems 17-2
The Sensory System 17-2
The Eye 17-3
Diagnosing Problems of the Eye 17-6
The Ear 17-7
Diagnostic Tests for the Inner Ear 17-10
Taste, Smell, and Touch 17-11
The Endocrine System 17-12

Diagnostic Tests for the Endocrine System 17-15
The Reproductive System 17-16
The Female 17-16
Diseases and Abnormal Conditions of the
    Female Reproductive System 17-19
Diagnostic Procedures for the Female Reproductive System 17-20
The Male 17-20
Diseases of the Male Reproductive System 17-22
Diagnostic Tests for the Male Reproductive System 17-23
Chapter Summary 17-23
Student Enrichment Activities 17-25

Chapter Eighteen
Basic First Aid **18-1**
Objectives 18-1
Key Terms 18-2
Skilled First Aid: It Saves Lives 18-2
Guidelines for Administering First Aid 18-3
The Primary Survey: Technique and Intervention 18-3
CPR for Adults 18-9
Foreign Body Airway Obstruction in the Adult Patient 18-10
Pediatric Basic Life Support 18-11
CPR for Children and Infants 18-12
Airway Obstruction in Children and Infants 18-15
Controlling Bleeding 18-17
The Secondary Survey: Patient Re-Assessment 18-19
Management of Shock 18-20
Seizures 18-22
Chest Pain 18-23
Shortness of Breath 18-24
Syncope 18-25
The Unconscious Patient 18-26
Poisoning 18-33
Burns 18-35
Sprains and Fractures 18-37
Epistaxis: Nosebleeds 18-39
Soft Tissue Injuries 18-40
Chapter Summary 18-42
Student Enrichment Activities 18-43

Chapter Nineteen
Healthful Living **19-1**
    Objectives 19-1
    Key Terms 19-2
    A Longer and Healthier Life 19-2
    Smoking: It Takes Our Breath Away! 19-3
    Hypertension 19-4
    The Use of Drugs and Alcohol 19-5
    Effective Stress Management 19-6
    The Healthy Diet 19-7
    A Word About Cholesterol 19-14
    The Value of Exercise 19-15
    Chapter Summary 19-17
    Student Enrichment Activities 19-19

Chapter Twenty
Career Planning **20-1**
    Objectives 20-1
    Key Terms 20-2
    Planning for Success 20-2
    Where Do I Start? 20-2
    Selling Yourself: The First Impression 20-4
    Writing the Resumé 20-7
    Organizing the Resumé 20-8
    Formatting the Document 20-10
    The Cover Letter 20-12
    The All-Important Interview 20-14
    The Ideal Employee 20-16
    Chapter Summary 20-18
    Student Enrichment Activities 20-19

Appendix A
Glossary .... **Appendix A-1**

Appendix B
The Manual Alphabet .... **Appendix B-1**

Appendix C
Bibliography .... **Appendix C-1**

Appendix D
Index .... **Appendix D-1**

Acknowledgements

The author would like to thank everyone who graciously contributed to the formation of this text. The contributions of the following are particularly appreciated.

Kay Cox-Stevens, RN, MA, Series Editor and Executive Director, for her "vision" for this series, and in particular, for her support, encouragement, and meticulous review and technical editing of the manuscript.

Valerie Harris, Project Coordinator and Senior Editor for this series, for her mechanical and substantive editing of the manuscript, as well as coordinating the production of the book.

Harold Haase, Publisher, and the rest of the staff at Career Publishing, Inc. for recognizing the need for proper entry-level training in the rapidly changing field of healthcare, and for responding to the need in such an enthusiastic manner.

The Staff of EMS Options Unlimited, for their time and expertise in staging many of the photographs, and particularly, Mr. Kenneth S. Garber, President, for his excellent photography and guidance.

Joan, Nancy, and Vikki for their sisterly support and never-ending encouragement. We're in perfect harmony!

And most of all, thank you to my loving family: my husband, Kenneth S. Garber, for his love, never-ending support, and professional knowledge; my children, Jennifer and Brian Taylor, for their love and support, and most of all, for their friendship; Mom and Dad, for "putting up" with all my questions, especially, "Why?" and "How come?" as I grew; and to my Father, for guiding and directing my life, and for always being the same.

Welcome to the Student!

Congratulations on your decision to become a team member of one of the most challenging and exciting professions available! WELCOME to the world of allied healthcare providers!

Caring for the sick and the injured is one of the most rewarding professions with which to be associated. The opportunities to provide care to patients, increase your skills and knowledge, and advance to other positions are virtually limitless.

As you begin your career as an allied healthcare worker keep in mind that whatever entry level position you select, it takes a special kind of person to join the team of dedicated allied healthcare workers. An allied healthcare worker must be reliable, trustworthy, trainable, skillful, flexible, and respectful of other people.

Remember, you are at the beginning of a satisfying and fulfilling career. The work will be hard and demanding; however, the satisfaction from knowing you touched the lives of others in a special way gives you THE reason to keep giving.

After you have mastered the concepts and technical skills offered in this course, you will be able to provide competent care and services that will be appreciated by everyone. BE PROUD OF YOURSELF! People involved in all areas of the medical field are very special people!

As you begin to study the concepts involved in delivering healthcare, be aware that feelings of anxiety, inadequacy, and even fear are common. However, as you explore and study the specific topics in this textbook, your self-confidence will increase.

As you examine the many different facets of allied healthcare, there will be other people available to you who have a wide range of knowledge and experience. They will be willing to assist you and answer any questions you may have. Do not be afraid to ask questions! THE FIELD OF HEALTHCARE IS NOT THE PLACE TO GUESS OR ASSUME ANYTHING! You are responsible for providing care to people who are depending on you for high quality, competent care!

The topics in this core text are included because they provide basic knowledge that is common to a variety of allied healthcare positions. Chapter objectives and key terms are provided for you at the beginning of each chapter. These will enhance your reading and highlight points that will help you in your health career. As you continue in this core text, concentrate on meeting the chapter objectives and on learning all the key terms and their definitions. By doing this, you will form the basis of a firm foundation in health occupations. To further assist you, words that appear in the glossary are in boldface type throughout the text.

This instructional series includes textbooks for specific allied healthcare positions. Those books are to be used in addition to the core text. Please ask your instructor if you have any questions about the textbook material or any of the allied healthcare positions.

Introduction

To work in the medical field is to make a real contribution to your fellow man. This is a career that will ask much of your mind and heart and give much in return. The satisfaction gained from calming a frightened child or brightening the day of a lonely patient will enrich you. The pride felt will be lasting when your observations and skills someday help to save a patient's life. This is a career where you can really make a difference!

Some of you have already made a decision to seek a career in some area of healthcare. Some of you are just exploring your options. Everything you learn will build a foundation of skills and knowledge, so learn well. Become competent in everything you are taught along the way and be your own task master. We all must be responsible for our own education. If at some point you discover you didn't learn a skill well enough, go back and practice until you do. Remember, some day a patient's life may depend on you and your mastery of what you are taught.

Today's healthcare industry places many demands on care givers. We must keep costs down, document everything we do, and have more knowledge and skills than ever before because of new technology. This textbook series was designed to help you build a sound foundation of knowledge and provide many opportunities for cross-training. This core textbook contains the skills and information we feel is common to all students. Each of the other textbooks provide training for a specific job title. The more you can learn, the better. Always remember, however, to practice the art, the science, and the SPIRIT of your new career. Good luck!

Kay Cox-Stevens, RN, MA
Series Editor

Contributors

About the Author

Debra L. Garber, RN, BSN, MICN, EMT-P received her Bachelor of Science in Nursing degree from California State University, Bakersfield in 1977. She has 28 years total experience in the Medical and Nursing fields since beginning her career in 1970 by serving as a candy striper. Mrs. Garber has served as a Charge Nurse in various hospital departments including Medical-Surgical, Telemetry, Intensive Care and Coronary Care Units, Pediatrics, Orthopedics, and the Emergency Department. Mrs. Garber is a Mobile Intensive Care Nurse with over 18 years experience. She continues to maintain her Public Health Nurse certification, performs as an expert witness, and performs as a legal nurse consultant.

Mrs. Garber also received recognition as an Outstanding Cardiac Educator from the Central California Heart Institute in 1992 and was nominated as *RN of the Year* in 1993. Currently, Mrs. Garber continues to work as a clinical nurse. She offers her professional services as an allied healthcare education consultant and personal tutor. She also provides clinical precepting services for students of allied health. In addition, Mrs. Garber has served as Chairperson of the California Rescue and Paramedic Association, CRPA, and is active with the American Heart Association for both Basic Cardiac Life Support and Advanced Cardiac Life Support.

About the Series Editor

Kay Cox-Stevens, RN, MA conceived this textbook series, and recruited and coordinated the authors in the development of each of their texts. She is the author of *Being a Health Unit Coordinator,* and the editor of a Medical-Clerical Textbook Series for Brady. Before entering education, she worked in medical/surgical and critical care nursing and in the inservice department as a clinical instructor.

Formerly a Professional Development Contract Consultant for special projects and curriculum development for the California Department of Education, Professor Cox-Stevens has also served as chairperson of the California Health Careers Statewide Advisory Committee, and been a Master Trainer for Health Careers Teacher Training through California Polytechnic University of Pomona. She also is a founding member of the National Association of Health Unit Coordinators. Professor Cox-Stevens is currently Program Coordinator of the Medical Assistant Program at Saddleback College in Mission Viejo, California, and operates her consulting business, Achiever's Development Enterprises.

Editor's Note

I would like to take this opportunity to thank the authors of this series. Their dedication and sense of mission made it a joy to work on this challenging project.

I would also like to express my sincere gratitude to the staff of Career Publishing, Inc. and most particularly to Valerie Harris, Senior Editor, for her professional and talented assistance throughout. I also would like to express my appreciation to Harold Haase, Publisher, for his enthusiasm for this project and for his humanistic approach to education.

Kay Cox-Stevens, RN, MA
Series Editor

Chapter One
Introduction to Healthcare Facilities

Objectives

After completing this chapter you should be able to do the following:

1. Define and correctly spell each of the key terms.

2. Name the most important aspect of quality patient care.

3. Briefly describe the historical perspective of healthcare facilities.

4. Identify at least two current trends in modern healthcare.

5. Describe at least three services offered by nonprofit organizations.

Key Terms

- acute
- asepsis
- chronic

- contagious
- hospitalis
- nonprofit agency

A Brief History of Healthcare Facilities

hospitalis:
a Latin word meaning a house or institution for guests

Perhaps the most familiar type of healthcare facility is the hospital. The term *hospital* comes from the Latin word **hospitalis**, which means a house or institution for guests. Now, of course, a hospital describes an institution where the sick and/or injured are given medical or surgical care.

Buddhists had established hospitals in India as early as 200 BC. During the early part of the Christian Era, hospitals were available for those who were crippled, sick, or weary from travelling.

In the beginning, hospitals served as places to care for those who were too poor or too ill to be treated at home. At that time, doctors provided care to patients in their homes or at the doctor's office. Doctors did not work in the hospitals.

asepsis:
a condition in which no pathogen, infection, or any form of life is present

Hospital construction increased in many European towns and cities during the 1700s. Early hospitals did not look like today's hospital facilities; most were dark, overcrowded, and dirty. The concept of **asepsis** was unknown at that time. Asepsis is vital to the prevention of infection. Because of the unsanitary conditions, poor people and those with **contagious** diseases were usually the only patients treated at the hospital. Back then, people who could afford it received their medical care in their homes because homes were much cleaner than the hospitals.

contagious:
capable of being transferred from one person to another, either directly or indirectly

In the 1800s, many medical discoveries greatly improved the quality of hospital care. For example, ether (an anesthetic) was used for the first time in 1842. During the latter part of the 1800s, asepsis increased the chances of recovery for patients in the hospital. In fact, asepsis became so much better in the hospital than in the home environment, the popularity of home healthcare began to decline.

In addition to the concept of asepsis, x-ray equipment began to be used in the hospitals beginning in the late 1890s. The x-ray machine takes a picture of a patient's body part, such as the hand, and produces a black and white picture that shows all of the bones and soft tissues (fleshy parts). This allows doctors to look inside the body and determine if, and where, a bone is broken, making it possible for doctors to provide more specific medical treatment to patients. These advances in patient care, along with the establishment of private rooms for patients, promoted additional hospital growth in the 1900s.

With the new century came more advancements. Health insurance plans, community health clinics, hospital-sponsored programs for alcohol and drug abuse, and ambulatory surgery centers all increased the quality and efficiency of healthcare. Furthermore, to reduce the problem of overcrowding in hospitals, the government provided grants for the construction of more hospitals.

Scientific progress has also improved patient care in several areas. For example, Intensive Care Units use electronically-advanced equipment to monitor **vital signs** and heart rhythms, and computers store voluminous records including medical, pharmacy, and laboratory test results. Additionally, hospitals now use *single use* items such as plastic syringes and needles, basins, bedpans, thermometers, and oxygen equipment. These items reduce the spread of germs because they are thrown away after a single use.

Due to the complexity of today's diseases, hospitals have had to purchase advanced diagnostic equipment such as a computerized tomography scanner, magnetic resonance imager, and ultrasonography. Some hospitals have become specialized in providing care to a particular type of patient (ie, children's hospitals, women's hospitals, and hospitals for the developmentally disabled).

Despite all the technical and scientific advances in the field of medicine, THE HEALTHCARE WORKER IS STILL THE MOST IMPORTANT ASPECT OF QUALITY PATIENT CARE. Patients are still people!

Types of Healthcare Facilities

This century has witnessed the establishment of many different types of healthcare facilities. This section will briefly describe several of the most common types.

Acute care facilities, usually hospitals, provide care to patients who require short-term healthcare. These types of patients have medical conditions that are **acute**, meaning that the symptoms are usually severe and the onset is frequently rapid. The length of a patient's stay in an acute care facility depends upon the diagnosis and the type of insurance he or she has. Sometimes, patients only require a few hours of treatment from these facilities.

acute:
sudden onset;
short duration

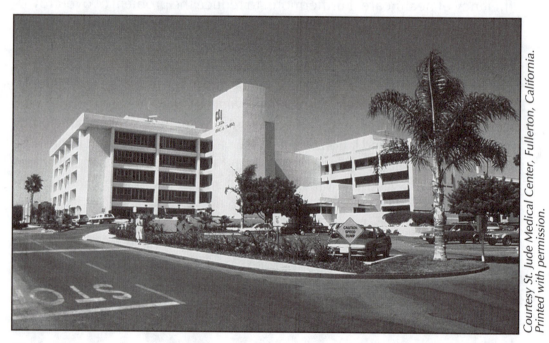

Courtesy St. Jude Medical Center, Fullerton, California. Printed with permission.

Figure 1-1: Acute care facilities offer many career opportunities in healthcare.

If a patient's condition requires extended medical care, then an **extended** or **long-term care facility** would be the appropriate healthcare facility. Usually, the majority of patients in this type of facility are elderly. Patients in a long-term care facility often have a **chronic** disease. This classification describes a disease that shows little change or that progresses slowly. Examples of long-term care facilities are **convalescent hospitals** (facilities where patients are admitted after the acute phase of an illness or injury for recovery), **rehabilitation facilities**

chronic:
slow to develop;
persisting for a
long time

(specialized facilities that assist patients in regaining maximum function and a level of independence after surgery, traumatic injuries, or illness), and **skilled nursing facilities**.

Patients in a skilled nursing facility require the availability of continuous services such as intravenous feedings, gastrostomy tube feedings, injections, or dressing changes. The services of skilled nurses are available at all times. A skilled nursing facility must have the following services: physician, skilled nursing, dietary, and pharmaceutical. The facility also must have an activity program.

Health clinics are usually formed by several doctors sharing a common building. Most counties have at least one clinic that provides healthcare services either free or for a relatively low fee. This clinic is usually associated with the Public Health Department of that county. Another type of clinic is called an **outpatient clinic**. This type of facility allows patients to be treated or have tests completed without being admitted to the facility. Outpatient clinics may be located in hospitals or surgery centers.

Medical offices provide medical care according to the doctor's specific type of education and training. For example, lung diseases are usually diagnosed and treated by a pulmonary specialist; kidney diseases are frequently treated by a nephrologist, and general health ailments are diagnosed and treated by a family practitioner, or general practitioner.

There are a variety of **community healthcare facilities**. Two of the most common types are **mental healthcare facilities** and **home health agencies**. Mental healthcare facilities provide care to people experiencing emotional and psychological dysfunction. The home health agency provides extended health-care and treatment to patients in their homes. Since today's patients are being discharged after minimal time in the hospital, the number of home health agencies is increasing rapidly.

Another important trend of healthcare today is the establishment of **urgent care centers**. These facilities offer non-emergency care for broken bones, sprains, colds, and flu. They also provide physical examinations for school, employment, and camp. These centers have relieved some of the burden from the hospital emergency departments, making them more able to treat patients with life-threatening problems.

Health maintenance organizations (HMOs) have existed for decades. However, in the 1980s, there was an explosion of insurance plans provided by HMOs. These insurance plans became popular because they offered employers a less expensive way to provide health insurance for their employees. HMOs provide prepaid comprehensive healthcare to enrolled members at a fixed rate, regardless of the utilization of services. When payment is made in this manner it is called **capitation**. This type of organization provides healthcare that is directed mainly toward the prevention of disease. Services include patient health education, basic medical services, physical examinations, and pharmaceutical services. Because health maintenance organizations are prepaid, costs to the patient are minimal or, in some cases, nonexistent. Examples of HMOs include Kaiser Permanente, FHP, Secure Horizons, and Health Net.

Nonprofit Organizations

nonprofit agency: an organization that is supported only by contributions

Nonprofit agencies are organizations that are supported only by contributions. They offer educational health services in the form of seminars, newsletters, classes, and literature at the national, state, and local levels.

Examples of nonprofit organizations include the American Heart Association, the American Red Cross, the American Lung Association, the American Cancer Society, the National Foundation of the March of Dimes, and Mothers Against Drunk Driving. Many of the hospitals are classified as nonprofit agencies. These agencies are devoted to research, raising funds for research, and promoting public education for a specific disease or societal problem. The specific organizations usually are involved with victims of that illness by purchasing medical equipment and supplies, assisting with treatment costs, and providing treatment centers.

Nonprofit organizations employ many volunteers and healthcare workers to assist in providing services to the public. These organizations are valuable resources for clinical healthcare workers!

Explore Your Options

Since there are so many types of healthcare facilities, today's healthcare workers have a lot of options available to them. And don't forget, these are just a few examples! There are other areas of healthcare to explore including Industrial Health, School Health, and more.

This instructional course will provide you with the information and skills that are necessary to be a clinical (direct patient caregiver), allied healthcare worker. There are other career options available which do not involve direct patient care, such as in the Medical Records Department, the Business Office, and various hospital departments doing reception and clerical work. The skills and the knowledge you gain from this course will be useful in a variety of the healthcare settings. Hospitals value workers who have multiple skills (cross-training), so continue to learn new things whenever you can.

Chapter Summary

The purpose of this first chapter was to provide you with a brief history of healthcare facilities, and to introduce you to several types of healthcare facilities. This chapter also furnished a brief description of nonprofit organizations, a valuable resource for clinical allied healthcare workers.

Name _____

Date _____

Student Enrichment Activities

Complete the following statements.

1. The term *hospital* is derived from the Latin word, _____, which means an institution for guests.

2. During the _____, most hospitals were dark, overcrowded, and dirty.

3. _____ is a condition in which no pathogen, infection, or any form of life is present.

4. X-rays were introduced in the late _____.

5. The _____ _____ is the most important aspect of quality patient care.

6. The _____ _____ _____ are hospitals that provide short-term healthcare to patients.

7. An extended care facility in which skilled nursing services are available at all times is called a _____ _____ _____.

8. Patients with a slow-progressing illness are often cared for in a _____ _____ _____.

9. _____ _____ _____ provide non-emergency care.

10. A prepaid healthcare plan that is directed toward healthcare prevention is called a _____ _____ _____.

11. Organizations that are supported only through contributions are

    _____ _____.

Unscramble the following terms.

12. TALHSIOPSI   _____

13. LICIYATF   _____

14. EMNATL TEHLAH   _____ _____

15. EIDCLMA FOFCEI   _____ _____

16. TRNOINPFO   _____

17. GRUINNS   _____

18. TRENGU   _____

19. ITEANNAMECN   _____

20. MUTYNOMIC   _____

21. TRAINONAZOIG   _____

22. PASSESI   _____

23. NYCAGE   _____

24. LKESILD USIGRNN   _____ _____

Chapter Two
The Acute Care Hospital

Objectives

After completing this chapter you should be able to do the following:

1. Define and correctly spell each of the key terms.

2. Explain the purpose of the organizational structure of a healthcare facility.

3. List and describe the main function of at least five types of acute care hospitals.

4. Briefly explain the main functions of four general classifications of hospital departments.

5. Identify at least six branches of Nursing Services and describe the type of care they provide.

6. Name two of the most serious infections to which healthcare workers may be exposed.

Key Terms

- chain of command
- critical care
- myocardial infarction

- rooming-in
- sterilization
- wellness

Understanding the Organizational Structure

This chapter will focus on the healthcare facility known as an **acute care hospital**. This type of facility commonly provides care to patients who have an **acute** health condition that requires short-term medical, nursing, and allied healthcare services. This chapter describes several types of acute care hospitals and discusses the organizational structure of a hospital. It is important to understand the general organizational structure of this type of facility because it helps you understand the **chain of command**. In other words, it shows you the person or department accountable for each area of responsibility. This way, if you have a question or a problem, you know who is in charge.

chain of command: the organizational structure of a given healthcare facility that indicates the person or department responsible for every aspect of the facility's day-to-day operations

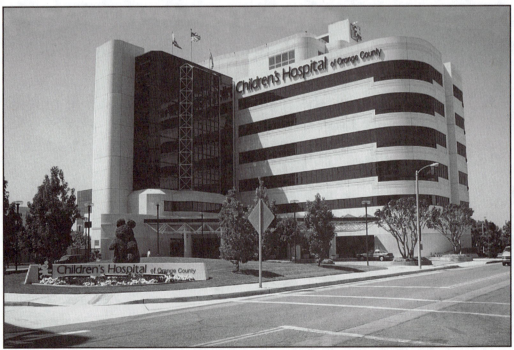

Courtesy Terry Whitener, Hacienda Heights, California. Printed with permission.

Figure 2-1: An Acute Care Hospital

Furthermore, a good understanding of the main function of each department will make you an asset to patient care and to the overall hospital operation, as well as provide you with insight regarding career opportunities.

If you are working in a large, complex facility, the organizational structure will also be complex. Similarly, a small facility is likely to have a simpler structure. The efficient healthcare worker makes a positive contribution to any hospital, regardless of its size or organization.

Types of Acute Care Hospitals

Most of the acute care hospitals in the United States are **general hospitals**. This type of facility provides care to people with all kinds of medical conditions regardless of their age. Many general acute care hospitals are educational institutions. These institutions often contain a school of medicine and provide a learning atmosphere for the students. These are frequently part of the state university system.

Providing medical care to a more specific group of people is a **women's hospital**. This type of facility offers childbirth services and provides care to females with **gynecological** diseases. These diseases may affect the uterus, ovaries, fallopian tubes, cervix, vagina, and the breasts. These specific anatomical and physiological terms are thoroughly discussed in Chapter Seventeen.

Pediatrics has become a very **specialized** area in medicine. The word *specialized* means that specific training, in addition to the general training, is recommended, or even required, in order to competently provide care in a particular area of medicine or nursing. Pediatrics usually refers to care given to patients from birth to 18 years of age. Today, however, an infant from birth to 1 month of age is called a **neonate.** Pediatric hospitals often provide a Neonatology Unit with specially trained personnel available to provide care to these very special patients.

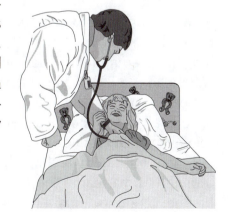

Cardiac intervention centers are a relatively new type of healthcare facility. They provide care to patients with cardiac disease. Cardiac diseases affect the heart and the heart vessels, frequently referred to as coronary vessels. Cardiac intervention centers usually include a Cardiac Catheterization Laboratory, a Critical Care Unit, a Transitional Care Unit, Cardiac Rehabilitation Services, and **surgical suites**. **Cardiac Catheterization Laboratories** usually perform procedures such as cardiac catheterization and a type of angioplasty. Both of these procedures involve the insertion of a catheter (a teflon tube), through a vein to the coronary vessels. Cardiac catheterization permits a doctor to see the number of coronary vessels that are occluded (blocked). Percutaneous transluminal coronary angioplasty (PTCA) allows the doctor to reach the area of occlusion and decrease the size of the blockage using a catheter with a balloon which is inflated directly against the occlusion. This actually *compresses* the occlusion, thereby opening that area of the vessel and permitting increased blood flow to the heart muscle. **Critical Care Units** contain special equipment and specially trained personnel to provide care to patients with diseases of the cardiac system. A **Transitional Care Unit** (TCU), which is also known as a Direct Observation Unit (DOU), is equipped to monitor a patient's heart rhythm and provide emergency cardiac care if needed. However, the patient is usually allowed to walk around and is frequently discharged from the hospital within a few days.

Cardiac rehabilitation is a service offered to cardiac patients that assists them with proper exercise therapy, dietetic counseling, and stress reduction. During the exercise phase, patients are observed by trained staff members who monitor their heart as they perform various exercises. Cardiac rehab, as it is frequently called, offers encouragement and hope to those who are recovering from open heart surgery or a **myocardial infarction (MI)**.

myocardial infarction: a heart attack; a condition caused by the blockage of one or more coronary arteries

In the 1980s, **trauma centers** were created. These facilities contain departments that employ highly skilled and trained personnel as well as advanced diagnostic equipment. They often provide a **helipad** for an air ambulance. A helipad is a landing area that is designed for a helicopter that transports patients to or from the trauma center. The helipad is constructed according to federal, state, and local rules and regulations. The trauma center also contains an **Emergency Department** (ED), also called an Emergency Room (ER), that has highly technical, lifesaving equipment and an appropriately trained trauma team. The Emergency Department is where patients with life-threatening or limb-threatening conditions receive medical care. Additional information on careers in the Emergency Department may be obtained from *The Emergency Department Technician* in this series.

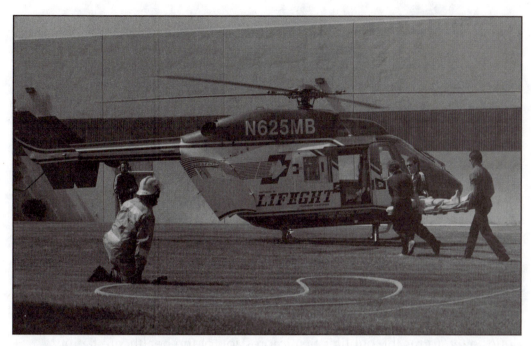

Figure 2-2: Helicopters are sometimes used to transport critically injured patients to a trauma center for care.

As medicine becomes more sophisticated and increasingly specialized, acute care hospitals that provide general medical, nursing, and allied healthcare services will become more rare. Instead, there will be an increase in the number and types of specialized acute care hospitals, designed and staffed to enjoy the benefits of advancing technology.

Hospital Departments

Different departments are responsible for specific areas of patient care and hospital function. These departments enable the healthcare facility to operate smoothly and efficiently.

At first, the organization of a hospital may seem complicated. However, you will find that each of the various departments can be grouped under one of the following general categories: Administration, Support Services, Diagnostic Services, Therapeutic Services, and Nursing. Analysis of these categories will help you understand how each department affects the efficiency of a healthcare facility.

Administration

Administrative Services include several specific departments: Admissions, Central Purchasing, Billing, and Collections. Each one provides a particular service concerned with the financial operations of the hospital.

One of the most important departments in the Administrative Services is the **Admissions**, or **Admitting**, **Department**. It is often the public's first contact with hospital personnel and procedures. Admitting personnel are responsible for obtaining such vital information as the patient's name, address, telephone number, admitting doctor's name, the admitting diagnosis, personal identification information (social security number), date of birth, and all insurance information. Frequently, Admissions also is responsible for patient room assignments. Whenever a patient is discharged, the Admissions Department does all the necessary paperwork to officially release the patient from the hospital. The efficiency with which the admissions clerk performs his or her duties often forms the public's first impression of the healthcare facility.

In some hospitals, the **Purchasing Department** is part of Administrative Services, or it may be included under Support Services. The primary purpose of this department is to buy and store all hospital supplies. It is important for all hospital personnel to be familiar with this department's ordering procedures.

Other branches in Administrative Services include the Billing and Collections Departments. These departments bill the patients for services rendered, interface with insurance companies, and make sure the money is collected.

Support Services

Several hospital departments fall under the heading of **Support Services**. Support Services provide maintenance and support for the overall function of the hospital. For example, the Business Office is a vital part of the hospital. It is through this department that monetary deposits are collected. In larger hospitals, this department is separate from the Admitting Office; however, in the smaller hospitals, both of these offices may be combined. Throughout the course of a normal day in the hospital, patients are often transported to different departments by the Transportation Department. Transporters take patients from their hospital room to departments such as X-ray, Physical Therapy, and other diagnostic or therapeutic departments. Transportation saves the nursing staff the time of moving the patient from one area of the hospital to another.

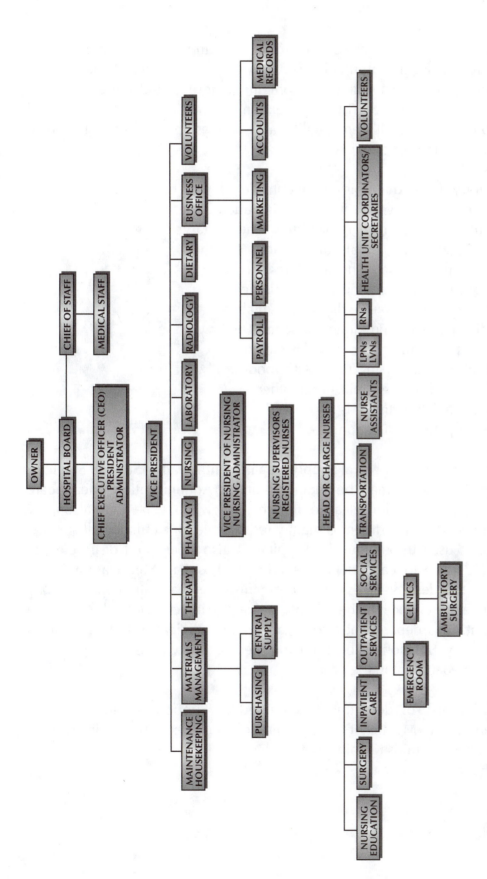

Figure 2-3: The Organizational Structure of a Large Acute Care Hospital

Every patient who receives services from a healthcare facility must have a medical record. Health Information Services (the Medical Records Department of the hospital) is responsible for compiling, storing, and retrieving every patient's medical record. This is an extremely important part of the legal operations of the healthcare facility and utilizes the services of clerical personnel and transcriptionists.

The **Dietary Department** is often considered part of Support Services; however, it may be included under Therapeutic Services in many facilities. The Dietary Department prepares meals and snacks for the patients of the hospital. The registered dietician frequently provides teaching and instruction to patients who are on a special diet such as diabetics, cardiac patients, and kidney patients. The Dietary Department is also responsible for stocking all of the nursing units with food items such as crackers, milk, and other beverages. This department is a valuable resource for patient education.

In some hospitals, the **Central Supply Department** is part of Support Services. In other facilities it may be included under Administration. Healthcare facilities cannot function at an optimum level without the Central Supply Department. This department is mainly responsible for sterilizing all surgical instruments used throughout the hospital. It also stocks and distributes all nursing supplies to each department in the hospital. **Sterilization** is the procedure that destroys all living microorganisms on that instrument. Sterilization reduces the chances of the patient receiving an infection from the use of the instrument. This department also organizes the surgical instruments into a particular combination to be used for specific procedures. This is a very important department in the hospital.

sterilization: the complete destruction of all forms of microbial life

Other examples of departments included in Support Services may be Engineering and Maintenance, Communications, Security, Environmental Services, and Grounds Keeping.

Diagnostic Services

The word **diagnosis** is defined as the use of scientific and skillful methods to establish the cause and nature of an individual's illness. With the data, or results, from diagnostic tests, a physician is able to provide a logical plan of treatment and care for the patient. **Diagnostic Services** includes many areas of the hospital; however, only a few will be discussed in detail.

The **Laboratory** is frequently one of the busiest departments in an acute care hospital. This important department provides valuable diagnostic information by analyzing blood, body secretions, and tissue samples. The Laboratory also obtains each patient's blood sample and performs specific tests on it. The Laboratory also is responsible for testing blood for blood transfusions. The data is then provided to the medical and nursing personnel providing direct care to that patient. Additional information on careers in the Laboratory may be obtained from *The Clinical Laboratory Assistant/ Phlebotomist* in this series.

The **Radiology**, or **Imaging Department**, provides valuable diagnostic information for the doctor by using **radioactive** substances such as x-rays and chemicals. A radioactive substance emits **radiation**; it releases rays of energy in different directions from a common point. X-rays use radiation to create a photograph of a targeted area of the body. The photograph can then be used to determine if a bone is **fractured** or broken. This diagnostic area is often referred to as the X-ray Department.

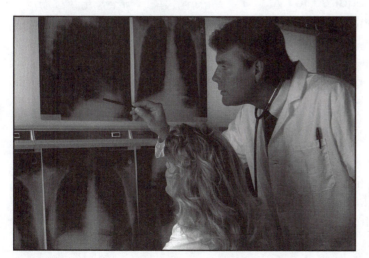

Figure 2-4: X-rays can be used to diagnose problems related to the bones and various internal structures.

Radiology, or Medical Imaging, may have a subspecialty area used for treatments such as **radiation therapy** for the treatment of cancer. Extremely high doses of radiation are used in the therapeutic control of cancer. Other divisions of the Radiology Department are **nuclear medicine**, computerized tomography and **magnetic resonance imaging** (**MRI**). These divisions provide the doctor with more in-depth diagnostic information than a simple **x-ray** can provide.

In some hospitals, several smaller departments are often included under Diagnostic Services. For example, personnel may perform tests such as **electrocardiograms**, called **EKGs** or **ECGs**, and **electroencephalograms**, or

EEGs. The electrocardiogram is a visual picture of the electrical activity of the heart. This test helps the doctor determine cardiac rhythm and detect myocardial damage. Another test that may be performed is the **stress test**. This test is a method of evaluating cardiovascular fitness. Usually, the patient rides a stationary bike or uses a treadmill during this test. (See Figure 2-5.) While the patient is exercising, his or her EKG is monitored, and the heart rate, blood pressure, and oxygen consumption are evaluated. If there are any abnormalities, the test is discontinued. Additional information about a career as an electrocardiograph technician may be obtained in *The Electrocardiograph Technician* in this series.

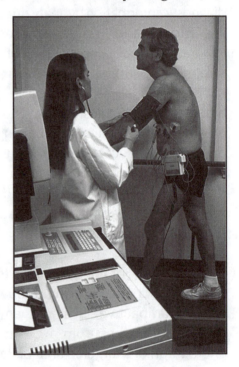

Figure 2-5: A stress test is one way of evaluating a patient's cardiovascular fitness.

Some patients may be required to wear a special portable heart monitor called a **Holter Monitor**. This evaluates a patient's heart activity for 24 hours. Then, the doctor can interpret the data, a continuous ECG showing the patient's heart activity during the course of the patient's normal day, and diagnose any abnormalities.

Electroencephalograms, or EEGs, provide the doctor with a visual picture of the electrical activity of the brain. They are often used to help the doctor determine why a patient may be having seizures and to localize lesions in the brain. There may be other tests available through this department too. Allied healthcare workers can learn a lot from this department.

Therapeutic Services

Departments included in Therapeutic Services provide a form of therapy for patients. These departments may vary between healthcare facilities. The **Physical Therapy Department** is one of the most widely prescribed forms of therapy for patients. It has become quite important to the recovery and **rehabilitation** of the patient. This area of rehabilitation deals with restoring function and preventing disability following disease, injury, or loss of a body part. A **physical therapist** is a trained individual who uses therapeutic treatments such as heat, cold, electricity, exercise, massage, and ultraviolet light to improve circulation, strengthen muscles, and improve the range of motion in joints. (Figure 2-6) Each of these methods can be used to help train or retrain a patient to perform his or her daily activities. Additional information on careers in Physical Therapy may be obtained from *Introduction to Sports Medicine and Physical Therapy: The Athletic Trainer, Personal Fitness Trainer and Physical Therapy Aide* in this series.

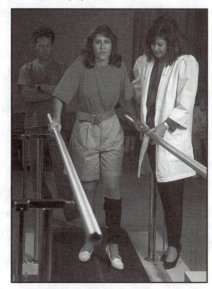

Figure 2-6: Physical therapy helps prevent disability following a disease or injury.

The **Respiratory Therapy Department** provides treatment to those for whom breathing is difficult. A **respiratory therapist** can give the patient breathing treatments in which he or she teaches the patient how to do specific breathing exercises. Often, the therapist can also provide a highly technical piece of equipment, called a **respirator**, for patients who are unable to breathe without mechanical assistance.

The **Pharmacy** provides the medications that have been prescribed by the patients' physicians. The **pharmacist** is an excellent resource when questions arise concerning types of medicine, dose, route of giving the medication, side effects, and **contraindications** of particular drugs. Throughout the day, a pharmacy clerk will deliver supplies to the nursing departments and perform other functions for the pharmacist. Physicians often use the services of the pharmacist throughout the treatment of the patient. Additional information on careers in the Pharmacy may be obtained from *The Pharmacy Aide* in this series.

Other areas of rehabilitation usually classified under Therapeutic Services may include Speech Therapy, Dietary Therapy, Cardiac Rehabilitation, and Occupational Therapy.

Nursing Services

Nursing Services includes all of the departments that provide direct nursing care to patients. A specific nursing unit is established to take care of the patients in each of these departments. One of the fastest growing areas in healthcare is **ambulatory surgery**, or *same day surgery*. This type of facility may be free standing or contained within an acute care hospital. Due to the high costs of a surgical hospital stay, many insurance companies are encouraging the use of ambulatory surgery centers. An ambulatory surgery center performs any surgery that can be completed within a short period of time and does not require the patient to stay in the healthcare facility overnight. Patients who use this type of facility must not have a pre-existing disease such as cardiac disease or a respiratory disease. They must also be at low risk of developing complications as a result of the surgery. Most patients who have **outpatient surgery** are admitted and discharged within a few hours. This way, the patient is allowed to recuperate in the familiar and comfortable surroundings of his or her own home.

There are many types of outpatient surgeries. The variety of surgeries depend, in part, on the equipment available and on the skill level of the practicing doctors. Examples of outpatient surgery include plastic surgery; eye surgery; ear, nose, and throat surgery; gastroenterologic surgery (procedures concerned with the esophagus, stomach, and intestinal tract), and urologic surgery (procedures involving the kidneys, ureter, bladder, and prostate gland). As the costs of healthcare continue to increase, many more ambulatory or outpatient surgery centers will be constructed.

The **Discharge Planning** and **Social Services Departments** of the hospital begin working with the patient and his or her family soon after the patient has been admitted to the hospital. These two departments work together very closely. The main function of the Discharge Planning Department is to make appropriate provisions for the patient after he or she leaves the acute care hospital. Many times this involves working together with a long-term care facility or a home health agency. The Social Services Department has the responsibility of assisting the patient and the family with social problems. Often this requires communication with agencies involved with child abuse, elderly abuse, monetary assistance programs, or food and shelter assistance. It may also involve informing the public health department of a hygiene problem. These departments can be valuable assets in the planning of care for patients.

Critical Care Units provide care to patients who are experiencing a life-threatening disorder. This includes diseases, surgeries, or surgical complications. Frequently, patients with chronic conditions require **critical care**; however, Critical Care Units also provide care to patients experiencing acute changes in their health status. This is an extremely stressful area of healthcare because the personnel must care for patients who are very sick, deal with frequent emergency situations, and be able to function quickly and accurately.

critical care: the rendering of care to patients with life-threatening conditions

The **Emergency Department** is one of the busiest departments in an acute care hospital. It is often part of the Critical Care Department. This department provides nursing and medical care to patients of all ages with life or limb-threatening problems. The nurses, doctors, and other ED personnel treat victims of myocardial infarctions (heart attacks), burns, severe cuts, drownings, traffic collisions, etc. Sometimes they deliver a baby. The people who work in the Emergency Department are highly trained and well-skilled in working with advanced equipment. Like the Admissions Department, the ED may be the first contact a person has with the hospital. This contact may be in a telephone conversation or in person. Remember that PATIENTS ARE PEOPLE; WE NEED TO BE CONSIDERATE AND UNDERSTANDING!

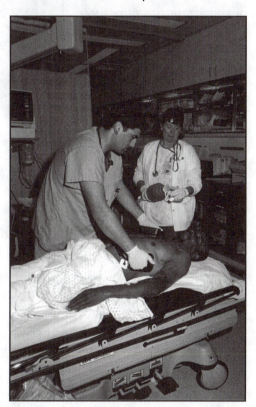

Figure 2-7: The Emergency Department provides nursing and medical care to patients of all ages with life-threatening problems.

The **Medical Surgical Nursing Unit** cares for patients experiencing general medical problems. This unit also gives care to those who have undergone general surgery, such as the removal of the appendix (an **appendectomy**), the removal of the gallbladder (a **cholecystectomy**), the removal of the uterus (a **hysterectomy**), and many other general surgical procedures. Medical disorders that frequently require hospitalization may include pneumonia; diabetes; or circulation problems. In this unit, allied health departments, such as Physical Therapy, Social Services, and the Dietary Department frequently are asked to provide patient education.

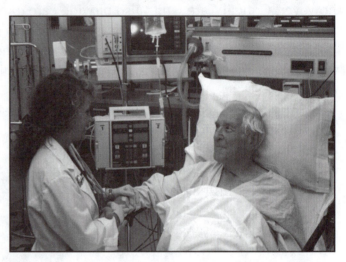

Figure 2-8: Patients recovering from surgery receive care in the Medical Surgical Nursing Unit.

Another specialized nursing unit is devoted to patients between the ages of 1 month and 18 years old. This unit is called **Pediatrics**. The nursing staff and the allied health workers must be highly skilled in technical duties and understand the psychological aspects of child development. It is important to remember that CHILDREN ARE NOT JUST SMALL ADULTS. Throughout the growing years, they experience physiological as well as psychological changes. **Physiology**, the study of the function of the body, refers to internal changes in the body. **Psychology** is the study of the mind and behavior patterns, both normal and abnormal. Sometimes, you will find that the child is not the only patient; the parents often need encouragement as well as education. Pediatrics is a challenging area in which to work!

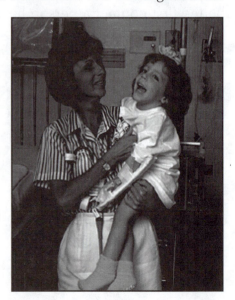

Figure 2-9: Working in Pediatrics requires knowledge of child psychology.

Labor and Delivery is frequently thought of as a very happy place to work. This is the nursing unit concerned with the delivery of babies. The word **labor** refers to the physiological process of delivering the fetus from the uterus through the birth canal and out of the mother's body. Mothers who are in labor may spend anywhere from a few minutes to several hours in this unit before being transferred to the delivery room. Generally, this is a pleasant area of the hospital; however, at times it is a very sad place because not all babies are born healthy. This unit can be very fast-paced.

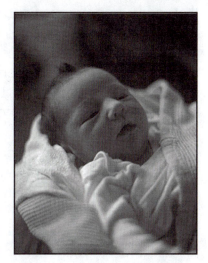

Figure 2-10: Labor and Delivery usually is a pleasant place in which to work.

After the baby has been delivered and the mother has been monitored by the staff for several hours, the mother is transferred to the **Post Partum Unit**. The baby is almost immediately transferred and admitted to the **nursery**. The Post Partum Unit provides care to the mother for several hours to a few days after the delivery. The new trend is for the mother and baby to be discharged home as soon as both patients are stable. Patient education is very important in this unit; especially for first time mothers. Most Post Partum Units offer mothers the option of **rooming-in** with their baby if a longer stay is necessary. This allows the baby to be in the mother's room during the mother's hospital stay, instead of in the nursery. This is a popular concept in many hospitals and birthing centers.

rooming-in: keeping the baby in the mother's post partum room instead of in the nursery

The **Oncology Unit** takes care of patients who have cancer. Oncology patients are often admitted to the hospital for special treatments called **chemotherapy**. Chemotherapy is a treatment with a special drug or drugs that are extremely **toxic** (poisonous) to the cancer. Some patients may need to have a special type of catheter inserted into a vein so that they may receive the chemotherapy without unnecessary needle punctures to their skin. Due to the chemotherapy treatments, there is considerable hazardous waste in this nursing unit. Be sure you are thoroughly familiar with the hospital's policy and procedure regarding the proper handling and disposal of the hazardous wastes. Because of the frequency of each patient's admission, the nursing staff and the clinical allied healthcare workers often know these patients by their first names. The families of these patients are also well acquainted with the nurses, doctors, and clinical health workers. This is a very intimate nursing unit with which to be involved.

Orthopedics is the department that deals with bone diseases and fractures. Many of the patients experience restricted movement due to the immobilization that results from **traction** and **casts**. Traction is a form of treatment that involves drawing or pulling on a bone in order to maintain proper body alignment of the bone ends. This allows the bone to heal in a straight line. A cast is a solid mold of a body part usually made of plaster or fiberglass. This cast is applied to the affected body part to hold the bone in proper alignment for healing. These patients often need assistance in moving; therefore, it is important to use proper **body mechanics** in order to prevent injury to yourself. Body mechanics are exercises and procedures that prevent and correct problems related to posture and daily activities. They will be thoroughly discussed in Chapter Seven.

Figure 2-11: Orthopedics is where fractures are treated using traction and casts.

Geriatrics is, perhaps, one of the fastest growing areas of medicine and nursing. This area is concerned with giving care to people over the age of 60 years. Geriatrics is concerned with all aspects of aging including social, health, psychological, and physiological issues. Like Pediatrics, this department has patients that require special areas of treatment. The United States Bureau of the Census reports that there are over 34 million people who are age 65 or older in the United States[1]. This is close to 13% of the total population. The United States Administration on Aging expects this figure to increase to 20% by the year 2030[2].

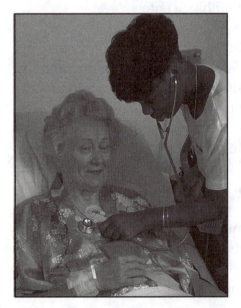

Figure 2-12: Like pediatric patients, geriatric patients need treatment that considers all aspects of aging including social, health, psychological, and physiological issues.

1. *Resident Population of the United States, Estimates by Age and Sex,* United States Bureau of the Census, http://www.fedstats.gov/index20.htm (27 Feb. 1998).

2. *Profile of Older Americans: 1997,* United States Administration on Aging, http://www.aoa.dhhs.gov (30 Nov. 1997).

Operating rooms, or surgical suites, are used exclusively for elective or emergency surgical procedures. **Elective surgery** means that the patient's condition permitted the doctor to schedule a date and time for the surgery. **Emergency surgery** indicates that the patient's condition either is, or could become, life or limb-threatening within a short period of time. Every person in the operating suite wears sterile gowns, hats, masks, gloves, and shoe covers.

Every piece of equipment used during the operation has been sterilized prior to the surgery. Sterilization means all germs have been killed through a special procedure. This area of the hospital is kept free of pathogens so that patients will not be exposed to germs and develop an infection. If you are working in this department, be sure to follow instructions concerning the areas you may

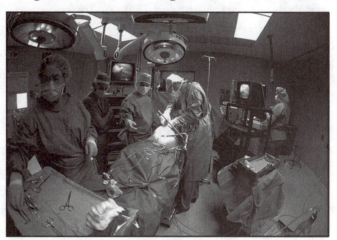

Figure 2-13: Operating suites must be kept free of pathogens to prevent infection in surgical patients.

or may not enter. Additional information on careers in the operating room may be obtained from *The Operating Room Aide* in this series.

After the patient's surgery has been completed, he or she is immediately transferred to the **Post Anesthesia Care Unit (PACU)**, or **recovery room**. It is

here that the patient is closely monitored for any breathing or bleeding problems that may develop immediately following the surgery. The patient usually remains in the recovery room close to one-half the time the surgery took to complete. The patient then will be taken to any of the areas previously described, depending on his or her condition.

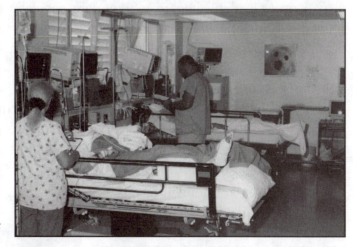

Figure 2-14: After surgery patients are taken to the Post Anesthesia Care Unit, where they are closely monitored.

The **Transitional Care Unit** may be referred to as the *Telemetry, Stepdown,* or *Direct Observation Unit.* This is the unit to which patients are frequently transferred after being discharged from the Critical Care Unit. Most of the patients on this unit have suffered a heart attack, or are recovering from surgery or **multitrauma** from an accident. These patients usually wear a small, mobile heart monitor that allows them to move around while the personnel at the desk watch their heart rhythm and rate on the monitors. There are many medications that may affect the heart. The doctor may decide to admit a patient to this unit because of the medication he or she may be taking. Make sure you understand exactly why the patient you are assisting is having his or her heart monitored before you do anything for the patient.

The **Infection Control Department** is responsible for developing policies and procedures concerned with reducing the risk of communicable diseases to both the staff and the patients. Two of the most serious health risks for the healthcare worker today are **acquired immune deficiency syndrome** (**AIDS**), and **hepatitis**. Two of the most serious infections that may be transmitted from the hospital employee to the patient are pneumonia and **staphylococcus aureus** (a bacteria commonly found on mucous membranes and skin). Follow the procedures regarding infection control so that patients do not experience any complications that could require an extended hospital stay. More information about infection control is provided in Chapter Nine.

Some of the hospitals have a **Psychiatric**, or **Mental Health**, **Department**. This is the area of medicine concerned with behavior and coping problems. There are many hospitals exclusively committed to providing care for the mentally ill patient. Mental healthcare workers are specially trained in handling crisis situations. Additional information on careers in the Psychiatric Department may be obtained from *The Mental Health Worker: Psychiatric Aide* in this series.

Substance Abuse, or **Chemical Dependency Units**, are frequently part of the mental health hospital; however, there are many acute care hospitals that also provide these services. This is a very challenging area of medicine. Since the level of stress in people's lives is getting higher, the need for these services is increasing. More and more employers now recognize this important aspect of healthcare and provide counseling services to their employees.

The **Education Department** of the hospital provides community and staff education classes. This is a valuable resource for research materials. Most of

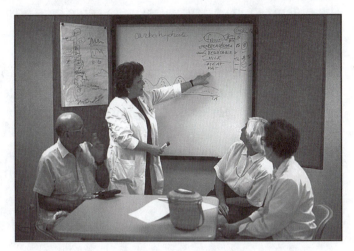

the staff education classes are open to any doctor, nurse, or allied health worker; however, be sure to specify your job title when inquiring about a class. The instructor will be able to direct you to the classes that will be most suitable for you. Be sure to explore any topic that sounds interesting to you. Education opens the doors to many career opportunities!

Figure 2-15: Anyone can benefit from the classes offered in the Education Department.

The Hospital Environment

All healthcare facilities are designed to promote **wellness**, or optimum health, for all people. The inside environment of a hospital should be clean, quiet, and free of all debris. Everything about the hospital environment is geared toward the patients' well-being; therefore, hospitals have become nonsmoking facilities. This means that all visitors and employees are permitted to smoke only in appropriately designated areas. After you become employed in a hospital, it is very important that you become aware of the smoking areas in that facility.

wellness: the state of optimum health

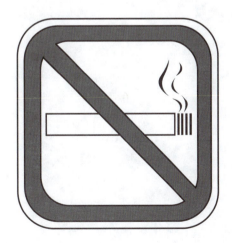

Chapter Summary

The organization and structure of an acute care hospital can be overwhelming and confusing. As a healthcare worker, familiarity with each department will enhance your confidence and increase your understanding of the function of the hospital. Understanding a hospital's organization gives you insight about the proper chain of command, and allows you to address the appropriate personnel with questions, complaints, or suggestions.

Your employment will begin with an orientation period. You should use this time to become familiar with each hospital department, the main function of each department, and the organization of the facility.

Name _____

Date _____

Student Enrichment Activities

Complete the following statements.

1. The organizational structure of a healthcare facility is indicated in the

    _____ _____ _____.

2. A general hospital is a type of _____ _____ hospital.

3. _____ is the branch of medicine that cares for infants, children, and

    adolescents to 18 years of age.

4. The _____ _____ is the department of the hospital

    that cares for patients with life or limb-threatening conditions.

5. The first contact the public may have with hospital personnel is usually with the

    _____ _____.

6. _____ is the release of rays in different directions from a

    common point.

7. The rehabilitation department that is concerned with the restoration of function and

    the prevention of disability is the _____ _____

    Department.

8. In addition to geriatrics, one of the fastest growing areas in healthcare is

    _____ _____.

9. The department of the hospital that treats bone diseases and fractures is

    _____.

10. Reducing the risk of communicable diseases to both the staff and the patients is the responsibility of the _____ _____ _____.

Unscramble the following terms.

11. NICAH FO MAMCOND   _____ _____ _____

12. LRATCICI RECA   _____ _____

13. CRAYOLADMI   _____

14. CRAFTINION   _____

15. GROOMNI NI   _____ _____

16. RTNSILITAZIOE   _____

17. SLEWSLEN   _____

Chapter Three
Hospital Employees and Medical Staff

Objectives

After completing this chapter you should be able to do the following:

1. Define and correctly spell each of the key terms.

2. Define the general term *doctor* and list at least three types of professional doctors.

3. Identify and discuss at least three clinical allied healthcare positions.

4. Define the phrase *irreversible brain death*.

Key Terms

- high risk
- infertility
- irreversible brain death
- neonate
- organ transplant
- pulmonary medicine
- rheumatology

Career Opportunities in Healthcare

There are a variety of occupations available for the clinical allied healthcare worker, offering numerous career options. This instructional course will introduce you to a number of the opportunities in the field of healthcare. Several of these positions are discussed briefly in this chapter.

Assistants

A well known clinical allied healthcare position is the **certified nursing assistant**. A course of training, including textbook material and clinical work, trains the student to provide bedside or basic patient care to patients under the direct supervision of a licensed nurse. The certified nursing assistant provides care to patients of all ages. They do not administer medications, receive doctor's orders, or do advanced patient care procedures such as giving injections. Several years ago, male nursing assistants were called orderlies. Today, however, both males and females who complete this training are known as certified nursing assistants (CNAs).

Medical assistants (MAs) work in doctor's offices, clinics, outpatient departments, and hospitals. They are trained in a classroom setting and complete clinical training under the supervision of a physician. Their duties include assisting the medical doctor with examinations and treatments. They perform certain procedures such as performing routine laboratory tests, taking electrocardiograms, drawing blood, and in some states, giving injections and administering other medications. Medical assistants are also trained in administrative duties.

Many departments of the hospital use assistants. These departments include Physical Therapy, Respiratory Therapy, Dietary, Health Information Services (Medical Records), Radiology, Mental Health, the Pharmacy, the Laboratory, and others. Duties will vary among departments and among healthcare facilities.

Nurses

Nurses make up the largest number of employees in most hospitals. There are several classifications of nurses with which you will be working. Most of the nurses you will come in contact with are classified as **registered nurses**, or RNs.

Registered nurses may be educated at several different levels. The associate degree RN attends a 2-year nursing program that includes the general education requirements, academic nursing courses, and clinical experience. At the end of the 2 years, he or she must take and pass the state examination given by the Board of Registered Nursing before it is legal to use the title *RN* after his or her name. The nurse is then subject to all the rules and regulations adopted by the Board of Registered Nursing concerning the registered nurse's scope of practice and licensing requirements.

The nurse who attends a 4-year program completes general education requirements and academic nursing courses, writes research papers, and has clinical experience. These programs are available through state colleges and universities.

At the completion of the fourth year, the nurse receives a bachelor of science degree in nursing. However, like the 2-year program candidate, he or she must complete and pass the state examination before the title *RN* may be used legally after his or her name. The advantage of a 4-year degree is that it helps prepare nurses for advancement into nursing administration and management.

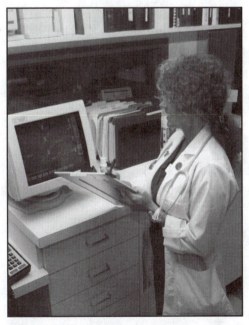

Figure 3-1: Registered nurses must pass the state examination given by the Board of Registered Nursing.

Registered nurses have many different kinds of responsibilities. They provide patient care such as administering medications, preparing patients for special diagnostic procedures, and admitting and discharging patients from the nursing unit. Nurses also inform doctors of the patient's progress and test results, and call doctors whenever the patient experiences a change in condition.

The nursing units organize patient care using either **primary care** or **team nursing**. Primary care nursing requires the registered nurse to provide all aspects of patient care, including tasks normally assigned to the nursing assistants, such as personal hygiene, bedchanges, and assistance with meals, as well as nursing responsibilities such as medication administration, and all types of wound care. Team nursing, on the other hand, means that the registered nurse is the team leader and supervises other nurses and allied healthcare workers while they provide direct patient care. The team leader is responsible for administering medication, admitting and discharging a patient from the nursing unit, and assisting the doctors. Most nursing units use the concept of team nursing to provide patient care.

Some RNs continue their education and expand their role by completing 2 additional years of schooling after receiving their 4-year degree. At the completion of the 2 years, they must pass a state examination. Depending on the course curriculum, the RN may then practice as either a physician's assistant or a nurse practitioner.

Another type of nurse that you will be in contact with is the **licensed vocational nurse** (**LVN**), or **licensed practical nurse** (**LPN**). This individual has received vocational training and performs many technical nursing duties. Training is usually 18 months in length and includes clinical training in a hospital setting. At the completion of this training, they must pass a state examination before the initials LVN or LPN after their name may legally be used. Many LVNs continue their education and advance through RN training.

The licensed practical nurse or vocational nurse performs limited nursing tasks when compared to the registered nurse. The licensed practical nurse is responsible for administering medications (mainly topically, orally, or through an injection), and providing wound care. This type of nurse may also administer solutions into a patient's vein, but they must be certified in that procedure first. The LPN often inserts special tubes into patients to either drain his urine or to provide a way to feed the patient.

Health Unit Coordinators

The **health unit coordinator**, **ward clerk**, or **unit secretary**, is another allied healthcare team member. Health unit coordinators perform clerical and receptionist duties in the nursing units. This position demands someone who is well organized, flexible, dependable, and able to work well under stress. There are considerable demands placed upon the health unit coordinator because he or she must constantly be attentive to the many needs of the doctors, nurses, patients, patient's families, and other departments in the hospital. The health unit

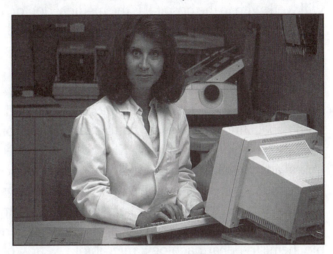

Figure 3-2: Health unit coordinators help the nursing units run smoothly and efficiently.

coordinator is the hub of the nursing unit. Health unit coordinators who have acquired national certification will have the initials CHUC after their name, which stands for Certified Health Unit Coordinator.

Doctors

The term **doctor** generally refers to a person who has received an advanced degree. There are various fields which grant the title of doctor, such as doctor of philosophy, doctor of education, and doctor of divinity. People with these degrees place the letters *PhD* or *EdD* after their names. Examples of doctors who specialize in different areas are medical doctors (doctors of medicine), doctors of osteopathy (doctors who are concerned with bone diseases and

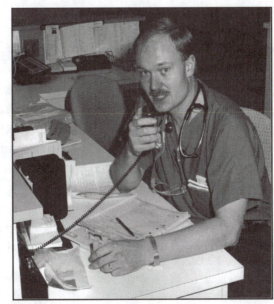

Figure 3-3: Medical doctors must be licensed by the state before they can treat patients without supervision from an experienced physician.

disorders), doctors of chiropractic (doctors who use spinal manipulation, as well as physical therapy, to correct common complaints such as headaches or back pain), and doctors of podiatry (doctors who are involved with the diagnosis, treatment, and prevention of conditions in human feet). The most common type of doctor you will work with in the hospital is the medical doctor, or MD, generally referred to as a physician. Medical doctors have advanced education and must pass specialized examinations. Once they have passed their examinations, they become licensed and may treat patients within their area of expertise.

The extent of a physician's education depends on the specific area of specialty. Some specialties require an additional 6 years of study. All physicians attend 4 years of premedical school. Most of the premedical students take courses in liberal arts as well as mandatory higher mathematics and advanced sciences such as chemistry, physics, biology, anatomy, and physiology. After acceptance into medical school, they begin 4 years of advanced training. These years consist of higher-level academic courses and direct patient care. The courses include biochemistry, pharmacology, microbiology, and pathology.

During these 4 years the student is known as an **intern** and uses the title *doctor*. The student participates in patient care decisions including prescribing medications and diagnostic tests. Interns are always directly supervised by licensed physicians.

After the internship has been completed, most physicians choose to specialize. This requires at least 1 year of advanced training. At this time, the student is known as a **resident** and cares for patients exclusively within his or her specialty. Interns and residents usually are assigned to teaching hospitals. After the term of residency has been completed, a written examination must be passed before being issued a license to practice medicine. With a license, a doctor can treat patients without supervision from experienced physicians. At this time, he or she may establish a medical office and begin treating patients.

Becoming a physician requires dedication, determination, and intellect. The study of medicine is very time-consuming and expensive. Physicians, therefore, should be respected for their extensive training.

Areas of Specialty

Because of scientific and technical advances in medicine, doctors and nurses have had to become more specialized in their areas of practice. Several specialties will be discussed briefly in the following pages. As you become familiar with these different areas, consider exploring the ones which are of interest to you.

Family practice is the specialized branch of medicine that focuses on providing care to the entire family unit. There are no age limits, nor is there any restriction to the type of disease that may be treated. Family practice uses medical knowledge from several different specialties such as internal medicine, geriatrics, pediatrics, general surgery, obstetrics, gynecology, and psychiatry. As with the other medical specialties, this doctor may become board certified in family practice. A closely related branch of medicine is **internal medicine**, which is the specialized branch of medicine that treats nonsurgical conditions of adults. For example, people who have gastroenteritis (nausea, vomiting, and diarrhea) may seek the medical care and advice of an **internist**. In large cities, most people will become established with an internist; it is then the responsibility of the internist to refer to other **specialists** if more specialized care is needed. Internists may not be available in small towns or more rural areas; general practitioners, or family practitioners, are more likely to treat patients in less populous areas. Nurses who take care of an internist's (or family practitioner's) patients are called **medical nurses**.

Cardiology is considered to be a specialty area; however, it is not unusual for an internist to also specialize as a **cardiologist**. Cardiology concerns itself with the diagnosis, treatment, and prevention of conditions of the heart and its blood vessels. Most people who are experiencing chest pain are seen and treated by a cardiologist. Cardiology nurses are known as **critical** or **coronary care nurses**.

Pulmonary medicine deals with disorders and diseases of the lungs. Patients with chronic obstructive pulmonary diseases such as asthma, chronic bronchitis, and emphysema will be treated by a pulmonary specialist. It is customary for a critical care nurse to care for this type of patient.

pulmonary medicine: the branch of medicine concerned with the diagnosis and treatment of disorders and diseases of the lungs

Over the past decade, **emergency medicine** has become a specialty in its own right. Emergency department physicians receive extensive training in emergency medicine, which includes internal medicine, pulmonary medicine, cardiology, pediatrics, obstetrics and gynecology, neonatology, urology, orthopedics, oncology, and dermatology. The nurses who specialize in this area are known as **emergency nurses** and often are classified as critical care nurses.

Gastroenterology, the area of medicine limited to diseases and disorders of the esophagus, stomach, and intestinal tract, is also a rapidly expanding field in medicine. Medical doctors who specialize in this area are also skilled in procedures involved with diagnosing disorders such as cancer of the stomach, esophagus, or intestinal tract, and ulcers. A nurse who specializes in this area is called an **endoscopy nurse** or **gastrointestinal nurse**.

Urology, the care of patients with dysfunction of the urinary tract system, is another area of specialty for doctors. Patients experiencing difficulty in urinating, those who have kidney stones, or those with diseases of the male reproductive system, often seek medical care and advice from a urologist. If these patients are hospitalized, the nurses in the Medical Surgical Unit provide the necessary nursing care.

Another area that relates closely to urology is **nephrology**. This branch of medicine is devoted exclusively to problems involving the kidneys. If a patient has severe kidney stones, then a nephrologist would provide care to that patient. The **medical surgical nurses** usually are responsible for the care of this patient.

Surgery is a broad classification with many subspecialties. It involves the use of manual and operative procedures to correct deformities and defects, repair injuries, and diagnose certain diseases. A **general surgeon** is a doctor who is not specialized in a particular type of surgery such as eye surgery or orthopedic surgery. A general surgeon performs procedures such as a cholecystectomy (the removal of the gallbladder) or an appendectomy (the removal of the appendix). Medical surgical nurses provide the necessary care for these patients.

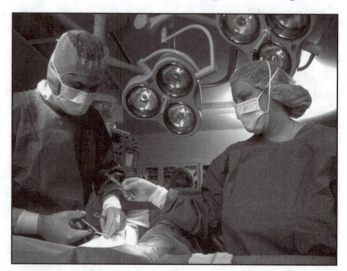

Figure 3-4: Surgery

Neurology is the branch of medicine concerned with the study of nervous system diseases, diagnosis, and treatment. A doctor in this specialty is called a **neurologist**. Neurologists provide care to patients who have had head injuries, seizures, and injuries to the nerves.

Cancer patients generally require the expertise of a physician who specializes in **oncology**, the study of cancer. This can be a very emotional area of medicine. Patients often are diagnosed and treated over a period of time by a physician until the time of their death. Healthcare workers often grow very close to their cancer patients and the family members. Nurses who specialize in this area are called **oncology nurse specialists**.

Gerontology is a rapidly expanding specialty. It is the field of medicine concerned with examining, diagnosing, and treating the elderly population. Elderly people represent the fastest growing segment of the American population. Nurses who specialize in care of the elderly are **gerontological nurse specialists**.

Rheumatology is another area in which doctors may concentrate their expertise. This is the branch of medicine concerned with the treatment of disorders and diseases of the joints of the body. Most rheumatology patients are cared for by **medical nurses**. However, as the number of citizens over the age of 60 increases, this may be a new area of specialization for nurses in the near future.

rheumatology: the branch of medicine concerned with the diagnosis and treatment of disorders and diseases of the joints of the body

Physicians who limit their area of practice to delivering babies and diagnosing and treating diseases and disorders of the female reproductive system specialize in **obstetrics** and **gynecology**. Obstetrics is the area devoted to caring for patients who hope to become pregnant, and for pregnant patients both before and six weeks after the delivery. Gynecology focuses on specific problems with the uterus, fallopian tubes, ovaries, cervix, vagina, and breasts. Frequently this area of medicine is abbreviated *OB-GYN*. **OB-GYN nurse specialists** provide care for these types of patients.

neonate: an infant from the age of birth up to 1 month old

Neonatology, the care of infants from birth to 1 month of age, is a very challenging area of medicine. It often includes caring for babies born before they are expected until the time of their discharge from the hospital. These infants, called **neonates**, are classified as **high risk**. They have an increased potential for developing life-threatening problems—often without previous warning to the untrained person. The **neonatology nurse** receives extensive training before caring for these infants.

high risk: a term used to describe patients who have increased potential for developing life-threatening problems, often without previous warning

infertility:
the diminished ability or inability to produce children

Some physicians practice medicine in the area of **infertility**. These doctors provide care and treatment to patients who desire children, but have been unable to conceive. Patients who seek medical care and treatment in this area are quite often discouraged by their problem. The doctor will do numerous tests on both the male and female. Sometimes surgery is a possible solution to the problem. Often, the condition of infertility can be reversed and the couple is then able to have children. **Obstetrical-gynecological (OB-GYN) nurse specialists** usually care for these patients.

Pediatrics is the area that cares for infants, children, and adolescents to 18 years of age. Special activities are frequently offered to the patients in this unit. For example, play rooms may be provided that are equipped with toys and equipment geared to specific ages. Frequently, an activities director will guide and direct the recreation time to create an atmosphere in which the patients can learn as well as have fun. The recreational room is kept very clean so as not to transmit disease causing germs to patients. **Pediatric nurse specialists** care for pediatric patients.

Many people have recognized the importance of caring for their skin. **Dermatology** is the branch of medicine concerned with disorders and diseases of the skin. Frequently, the doctor who specializes in dermatology, the **dermatologist**, is also trained in cosmetic surgery. They often perform surgical procedures on the face and other sensitive areas of the body where minimal scarring is desired. A medical surgical nurse usually provides nursing care for this type of patient.

Cosmetic and reconstructive surgery is a specialty devoted to very intricate procedures that often involve delicate surgery. Examples of cosmetic, or plastic, surgery include face lifts, eyelid lifting, breast reduction and augmentation (enlargement), and tummy tucks. The term *plastic* actually means capable of being molded. Reconstructive surgery may include skin grafts for burned areas on the body, or procedures to correct birth defects. These procedures are frequently completed as outpatient procedures in the physician's office. A **surgical**, or **operating room nurse**, will be in attendance.

Physicians dedicated to the diagnosis and treatment of diseases and disorders of the eye specialize in **ophthalmology**. They not only examine eyes and prescribe glasses, but are also trained to diagnose and treat disorders of the eyeball and surrounding tissues. Ophthalmologists also may be trained in plastic surgery. These doctors will treat scratches of the eye, infections of the eye, eye muscle disorders, cataracts, and glaucoma. Usually a surgical nurse cares for these patients.

The **orthopedic specialist** diagnoses and treats diseases of and problems with the bones of the body. Orthopedists make extensive use of casts and traction to treat broken bones and infections of the bone. This type of doctor also specializes in surgery of the bone. A medical surgical nurse who has additional training in orthopedics provides care for these patients.

Because of the vigorous and extensive training to which athletes are subjected, another area of specialty, known as **sports medicine**, has emerged. Sports medicine deals with the prevention and treatment of athletic injuries. Under the direction of the prescribing physician, physical therapists provide most of the treatment to the athlete. This type of patient receives care from an **orthopedic nurse specialist**.

Mental health is a rapidly expanding area of medicine. This branch of medicine deals with the diagnosis, treatment, and prevention of mental illness. A physician who specializes in mental health is called a **psychiatrist**. A clinical psychologist is one who has received training in psychological analysis, research, and therapy. Some nurses also receive extensive training in mental health and are called **psychiatric nurse specialists**. Examples of mental illness are depression, schizophrenia, and suicidal tendencies. Specific behavior problems also are included in this category of illness. **Counseling centers** are healthcare facilities that specialize in behavioral disorders.

One of the newest and most controversial branches of medicine deals with **organ transplants**. Because of the nature of this specialty, there are many ethical questions being asked by medical experts. This area of medicine involves the harvesting, or surgical removal, of transplantable organs from a donor who has suffered **irreversible brain death** to a recipient who is experiencing failure of a vital organ. Irreversible brain death means that brain-specific tests, such as electroencephalograms, have shown that the donor's brain cells have died, and therefore, the brain is inactive and has no chance for recovery. There are many documented incidents of one person's life being extended due to the decision by a family to donate the organs of a loved one who has died.

Many people may not be able to cope with having to make a decision to donate an organ. It is difficult for people to accept the loss of a loved one; however, the decision to release the organs of a loved one who has died must be made quickly. Therefore, the transplant team and the critical care nurses explain the need for organs to the family and offer support for whatever decision they may make. Many factors can affect the decision to donate an organ for transplant. For example, state laws, power of attorney, and living wills can all affect the outcome of a potential organ donation.

organ transplant: a surgical procedure in which a vital organ provided from a donor is transferred to a recipient who is suffering from failure of that organ

irreversible brain death: a condition in which brain-specific tests show that the patient's brain cells have died, and therefore, the brain is inactive and has no chance for recovery

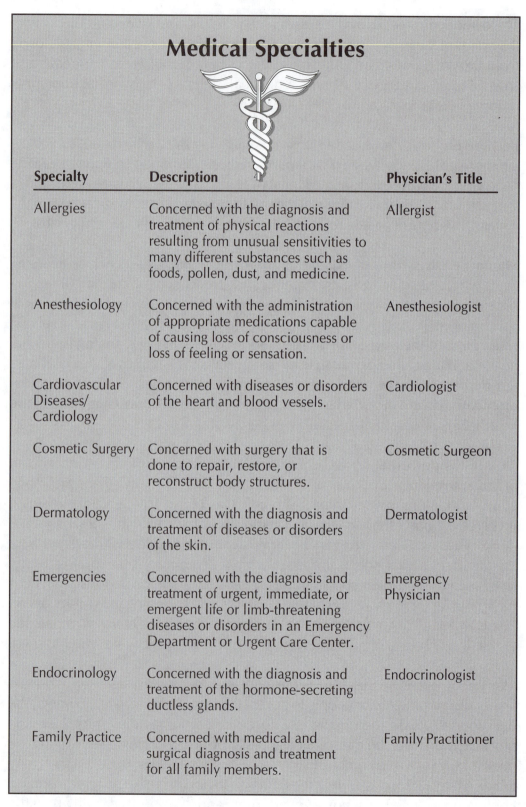

Medical Specialties

Specialty	Description	Physician's Title
Allergies	Concerned with the diagnosis and treatment of physical reactions resulting from unusual sensitivities to many different substances such as foods, pollen, dust, and medicine.	Allergist
Anesthesiology	Concerned with the administration of appropriate medications capable of causing loss of consciousness or loss of feeling or sensation.	Anesthesiologist
Cardiovascular Diseases/ Cardiology	Concerned with diseases or disorders of the heart and blood vessels.	Cardiologist
Cosmetic Surgery	Concerned with surgery that is done to repair, restore, or reconstruct body structures.	Cosmetic Surgeon
Dermatology	Concerned with the diagnosis and treatment of diseases or disorders of the skin.	Dermatologist
Emergencies	Concerned with the diagnosis and treatment of urgent, immediate, or emergent life or limb-threatening diseases or disorders in an Emergency Department or Urgent Care Center.	Emergency Physician
Endocrinology	Concerned with the diagnosis and treatment of the hormone-secreting ductless glands.	Endocrinologist
Family Practice	Concerned with medical and surgical diagnosis and treatment for all family members.	Family Practitioner

Figure 3-5: Medical Specialties

Medical Specialties (Cont.)

Specialty	Description	Physician's Title
Gastroenterology	Concerned with the diagnosis and treatment of disorders and diseases of the digestive tract.	Gastroenterologist
General Surgery	Concerned with the diagnosis and treatment of disorders and diseases of all body systems by surgical intervention.	Surgeon
Gerontology	Concerned with the diagnosis and treatment of the elderly.	Gerontologist
Gynecology	Concerned with the diagnosis and treatment of disorders and diseases of the female reproductive system.	Gynecologist
Internal Medicine	Concerned with the diagnosis and nonsurgical treatment of disorders and illnesses.	Internist
Neonatology	Concerned with the diagnosis and treatment of infants from birth to one year of age.	Neonatologist
Nephrology	Concerned with the diagnosis and treatment of disorders and diseases of the kidneys.	Nephrologist
Neurology	Concerned with the diagnosis and nonsurgical intervention for illnesses involving the brain, spinal cord, and nerves.	Neurologist
Obstetrics	Concerned with the diagnosis and care given to women during pregnancy, childbirth, and 6 weeks after delivery.	Obstetrician
Oncology	Concerned with the diagnosis and treatment of cancer.	Oncologist
Ophthalmology	Concerned with the diagnosis and treatment of disorders and diseases of the eye and surrounding tissue including prescriptions for eyeglasses.	Ophthalmologist

Figure 3-5: Medical Specialties (Cont.)

Medical Specialties (Cont.)

Specialty	Description	Physician's Title
Orthopedics	Concerned with surgical and non-surgical intervention for diseases and disorders involving the muscular and skeletal system.	Orthopedist/ Orthopedic Surgeon
Otolaryngology	Concerned with the diagnosis and treatment of diseases and disorders of the ears, nose, and throat.	Otolaryngologist
Pathology	Concerned with the diagnosis of the cause of disease including change in structure and function.	Pathologist
Pediatrics	Concerned with the provision of medical care to children as well as the diagnosis and treatment of disorders and diseases affecting children.	Pediatrician
Physical Medicine and Rehabilitation	Concerned with the treatment of sports and other injuries and the recovery of most, if not all, muscle strength and function and joint range of motion.	Physiatrist
Proctology	Concerned with the diagnosis and treatment of diseases and disorders of the rectum.	Proctologist
Psychiatry	Concerned with the diagnosis and treatment of mental disorders.	Psychiatrist
Radiology	Concerned with the diagnosis of disorders and diseases using radiant energy.	Radiologist
Therapeutic Radiology	Concerned with the use of radiant energy in the treatment of cancer.	Radiologist
Thoracic Surgery	Concerned with the operative treatment for medical problems of the heart and large vessels of the chest cavity.	Thoracic Surgeon
Urology	Concerned with the diagnosis and treatment of dysfunctions of the urinary tract and the male reproductive system.	Urologist

Figure 3-5: Medical Specialties (Cont.)

Chapter Summary

From the preceding discussion, it is easy to understand why careers in medicine and allied health are fascinating and challenging to pursue. There are numerous specialties already, and as the technology, skills, and knowledge become more complex, more branches of medicine will evolve.

Know the definition of each specialty. You will be a positive asset to the hospital and the patients as your skills and knowledge increase! Skillful and knowledgeable employees are one of the key elements in the efficient operation of the healthcare facility.

Name _____

Date _____

Student Enrichment Activities

Complete the following statements.

1. The two types of nurses with whom you will be in contact are _____
    _____ and _____ _____ _____.

2. MD is the accepted abbreviation for _____ _____.

3. A closely related branch of medicine to Family Practice is _____
    _____.

4. Emergency nurses are also called _____ _____ _____.

5. Asthma is a disease that is classified under the branch of _____
    _____.

6. Endoscopy nurses specialize in the field of _____.

7. The branch of medicine concerned with the study of disorders and diseases of the
    joints of the body is called _____.

8. OB-GYN is an accepted abbreviation for _____ and
    _____.

9. Infants younger than the age of 4 weeks are cared for by a specialist in
    _____.

10. The term *plastic* actually means _____ of being _____.

11. Counseling centers specialize in providing assistance to patients with

    _____ _____.

12. An area of medicine that often raises many ethical questions deals with

    _____ _____.

Unscramble the following terms.

13. RONCAROY   _____

14. IHHG SIRK   _____ _____

15. TINYFLIRTIE   _____

16. BNRIA EADHT   _____ _____

17. TENAEON   _____

18. STARTNPLAN   _____

19. RONPLAYUM   _____

20. OHGLUEMATORY   _____

Chapter Four
The Allied Health Worker, the Law, and Professional Ethics

Objectives

After completing this chapter you should be able to do
the following:

1. Define and correctly spell each of the key terms.

2. Name and describe both allied health professional organizations.

3. Explain the term *ethics*.

4. Describe the Patient's Bill of Rights.

5. Name and explain each of the four parts of the
    patient/healthcare provider contract.

6. Identify and describe at least four kinds of intentional torts.

7. Identify at least seven ways to decrease your chances
    of being sued.

8. Identify at least four guidelines to follow when witnessing
    a consent.

9. Describe the legal aspects of AIDS and confidentiality.

10. Define and state the purpose of advance directives.

Key Terms

- abandonment
- advance directives
- battery
- breach of duty to act
- contract
- damages
- duty to act
- ethics
- healthcare provider

- Health Occupations Students of America (HOSA)
- malpractice
- negligence
- patient advocate
- Patient's Bill of Rights
- privileged information
- proximate cause
- scope of practice
- tort

Patient Trust

One of the most rewarding privileges of being a healthcare worker is the trust patients place in your actions, suggestions, and decisions. The overall safety and well-being of the patient is the primary obligation of the healthcare worker. Healthcare workers act as **patient advocates** and therefore, must take great care in what they say and do.

patient advocate: an individual who supports and pleads the cause of the patient

Since the early 1980s, there has been an astounding increase in the number of lawsuits against healthcare workers. It is important for professional healthcare workers to be currently educated and precisely skilled. They must NEVER exceed their **scope of practice**. Although there are no guarantees that you will never be sued, proper education and adherence to procedures will help build a strong defense for you in case you are named as a defendant.

scope of practice: a legal description of what a specific health professional may and may not do

This text provides introductory information about medical law and ethics. It is not intended to provide legal advice. The healthcare facility you work for will have attorneys available to handle questions concerning patient care and patient outcome. Each state and hospital manages legal inquiries according to established **protocol**. Protocols are the established rules for a particular procedure. If there are any questions concerning the care you gave to a patient, consult your supervisor regarding what action you should take.

Scope of Practice

Every state has written laws, called **statutes**, that define certain categories of work that healthcare workers legally may and may not do. This is called the scope of practice. All licensed and certified personnel have a scope of practice. Unlicensed healthcare workers must perform within their hospital job description and be careful not to do tasks or procedures for which they have not been trained or are not legally permitted to perform. Medicine is closely governed through licensing and certification. State boards or agencies regulate the **licensee** and generally have the authority to remove the license or certificate. Emerging healthcare workers, though not licensed by the state, have state and national organizations that work toward identifying educational requirements, accrediting schools, establishing a scope of practice, and/or developing a **Code of Ethics**. Most of these professional organizations provide educational seminars for their members.

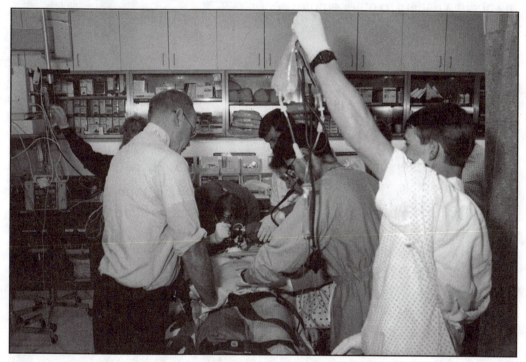

Figure 4-1: A healthcare worker must never exceed his or her scope of practice or job description. Never attempt to perform a task or procedure unless you have been properly trained to do so. If you are unsure how to do something, ask for assistance.

Ethics

ethics:
principles of conduct that establish standards and morals that govern decisions and behavior

Ethics set principles even higher than the law. As a healthcare worker, there will be many times when your understanding of ethics will be tested. For example, you will be asked to either assist with, or fully manage, a patient's valuables and belongings. Some patients will have expensive jewelry or large sums of money that might be entrusted to your care. All hospitals have a policy and procedure for securing a patient's belongings and valuables. You will need to be familiar with the documents that must be completed and signed by the patient and the

healthcare worker, and know which department is responsible for placing the possessions in the hospital safe. Then you must follow the procedure exactly! Other examples of ethics include going to work when you don't feel like it; being dependable; using **discretion** when talking about a patient to other employees or patients, etc.

Ethical decisions involve integrity, honesty, and a strong sense of right and wrong. At the end of each day you should ask yourself, "Did I do unto others as I would have others do unto me?" If the answer is yes, then you can comfortably return to work to provide care for the people who depend on you—the patients.

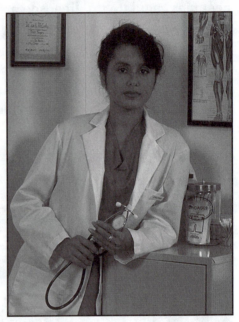

Figure 4-2: Patients depend on you to make ethical decisions.

The Patient's Bill of Rights

The patient has a right to expect certain things to be done for his or her safety and well-being. Patients have a right to expect, and RECEIVE, this level of care from ALL healthcare workers. The California Administration Code, Section 70707 has established guidelines for healthcare facilities in the state of California identifying legal rights a patient can expect to receive while a patient in that facility. This document is called the **Patient's Bill of Rights**. It is posted in all hospitals in a place that is readily visible to patients. Each patient receives a copy of these rights upon being admitted to the hospital. An example of the *Patient's Bill of Rights* follows.

Patient's Bill of Rights:
a document that identifies the basic rights of all patients

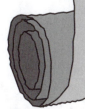

Patient's Bill of Rights

1. The patient has a right to considerate and respectful care.

2. Patients have the right to obtain from their physician complete current information concerning their diagnosis, treatment and prognosis in terms they can be reasonably expected to understand.

3. An informed consent should include knowledge of the proposed procedure, along with its risks and probable duration of incapacitation. In addition, the patient has a right to information regarding medically significant alternatives.

4. The patient has the right to refuse treatment to the extent permitted by law, and to be informed of the medical consequences of his action.

5. Case discussion, consultation, examination, and treatment should be conducted discretely. Those not directly involved must have the patient's permission to be present.

6. The patient has the right to expect that all communication and records pertaining to his care should be treated as confidential.

7. The patient has the right to expect the hospital to make a reasonable response to his request for services. The hospital must provide evaluation, service, and referral as indicated by the urgency of the case.

8. The patient has the right to obtain information as to any relationship of his hospital to other healthcare and educational institutions, insofar as his care is concerned. The patient has the right to obtain information as to the existence of any professional relationships among individuals, by name, who are treating him.

9. The patient has the right to be advised if the hospital proposes to engage in or perform human experimentation affecting his care or treatment. The patient has the right to refuse to participate in such research projects.

10. The patient has the right to expect reasonable continuity of care.

11. The patient has the right to examine and receive an explanation of his bill regardless of the source of payment.

12. The patient has the right to know what hospital rules and regulations apply to his conduct as a patient.

Figure 4-3: A Patient's Rights

Contractual Relationships

contract:
an agreement by all people involved to perform certain obligations

The relationship between the hospital and the patient is contractual. A **contract** implies that everyone involved has agreed to do something. In order for the contract to be valid, there must be an offer for services, an acceptance of the offer, and then compensation for the services (such as money). The contract may be implied or expressed. For instance, presenting yourself at a physician's office for healthcare is implied consent, whereas signing a written document, such as a financial agreement, is consent that is expressed.

There are four parts of this contract; omission of any part is a **breach of contract**. These are the four parts.

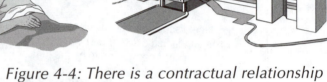

Figure 4-4: There is a contractual relationship between the hospital and the patient.

healthcare provider:
a professional (such as a physician or advanced practitioner) or institution that provides healthcare

1. DUTY TO ACT: As an employee of the hospital or other **healthcare provider**, the healthcare worker has a legal duty to provide care to a patient within his or her legal scope of practice.

2. RELEVANCE: The contract must be relevant to the subject matter. For example, the doctor must provide medical care to the patient.

3. COMPENSATION: There must be compensation for the services provided (ie, money).

4. MUTUAL AGREEMENT: There must be a mutual agreement between the parties concerning the obligation to provide pertinent services for the compensation.

ALL FOUR OF THESE MUST EXIST IN A VALID CONTRACT.

If one of the parties feels there is a breach of contract, four items must be proven:

1. **duty to act**

2. **breach of duty to act**

3. **proximate cause**

4. **damages** (recoverable)

If any one of these cannot be proven, there is no lawsuit!

The two parties involved in this contract are the healthcare provider and the patient. The patient is obligated, by law, to pay for the services received from the healthcare provider. On the other hand, the healthcare provider is obligated to provide a standard of care that is the same as that provided by other healthcare providers under the same circumstances and with similar training. Consideration is given to what the majority of doctors, nurses, or assistants would have done using their best judgement. Every person is entitled to the same standard of care regardless of insurance status, finances, race, religion, sex, or age.

As soon as the patient seeks care, consent for treatment is implied. Consent for treatment must be given by a legal adult (or guardian, if the patient is a **minor**) who is mentally competent and has not been coerced into consenting. This is the beginning of the contract, and means that the patient has agreed to be treated by the healthcare provider. If care is not properly provided, this duty to act has been breached. Whenever the breach of duty to act results in an injury, serious illness, or death, the third part of a lawsuit has been fulfilled (proximate cause has occurred). The results of the breach of duty to act and the proximate cause must be damages that are recoverable in terms of money in order for a lawsuit to go to court. There are many instances in which there is proven to be a duty to act, breach of that duty to act, and proximate cause, but there are no recoverable damages. If there are no recoverable damages, the case will not go to trial. (There is no lawsuit).

If there ARE recoverable damages, they are awarded to the plaintiff in terms of money. The size of the award depends on the amount of money that is estimated to be equivalent to the amount of loss or injury that has been sustained. This award is referred to as *compensatory damages*, because the money is supposed to compensate for the plaintiff's loss.

duty to act: the legal duty to provide care within the scope of practice

breach of duty to act: the omission of care

proximate cause: a legal concept meaning that an aspect of care that was omitted or committed directly caused a patient's injury or death

damages: a degree of loss that has occurred due to injury to person, property, or reputation

There are two specific types of lawsuits that are common to the healthcare field.

negligence:
the failure to give reasonable care or to do what another prudent person with similar experience, knowledge, and background would have done under the same or similar circumstances

1. **negligence:** the failure to give reasonable care or to do what another prudent person with similar experience, knowledge, and background would have done under the same or similar circumstances.

2. **malpractice:** professional misconduct or lack of professional skill that results in injury to the patient; negligence by a professional, such as a physician or nurse.

malpractice:
professional misconduct or lack of professional skill that results in injury to the patient; negligence by a professional, such as a physician or nurse

Intentional Torts

Acts of negligence are classified as either intentional **torts** or unintentional torts. There are specific examples of intentional torts that occur in the healthcare field.

tort:
a private or civil wrong against another person or his property

- **battery:** the unlawful touching of an individual without consent (eg, performing a blood draw after the patient has refused).

- **assault:** the threat of an immediate harmful or offensive contact, without the actual commission of the act.

- **false imprisonment:** restraining a person against his or her will, either physically or with verbal threats.

- **abandonment:** the termination of supervision of a patient by a physician without adequate written notice or the patient's consent.

battery:
the unlawful touching of an individual without consent

- **invasion of privacy:** public discussion of private information (eg, release of medical information without the patient's written consent).

- **defamation of character:** discussion of a person by another either in writing (libel) or verbally (slander) that damages that person's reputation.

- **fraud and misrepresentation:** the intentional withholding of information from a patient to cover up mistakes.

abandonment:
the termination of supervision of a patient by a physician without adequate written notice or the patient's consent

The most common patient complaints concern the fact that their physician did not spend enough time with them and did not keep them informed of their treatment, results, and progress. Everyone must make an effort to provide the highest quality of care because lawsuits are better prevented than defended.

The following are some guidelines to decrease your chances of being named in a lawsuit.

1. Be kind and courteous to every patient.

2. Do not give your opinion concerning the actions of another healthcare worker.

3. Do not use the word *cure.*

4. Do not use the word *mistake.*

5. Always take time with your patient.

6. Explain procedures, policies, and treatments using terms the patient understands.

7. Include the patient's family or significant other in the patient's care UNLESS THE PATIENT DOES NOT WANT YOU TO.

8. Attend educational inservices or seminars.

9. Maintain fluency in performance of procedures.

10. Never leave a patient unattended who might be in danger of falling.

11. Follow the hospital policies and use good judgement concerning the use of siderails.

12. Do not routinely restrain a patient with soft restraints unless there may be an increased chance of the patient injuring themselves.

13. Do not practice outside of your scope of practice, or job description.

14. Treat patient information as confidential and discuss it only with those directly involved with patient care.

Consent

The consent that is established between the patient and the healthcare provider must be written. The law states that each and every patient has the right to determine what shall or shall NOT be done with his body. To be legal, consents must be **informed**. The patient must not only understand what the treatment will be but the risks and alternatives as well. All consents require a witness. This witness should be someone who is of legal age; and someone who is not going to perform the procedure; however, it should be someone who is qualified to determine if the patient understands all aspects of the procedure. Here are some general guidelines to follow when witnessing a consent.

1. Always use black ink.

2. Do not use abbreviations—be sure to spell everything correctly and completely.

3. Accepting telephone consent requires two people to listen at the same time and accept the verbal consent for treatment.

4. State laws differ concerning consent for treatment of minors. A minor is someone who is not of legal age. An emancipated minor is one who is not of legal age, but who is single, married, or divorced, living on his or her own, and is self-supporting, AND has legal documents affirming that fact. Be sure and learn your state's laws concerning the treatment of minors and emancipated minors.

Advance Directives

advance directive: a legal document prepared when an individual is alive, competent, and able to make decisions. It provides guidance to the healthcare team if the person is no longer able to make decisions.

In 1991 a law known as the Patient Self-Determination Act went into effect. This act requires hospitals and other healthcare facilities who participate in Medicare or Medicaid reimbursement to ask each patient who is of legal age if he or she has an **advance directive**. The law also requires that these facilities make available to patients written information about their state's laws regarding advance directives and the patient's right to refuse treatment.

An advance directive is a legal document prepared when an individual is alive, competent, and able to make decisions. It provides guidance to the healthcare team if the person is no longer able to make decisions.

Confidentiality

Working in a hospital exposes the healthcare worker to special information about patients. This information is called **privileged information**. It includes all medical and personal details provided in the medical records and information the patient has personally disclosed to the healthcare worker. Everything that is heard, written, and discussed in the hospital STAYS AT THE HOSPITAL!

privileged information: confidential data; all data concerning a patient that is disclosed within the hospital

Respect the patient's privacy! Do not discuss patients' cases in the cafeteria, gift shop, parking lot, grocery store, at social gatherings, in the elevators, in the hallway, or in other departments. Conversations can be, and often are, overheard! Do not discuss the patient with anyone not directly involved in his or her care.

AIDS and Patient Confidentiality

Acquired immune deficiency syndrome (AIDS) is a major concern in hospitals today. The disease is transmitted through sexual contact or contaminated blood and blood products. At this point, AIDS is incurable, but preventable. The spread of AIDS has reached epidemic proportions throughout the world. This has led to many laws and regulations concerning disclosure of medical information about a patient with AIDS or who is **HIV positive**. A person who is HIV positive is positively infected with the virus, but may not have displayed any outward signs or symptoms of the AIDS disease.

The following guidelines are based on the state of California's approved legislation. Be sure to become familiar with the guidelines issued by your state.

1. Testing by blood banks and plasma centers is mandatory.
    Every donation of blood is tested for HIV prior to distribution.

2. Testing sites are available to detect the presence of the HIV virus.
    This is a free service.

3. All confirmed cases of AIDS must be reported by hospitals and
    physicians to the state and county health departments. Blood tests
    indicating HIV positive results do not have to be reported.

4. State and county health officials are required to contact those patients
    who test positive for follow up care, treatment, and to instruct them
    not to donate blood.

5. A written, signed consent must be obtained from the patient who
    is going to be tested for HIV. Become familiar with the consent
    used in the hospital and with the exceptions to this rule.

6. The patient must provide the healthcare worker with written
    permission to release the test results before the results can be given
    to anyone else. The person to whom the results will be given must
    be indicated on the consent form.

7. Unauthorized releases of test results can result in either penalties
    or imprisonment.

8. Employment and insurance cannot be denied solely on the basis of
    HIV positive test results.

AIDS confidentiality and testing remains extremely controversial. For your
protection and the protection of patients, follow the guidelines established by
the Centers for Disease Control and Prevention, your hospital, and state laws
concerning **Standard Precautions**.

Legal Terms

Here are some legal terms with which healthcare workers need to be familiar.

- **civil law:** a statute that provides for the protection of one's private rights and stipulates one's liabilities.

- **defendant:** a person named in a lawsuit; the accused.

- **deposition:** testimony given under oath concerning the events of a particular incident. (Usually conducted in an attorney's office.)

- **felony:** a major crime that is punishable by a greater means than a misdemeanor.

- **incompetent:** lacking skills; not mentally able.

- **judgement:** the final decision from a court.

- **litigation:** a lawsuit.

- **misdemeanor:** a minor crime; a crime less serious than a felony.

- **plaintiff:** the person filing a lawsuit; the injured person in a lawsuit.

- **res ipsa loquitor:** Latin for it speaks for itself; a legal concept that is used to determine negligence in cases in which a patient is injured while under the care of a healthcare provider.

- **respondeat superior:** a Latin phrase meaning the employer is responsible for the acts of its employees. Literally, *let the master answer.*

- **statute:** a law approved by the legislative branch of a government.

- **statute of limitations:** the particular length of time during which a lawsuit can be filed for a certain issue.

- **subpeona:** a document that requires a witness to appear at a trial or other proceeding to provide testimony.

- **testimony:** a statement, given under oath, providing details of a particular incident.

National Student Health Organizations

Professional organizations can play an important role in your career. There are two national student healthcare organizations that provide membership opportunities for students enrolled in allied healthcare classes:

Health Occupations Students of America (HOSA): a professional organization for students of health occupations

1. **Health Occupations Students of America (HOSA).** This organization is specifically designed for students who are interested in health careers. HOSA is directed toward the students of secondary, postsecondary, and approved pre-vocational educational programs. HOSA provides activities such as state-level competitions that focus on the needs of health occupations students. These particular activities encourage personal growth, promote career exploration, assist in developing leadership skills, and promote involvement in health-related community affairs. HOSA also publishes newsletters focusing on issues that are relevant to students in the field of allied health. More information can be obtained by writing to the following address:

   National HOSA Office
   P.O. Box 610755
   Dallas-Fort Worth, Texas 75261-0755

2. **Vocational Industrial Clubs of America (VICA).** This is a national organization that emphasizes respect for the dignity of work, high standards in work ethics, workmanship, scholarships, and safety. VICA is for students who are enrolled in various areas of study; namely, technical, industrial, trade, and health occupations programs. More information can be obtained concerning this organization by writing to the State Department of Education of your state:

   State Supervisor, Trade and Industrial Education
   State Department of Education
   State Capitol
   Street Address
   City, State Zip Code

One function these organizations have in common is the development of a Code of Ethics. The importance of this code in the healing arts is recognized by all areas of medicine.

Chapter Summary

Over the last decade, there has been an alarming increase in the number of lawsuits concerning the care patients have received from healthcare providers. The most frequent complaints concern the lack of time the healthcare provider spent with the patient and the lack of information provided to the patient by the healthcare provider.

Patients have a right to expect competent, high quality healthcare. As the patient advocate, you have the responsibility to keep yourself educated and well-skilled. Although there are several areas in which lawsuits can occur, treating patient's with kindness, consideration, and respect may greatly decrease your chances of being named as a defendant!

Providing hands-on care, documenting care given to patients, obtaining legal consent, caring for patients with a diagnosis of AIDS or HIV positive, and maintaining confidentiality are some of the areas in which lawsuits occur. Proper education regarding your job description or legal scope of practice and the hospital's policies and procedures can help make you a competent patient advocate.

Name _____

Date _____

Student Enrichment Activities

Complete the following statements.

1. Healthcare workers act as the _____ _____.

2. Healthcare professionals must never exceed their legal _____ _____ _____.

3. Principles and moral decisions are determined by one's _____.

4. The document that identifies the basic rights of all patients is the _____ _____ _____ _____.

5. The professional relationship between the healthcare provider and the patient is a _____.

6. The four items that constitute a breach of contract are:
    _____, _____, _____, and _____.

7. The two types of lawsuits common to the healthcare field are _____ and _____.

8. A private or civil wrong against another person is a _____.

9. Healthcare workers know special information about patients. This information is _____.

10. _____ confidentiality and testing remains controversial.

Unscramble the following terms.

11. STICHE   _____

12. TRAMICPLACE   _____

13. CROCTNAT   _____

14. APTNIET AVDCOTAE   _____ _____

15. ROTT   _____

16. TRAYBET   _____

17. ILENGCENGE   _____

18. SLATUSA   _____

19. ILCIV LWA   _____ _____

20. STIEPOINDO   _____

Chapter Five
Understanding the Patient as a Person

Objectives

After completing this chapter you should be able to do the following:

1. Define and correctly spell each of the key terms.

2. List the seven life stages.

3. Identify the four aspects of growth and development affected in each life stage.

4. List at least four characteristics of each life stage.

5. Identify at least three causes of stress that may affect an individual.

6. Describe the steps that may lead to a crisis situation.

7. List and describe the five stages in the dying process.

8. Explain hospice care.

9. Define the phrase *right to die.*

Key Terms

- Alzheimer's disease
- coping mechanisms
- culture
- custom
- death

- Elisabeth Kubler-Ross
- hospice
- life stage
- palliative
- right to die

The Challenge: Understanding Your Patient

The main focus of this chapter is to acquaint the clinical allied healthcare worker with the patient. Throughout a person's life, changes occur that affect the physical, psychological, and spiritual aspects of that particular person. In the clinical environment, you will be in contact with people from different ethnic and religious backgrounds who are at various stages of physical and emotional development. This is perhaps the most challenging aspect of providing healthcare. At each and every stage of treatment IT IS VITALLY IMPORTANT TO REMEMBER THAT THE PATIENT IS A PERSON!

From Infancy to Geriatrics

Learning to provide care for the public has become an increasingly complex medical, social, and ethical issue for the healthcare worker. According to the United States Bureau of the Census, there are over 34 million people aged 65 or older. That's almost 13% of the current population. The United States Administration on Aging expects this number to increase to 20% by the year 2030. The health of the aged is an area of growing concern to most people. For example, it would not be unusual for a person over the age of 85 to spend 50% of his or her personal income on healthcare. Because of the increasing numbers of people over the age of 65, it is important to have an understanding of the stages of growth and development that occur throughout a person's life. These stages will be briefly discussed in this chapter.

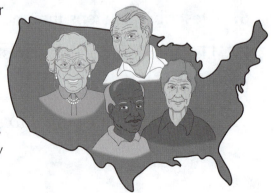

Development generally refers to successive changes in the process of one's natural growth. It occurs through the maturation of physical and mental capacities and learning. **Growth** generally refers to changes in the structure or size of a living organism. Human growth and development is an ongoing process; it begins at birth and does not end until death. Individual's have needs that must be met in every stage of growth and development. As a healthcare worker, you must be familiar with each stage in order to provide competent and high quality healthcare to the patient and his or her family.

Studies have demonstrated the influence heredity and environment have on the development of all people. Almost every person advances through a predictable and continuous development pattern consisting of particular stages that occur at specific ages in one's life. These development stages are commonly referred to as **life stages**. The following seven classifications are usually used to describe the various life stages.

life stage:
a segment of one's life that spans specific ages, and in which a predictable pattern of growth and development occur

- **infancy:** birth to 1 year old

- **early childhood:** 1 to 6 years old

- **late childhood:** 6 to 12 years old

- **adolescence:** 12 to 20 years old

- **early adulthood:** 20 to 40 years old

- **middle adulthood:** 40 to 65 years old

- **late adulthood:** 65 and older

These are the four aspects of growth and development that are affected by each life stage.

- **physical:** refers to the growth of the body.

- **mental:** refers to the development of the mind, such as solving problems, judgements, and decision making.

- **emotional:** refers to one's feelings.

- **social:** refers to a person's interactions and relationships with other members of society.

You will be able to provide much better care to your patients if you understand the developmental processes that occur in each of the seven life stages.

Infancy

The first year of life produces the most rapid and dramatic changes in a person's life. The most obvious changes occurring in infancy include physical changes in height and weight. Muscular and neurological changes also occur rapidly. Infants' motions progress from uncoordinated movements of the head and extremities to the development of fine motor coordination. The ability of an infant to pick up objects and put them in his mouth is an example of motor coordination. Infants are usually born without teeth; however, by their first birthday, they may have as many as twelve teeth. The newborn's vision is poor at birth and probably limited to black and white. However, as the first year of life progresses, vision greatly improves and so does his ability to see colors. By the time they are 1 year old, infants can focus on small objects and their eye movements are coordinated.

Mental, emotional, and social development also occur at a rapid pace. An infant's vocabulary increases from mere sounds to actual words by the age of 6 months. Emotions, and the expression of them, expand from simple excitement to distress, anger, fear, and affection. From birth to approximately 4 months of age, the infant's social skills are limited to being self-centered. By 4 months old, the infant recognizes the primary care giver, often smiles, and may frequently stare at others. Between the ages of 6 and 12 months old, the infant watches the activity of others, shows signs of possessiveness, withdraws from strangers, socializes freely with familiar people, and imitates facial expressions, gestures, and sounds. Infants are totally dependent on others for all of their physical, mental, emotional, and social needs. Infants who are ill must have these needs met in the hospital environment!

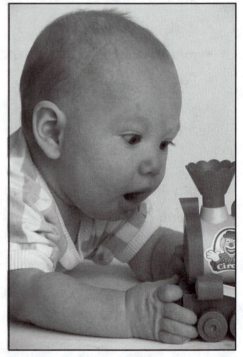

Figure 5-1: Infants undergo rapid developmental changes.

Early Childhood

Early childhood includes children from 1 to 6 years old. During this stage of development, the child's physical appearance begins to resemble that of an adult. The physical growth is slower than during the infancy stage. Muscles become larger, enabling the child to run and climb more freely. Most children start walking around their first birthday, and between the ages of 2 and 3 they learn how to control bowel and bladder functions. Children in this stage are able to eat adult food due to the maturation of the digestive system, and are learning to read, write, and draw.

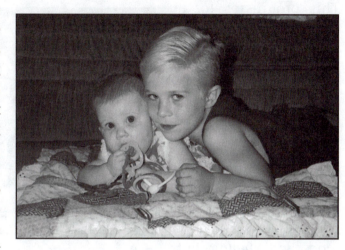

Figure 5-2: Early childhood describes children between the ages of 1 and 6 years.

Mental and emotional developments continue to occur rapidly. The vocabulary increases from the use of several small words to 2500 or more words by the age of 6. Although the attention span of the 2-year-old is very short, they express interest in many different activities. Emotionally, children between the ages of 1 and 2 are more aware of themselves and the effect they may have on others than when they were infants. The 4-year-old frequently asks questions and may be able to recognize words and letters. The typical 4-year-old is also beginning to form the basis of logic and usually attempts to make decisions by trial and error. Children in this stage may accept or defy the limitations and guidelines that are being established. Temper tantrums are an expression of frustration at not being allowed to perform as desired. Routine is especially important to a child of this age. If the routine is interrupted, for example due to illness, anger and stubbornness may be evident in the child's behavior. Children begin to gain control over their emotions by the age of 6 years. They are also less anxious when their routine is interrupted.

Children progress from the self-centered infancy stage to being more sociable with other children. They begin to enjoy the company of others; however some children in this stage may still be very attached to their parents. Slowly, they begin to develop social skills by playing with other children. This progresses to an actual interest in playing with others. Friends usually have become very important to children by the time they reach the age of 6.

Children in early childhood are still dependent on others for the basic needs of love, security, food, and shelter; but, they are gaining independence. This independence

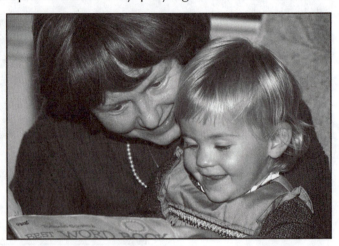

Figure 5-3: Children in early childhood need guidance and supervision from their parents.

is important, but they still need consistency and routine in their daily lives. Responsibility and conformity to guidelines can be taught to the child by making reasonable demands based upon the child's ability to comply.

Late Childhood

The stage of growth and development known as late childhood is commonly referred to as preadolescence. Children in late childhood are between the ages of 6 and 12. Physical development and changes occur at a slow but steady pace. It is during this stage of development and growth that the child enters the world of his peers. Both the large and small muscles are well-developed and enable the child to participate in physical activities that require complex motor-sensory coordination. Children have usually acquired most of their permanent teeth by the end of this stage, and visual acuity has matured to its best. In some children, sexual maturation may begin as early as the age of 9.

Changes continue to occur in **mental**, **emotional**, and **social** capacities. Mental maturation increases rapidly since most of their lives are centered around school and their peers. It is during this phase of development that speech, reading, and writing skills develop more completely. Memory is more complex, and children are learning how to use abstract information to solve problems. It is during this **life stage** that children are learning their morals and values.

Emotional changes occurring at this time of growth and development seem to assist the children in fully developing their independence. As preadolescents progress through school their self-confidence increases, enhancing their ability to cope with life's challenges. Between the ages of 9 and 12, sexual maturation and changes in bodily functions often lead to times of confusion and depression followed by periods of happiness and joy.

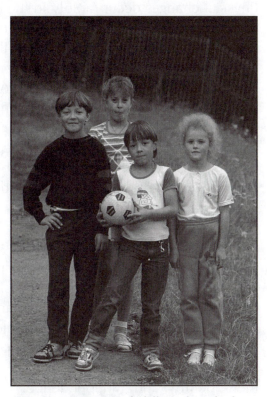

Figure 5-4: Late childhood includes those between the ages of 6 and 12 years of age.

Social skills increase between the ages of 6 and 12. Children progress from independent activities to group activities with members of the same sex. However, by the end of this life stage, children are becoming more aware of members of the opposite sex. They are learning how to accept the opinions and ideas of others, conform to guidelines, and mold their behavior according to their peers. Peer pressure is evident at the end of this life stage as acceptance by their peers is very important to the child. Parental approval and reassurance are the basic **needs**; however, peer pressure often causes mental and emotional confusion for the child. Children in this stage should be encouraged to make their own decisions.

Adolescence

Adolescence includes young people between the ages of 12 and 20. This can be a very traumatic life stage for both the child and any authoritative figure. Physical changes occur rapidly in the early years of this life stage; however, muscle coordination does not occur as quickly. This can make the child clumsy and awkward. It is during this time that **puberty** occurs. Puberty involves changes that enable members of both sexes to become functionally capable of reproduction. These changes usually provide the most obvious physical changes during this life stage. Girls will experience the onset of menstruation; boys will begin producing sperm and semen. Secondary sexual characteristics also occur. For example, the boy's voice deepens, facial hair begins to grow, muscle mass increases, and the shoulders broaden. Girls will acquire the familiar shape of the adult female—their hips will widen, breast size increases, and body fat is redistributed.

Since the basis for making decisions has already been established, adolescents learn to be accountable and accept responsibility for their actions. Education, morals, and values need to be emphasized through communication between the adolescent and their parents. Perhaps the greatest challenges in life are the conflicts that may arise between childhood and adulthood. Emotions run high. For example, adolescents are concerned about their appearance, relations with their peers, and their abilities. Adolescents are attempting to establish their identity and independence. Feelings of uncertainty, inadequacy, and insecurity may surface—sometimes in confrontation with authority. Near the end of this life stage, they have gained self-confidence and direction for their life. This leads to emotional maturity and a decrease in conflict and confrontations.

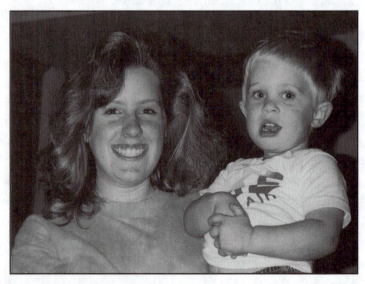

Figure 5-5: As adolescents mature, responsibilities increase, and may include caring for young children.

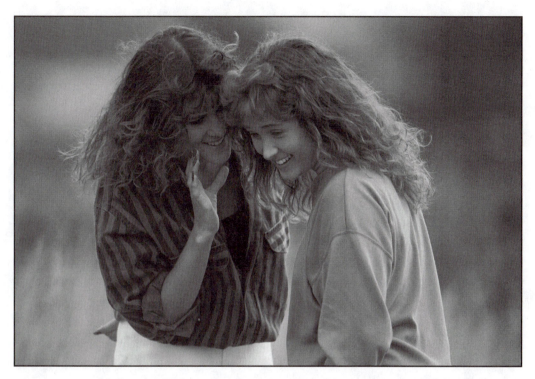

Figure 5-6: Adolescents thrive on approval and acceptance of their peers. Social activities begin to increase at this age.

Social skills become enhanced through association with peer groups who are frequently experiencing similar feelings and problems. Approval by their peers promotes self-confidence, thereby allowing the adolescent to become more satisfied and secure. As they near the end of this stage they begin to develop behavior patterns that are associated with adult behavior.

If the adolescent is exposed to excessive feelings of inadequacy and insecurity, certain behavior disorders may develop. Some of these disorders may be exhibited through physical problems. Eating disorders may stem from excessive concern regarding one's appearance. **Anorexia nervosa** usually finds its roots in an obsessive fear of becoming obese. However, this fear of obesity may continue even after substantial weight loss has occurred. This illness can be life-threatening. Treatment usually includes psychiatric therapy. Another psychiatric eating disorder is **bulimia**. It is characterized by binges of overeating followed by voluntary vomiting, fasting, or induced diarrhea. This can also be a life-threatening disorder. People with these types of disorders need immediate psychological intervention.

Substance abuse and suicide are enormous problems during this life stage. Although substance abuse can occur during any life stage, it frequently starts during adolescence. Substance abuse is the excessive use of chemicals, drugs, or alcohol in order to cope with daily problems. Substance abusers are emotionally addicted to these substances and, if not treated, will become physically dependent.

Suicide is the voluntary ending of one's life. It is one of the leading causes of death in adolescents. Suicide may stem from depression, low self-esteem, failure in school, lack of acceptance by family and peers, grief over a loss or love affair, or the inability to meet expectations. Usually, warning signs are given by the person contemplating suicide. These signs include: changes in sleep habits or appetite; withdrawal or mood changes; loss of interest in hobbies or other areas of life; and comments like, *I'd rather be dead*, or, *You'd be better off without me.* THESE INDIVIDUALS NEED IMMEDIATE HELP! Their cries for help should not be ignored.

Early Adulthood

People between the ages of 20 and 40 are considered to be in early adulthood. This is usually the most productive stage in one's life. Physical development is complete and motor coordination is at its peak. Mental development continues however, and often creates a desire for additional education. Individuals are involved with establishing a career, selecting a marital partner, and determining a particular lifestyle.

Emotional maturation continues to develop in this stage. Young adults are subject to many emotional stresses during this phase of their life; however, they usually have learned to accept responsibility for their actions, accept criticism, and how to profit from their errors. Socially, they have progressed from peer groups to associates with similar ambitions and desires, regardless of their age.

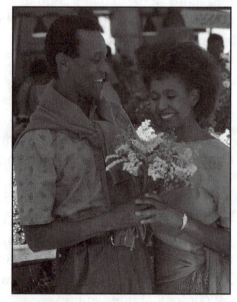

Figure 5-7: Early adulthood includes people between the ages of 20 and 40 years of age.

Middle Adulthood

Middle adulthood includes individuals who are between the ages of 40 and 60 years old. As with infancy, noticeable physical changes occur during these years. For example, the hair usually begins to thin and gray, wrinkles appear, muscles may lose their tone and strength, and hearing and vision may decrease. It is during this phase that weight sometimes begins to increase and become a problem. Hormones begin to change in both sexes and body changes reflect those hormonal variations.

Education may continue to be an important goal. Since individuals in middle adulthood often have acquired quite an understanding of life's problems, they sometimes are excellent at analyzing situations. From an emotional standpoint, this period of life may be filled with contentment or distress. Events concerning one's health, job security, children, aging parents, and the fear of aging during this period significantly affect the emotional status of the individual. Many people in this age group experience the death of one or both of their parents. Relationships with family members may change as offspring begin making families of their own. Marriages may become stronger or may end in divorce. Statistically, the divorce rate is high within this age bracket. Friendships are usually established with those who share the same or similar interests and lifestyle. As with the other life stages, love and acceptance continue to play major roles in the lives of these individuals.

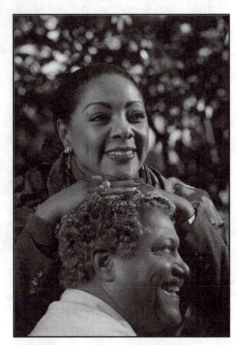

Figure 5-8: Mid-adulthood includes those between the ages of 40 and 60 years old.

Late Adulthood

Individuals over the age of 65 may be referred to as *elderly*, *senior citizens*, or *retired citizens*. Because of the increased life-span most individuals can expect today, this is the fastest growing age bracket of society. Individuals in this stage experience continued physical deterioration; bones become brittle, hair thins, skin becomes dry and wrinkled, and muscles lose their tone and strength, leading to poor coordination. Generally, all body systems are affected by advancing age. However, if the individual has been in overall good health, these changes usually occur slowly over a period of time. If this is the case, then these physical changes may not become apparent until the age of 80 or older.

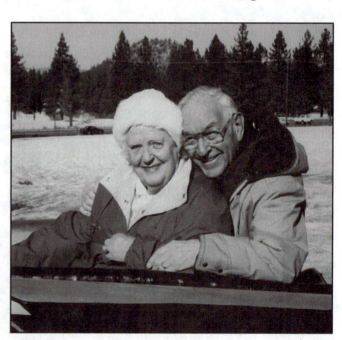

Some people in this age bracket may experience memory problems; however, individuals well into their 90s may exhibit no memory deficiencies at all. **Alzheimer's disease** is an illness that causes irreversible memory loss in many people in this stage. It is estimated that within the next ten years, one out of

Figure 5-9: Late adulthood includes those over the age of 65.

Alzheimer's disease: a neurological disease that causes irreversible memory loss and physical deterioration, which eventually leads to the complete loss of intellectual and physical functions

two people over the age of 80 will be affected by some stage of Alzheimer's disease. This is a serious problem for both its victims and their families because there is no known cure.

Social contacts remain important during late adulthood. With retirement often comes a loss of identity. Loss of a spouse or friends often leave the elderly feeling lonely and unimportant. It is important for individuals within this age bracket to remain active in organizations such as churches and community centers. The needs of the elderly are the same as the other life stages: a feeling of acceptance, love, self-esteem, and financial security.

Stress and the Patient

Illness, disease, and hospitalization are likely to be causes of **stress** for any patient. Stress simply refers to any event or situation that is perceived by a person to be threatening, and which disturbs his or her state of balance, or equilibrium. Each person's equilibrium involves his or her physical well-being, mental health, and spiritual life. It is essential that each of these aspects be fulfilled in the proper proportion. If they are not, that person's ability to deal with certain situations becomes impaired, and the situation seems overwhelming.

Stress, initially, is not always harmful to a person. However, when something occurs that interferes with one's ability to cope, then stress becomes harmful. There are times when a person feels threatened by something that is anticipated, such as surgery, or he may feel threatened by something he has only imagined. For example, a patient might imagine that he has a terminal illness when, in fact, he does not. Once an event or situation has been perceived as stressful to an individual, his or her equilibrium is threatened and tension begins to mount. Since tension causes discomfort, individuals try to reduce this tension using their normal **coping mechanisms**. A coping mechanism is a psychological or physical method that helps a person adjust or adapt successfully to a challenge. If these are not available, for example due to hospitalization, the tension remains unrelieved and, in fact, increases. As the tension continues to increase, the patient will become frustrated, and frustration will increase the patient's growing distress. This situation can deplete the patient's energy to the point that he or she may not be able to deal effectively with the problem. At this point, the patient is in a crisis and needs immediate help. As a healthcare worker, it is important to be sensitive to the needs of the patient.

coping mechanisms: defense mechanisms; the psychological or physical methods by which an individual adjusts or adapts to a challenge or stressful situation

Hospitalization can be stressful for the patient and his or her family members. Since each person reacts differently to this situation, all healthcare workers need to be aware of the signs and symptoms of severe stress. It is important to make each and every contact with the patient a meaningful encounter.

Certain concerns may increase the level of stress and frustration for the patient and his or her family. These areas include ethnic customs and religious beliefs. As a healthcare worker, be aware of these areas as they may illicit an irrational response from the patient. There are numerous studies that show stress can interfere significantly with the healing process.

custom:
a tradition or usual practice of a particular people or social group

culture:
the skills and arts of a given people at a given time

Ethnic **customs** and **cultural** differences may promote stressful situations for the patient and his family. Religious practices may need to be altered during an individual's hospitalization. This could be a source of stress for some people. It also may be difficult for some groups of people to be under the authority of a healthcare worker. Although the desires of the patient are not to be overlooked, the long term well-being of the patient is the ultimate goal. It is the responsibility of the healthcare worker to promote an atmosphere that is conducive to the overall healing of the patient. At times this may conflict with certain ethnic and religious customs and beliefs. As much as possible, allow the patient and their family the privilege of continuing their lifestyle in the hospital. This may reduce stress and promote the well-being of the patient.

As there are differences in religious beliefs and cultural customs, coping mechanisms vary between the different ethnic groups. It is important for the healthcare worker to display patience and understanding when differences are encountered. As a clinical allied healthcare worker, differences in religious beliefs and cultural customs must be dealt with in a mature manner. Effective listening skills, verbal and nonverbal communication, and reflective questioning are communication skills that will be valuable in promoting the overall healing of the patient. These skills will be addressed in Chapter Six.

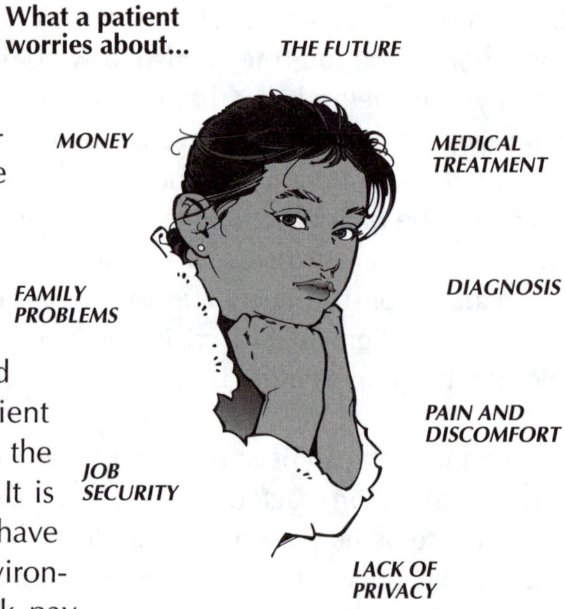

Other concerns that may compound a stressful situation for the patient are family matters, finances, and the diagnosis of the illness or injury. It is important to remember that patients have lives outside of the healthcare environment; they have relatives, go to work, pay bills, and go shopping. Sometimes, healthcare workers are so busy with their tasks they forget the patient may have other responsibilities on his or her mind. For example, the patient already may be burdened with bills at home, and now he or she must deal with medical bills too. Many patients are concerned about their children. If the patient is a single parent, child care will be a major concern.

What a patient worries about...

THE FUTURE

MONEY

MEDICAL TREATMENT

DIAGNOSIS

FAMILY PROBLEMS

PAIN AND DISCOMFORT

JOB SECURITY

LACK OF PRIVACY

Figure 5-10: A patient's concerns

Hospitalization does not put the patient's life on hold. Since the patient may not physically be able to do anything about his or her concerns, the mental burden can become increasingly heavy. Social Services and Discharge Planning are departments that may be valuable resources during these times of stress.

Death and Dying

One of the most stressful subjects for anyone to deal with is **death**. The prospect of death creates stress for everyone involved: the patient, his or her family, and the healthcare workers. As a healthcare worker, you must examine your own feelings and beliefs concerning death and dying; undoubtedly, you will be part of this very emotional experience at some point in your career.

Death is defined as the permanent cessation of all vital functions; the loss of brain stem and spinal reflexes, and flat EEGs over at least 24 hours. People react to death and dying in predictable stages; however, the initial stage and the length of each stage may vary. Each stage of the dying process will be discussed briefly in the next section.

Extensive research concerning death and dying and its effects on people has been completed by Doctor **Elisabeth Kubler-Ross**. She is considered to be a leading expert in this area. As a healthcare worker, it is important to have a basic understanding of each of the stages people will experience. In the past, patients were not usually told when they were dying. It was felt that the news might cause them to stop fighting for life, thereby hastening their death. Because of Doctor Kubler-Ross's extensive work, patients now are often informed of their impending death; however, patients should be left with as much positive information as possible. If a patient has been diagnosed with a **terminal** illness, it is imperative that the staff members know exactly how much information has been given to the patient and how the patient reacted to that information. Do not offer information to the patient or family concerning the illness without consulting the primary caregiver.

Doctor Kubler-Ross identified five stages of dying that all dying patients and their families and friends will experience. These stages may not occur in the same order. Stages may overlap, be repeated, or be concurrent. Of course, some patients may die before experiencing some of the stages. No matter how the patient responds, respect both the patient and the family's reaction.

death:
the end of life as indicated by the permanent cessation of all vital functions; the absence of brain stem and spinal reflexes, and flat EEGs over at least a 24 hour period

Elisabeth Kubler-Ross:
a leading expert in the area of death and dying; the first to identify the five stages of the dying process

DENIAL

Denial is referred to as the first stage of the dying process. The patient or family typically responds with statements resembling, "What do you mean I'm dying?" or, "There must be a mistake in the tests, I'm too young to have cancer," or "That's impossible, there's no way I could have gotten AIDS." Statements such as these indicate nonacceptance of the truth either by the patient, the family, or both. Patients will frequently seek another medical opinion. As a healthcare worker, the patient should be encouraged to share his feelings. Do not confirm nor deny; statements such as, "It must be hard on you," or, "Do you feel that seeing another doctor will help?" may help the patient express his or her feelings. Some patients may refuse to mention the disease. These people need support and encouragement. Once the patient has accepted the diagnosis and its implications, the second stage of the dying process will often surface.

ANGER

The second stage is identified as **anger**. Patients or family members will often strike out at anyone who happens to come in contact with them. Hostility and bitterness become apparent. It is important for the healthcare worker to remember that this reaction of the patient or family member is not a personal attack on the staff member; but an attack on their personal situation. Once again, as a healthcare worker, you should provide support, understanding, and excellent listening skills. Frequently, the patient will be demanding during the anger stage. Make every attempt to respond to the patient's demands as quickly as possible and with kindness. Never forget that the patient is a person!

BARGAINING

Usually after the patient has accepted death, the third stage of dying becomes evident. This stage is commonly referred to as **bargaining**. The patient now realizes that death is certain; however he wants more time so that certain goals might be attained. This is usually the time when the patient and/or family members look for spiritual strength. For example, the patient may try to bargain with God. For example a patient might pray, "Let me live so I can see my child get married," or, "I just want to see my new grandbaby." Healthcare workers must be attentive listeners and, whenever possible, help the patient achieve those goals.

DEPRESSION

As the patient realizes that death is imminent, **depression** will inevitably set in. Doctor Kubler-Ross has identified this as the fourth stage of dying. It has occurred to patients that they will no longer be with their families or their goals may not be completed. Patients may exhibit several different types of behavior. They may talk about their depression, become quiet and withdrawn, or deny that anything is wrong. During depression, the patient experiences great sadness and, at times, overwhelming despair. You will need to let the patient and the family know that it is both acceptable and expected to be sad. These are normal and natural emotions. Allow the patient and his or her family the liberty to cry and express those emotions. Be supportive; often a simple touch is all that is needed. It is alright to cry with the patient; after all, it is often the most difficult stage for the healthcare worker too. However, it is important to use self-control.

ACCEPTANCE

The final stage of the dying process is **acceptance**. When the patient and the family enter this stage, completing *unfinished business* will be the priority for the patient. When death is accepted, the patient may begin to help the survivors deal with the finality of death. As with the other stages, it is important to be supportive. Letting the patient and the family members know that you understand and care for them during this time of need is often the best therapy of all.

Working with dying patients and their families is a challenging aspect of healthcare. It is also an area that cannot be avoided. Patients are going to die while you are caring for them. To be supportive to the patient and the family, you must first evaluate and understand the patient's personal feelings about death and dying. Fear, frustration, sadness, and uncertainty may surface. These, in turn, may make you to want to avoid patients who are dying; but, you must come to terms with these feelings. After all, health-care workers are meant to be an ASSET to the patient and the family. As you gain experience with death and dying, you will be able to provide the appropriate supportive care.

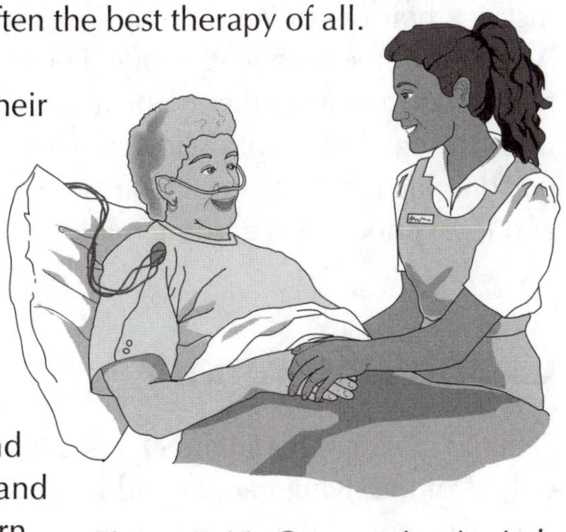

Figure 5-11: Compassion is vital when dealing with patients and their loved ones.

hospice:
a supportive agency offering care and counseling to dying patients and their families; a program consisting of palliative and supportive services

palliative:
care which relieves or eases, but does not heal

right to die:
a controversial issue concerning the right of a terminally ill patient to request that no life-sustaining measures be taken

Current medical costs are encouraging new methods of treatment and earlier discharges from the hospital environment. An increasing number of patients are in their homes when death occurs. An important supportive service offering care and counseling to dying patients and their family is **hospice** care. This care can be offered in a medical care facility or in the patient's home. The main philosophy of hospice is to allow the patient to die with dignity. Hospice is a program consisting of **palliative** and supportive services. Psychological, financial, social, and spiritual counseling are provided through the agency. Home health aides give personal care to the patient. The specially trained aide will often attend to the patient while other family members leave the home for brief periods of time. This service also relieves the family of the sole responsibility of providing care to a dying loved one. It is vital to remember the individual needs of the family members during this time.

Another healthcare issue that has received a great amount of attention over the last decade concerns a person's **right to die**. With advanced medical technology capable of sustaining life, allowing patients to die can be an area of great conflict in a profession that is concerned with preserving and sustaining life. Results of recent studies and surveys have shown that a growing percentage of the general public and health professionals feel that patients with a terminal illness should be allowed to die as peacefully as possible. Because of this, almost all states now have laws that provide mentally competent adults to instruct their physician, in writing, to withhold life sustaining measures. (See Advance Directives in Chapter Four.) This means that using pacemakers, respirators, and any other medical device or form of treatment used to prolong life can legally be withheld. However, deliberately taking action to end a person's life is still against the law. Legislation continues to explore the ethical and legal concerns regarding the issue of a person's right to die.

Chapter Summary

Death is a natural part of life. As healthcare workers understand the needs and desires of the dying patient and his or her family, supportive care becomes a natural response. Understanding the seven life stages that all people experience enhances the ability of the healthcare worker to more clearly understand the actions and reactions of the patient and/or the family. The five stages of the dying process, along with the seven life stages, paint a complex picture of people. Always remember that patients are people, and basic needs and life's responsibilities do not end with hospitalization! Be as supportive and understanding as possible; after all, you may be a patient one day.

Name _____

Date _____

Student Enrichment Activities

Complete the following statements.

1. It is not unusual for the elderly to spend approximately _____ of their income on healthcare.

2. There are _____ different life stages throughout one's life span.

3. In a healthy life span, total dependency on others for all physical, mental, emotional, and social needs usually occurs during _____.

4. It is estimated that within the next 10 years, 1 out of 2 people over the age of 80 will be affected by some stage of _____ _____.

5. During the _____ _____ stage, the social skills are influenced by both the parents and the peers.

6. Substance abuse and suicide can be enormous problems during _____.

7. Establishing a career, selecting a marital partner, and determining a particular lifestyle often occur during _____ _____.

8. Inadequate coping mechanisms result in a negative occurrence of _____.

9. Two hospital departments that may be valuable resources during times of stress are _____ _____ and _____ _____.

10. _____ _____ _____ is a well-known authority on death and dying.

11. An important supportive service offering care and counseling to dying patients and their families is _____ _____.

12. A controversial issue concerning the rights of patients is the _____ _____ _____.

Unscramble the following terms.

13. FILE TESAGS   _____ _____

14. GIRTH OT IDE   _____ _____ _____

15. LIVEATALIP   _____

16. SHOPICE   _____

17. LIZAREMESH SEASIDE   _____ _____

18. TRUELUC   _____

19. UBPRETY   _____

20. GINPCO SCHEMAMIN   _____ _____

Chapter Six
Communication Skills

Objectives

After completing this chapter you should be able to
do the following:

1. Define and correctly spell each of the key terms.

2. Identify examples of verbal and nonverbal communication skills.

3. Name at least three factors that influence the transmission of a message.

4. Name at least three factors that influence the receipt of a message.

5. Describe each of the five levels of Maslow's Hierarchy of Needs and the factors that may affect each level.

6. Describe at least three defense mechanisms and give examples of each.

7. List five rules of proper telephone etiquette.

Key Terms

- Abraham Maslow
- communication
- defense mechanisms
- Maslow's Hierarchy of Needs
- need

- nonverbal
- receiver
- sender
- significant other
- verbal

The Need for Effective Communication

communication:
the verbal or nonverbal exchange of messages, ideas, thoughts, feelings, and information

The establishment and growth of a lasting, meaningful relationship depends on effective communication. **Communication** is the verbal or nonverbal exchange of messages, ideas, thoughts, feelings, and information. The art of communication involves the mastery of specific skills. Learning, developing, and using these techniques promotes a positive, healthy relationship between people.

significant others:
people who are emotionally concerned for or attached to the patient

This concept is vitally essential to the initial and ongoing relationship between the healthcare worker, patient, and **significant others**. A significant other may be a spouse, relative, or friend. Legalities concerning release of information regarding the patient are discussed in Chapter Four.

This chapter deals with the development and implementation of communication techniques and the effects they have on the healthcare worker-patient relationship. Effective use of these specific skills will promote a healthy environment for the recovery of the patient.

sender:
the person who attempts to transmit information to another person or a group of people

Senders and Receivers

receiver:
the person or group of people for whom information is intended

In order for effective, valuable communication to occur, at least two people must be involved—the sender and the receiver. The **sender** is the person who desires to transmit information to another person or group of people. The **receiver** is the person, or group of people, for whom the information is intended. The **message** is the information that must be transmitted. Without the sender, message, and receiver, communication cannot occur.

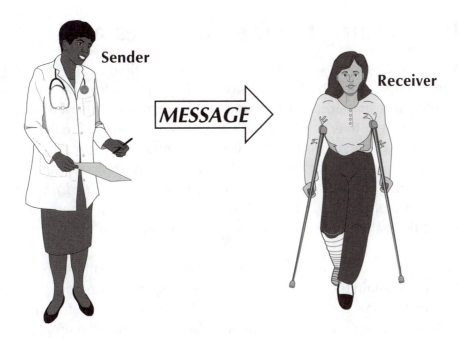

Figure 6-1: The Elements of Communication

Verbal and Nonverbal Communication

Information can be transmitted verbally or nonverbally. **Verbal** communication involves the use of spoken words. **Nonverbal** communication involves body language, tactile stimulation (touch), and facial expressions. Both the sender and the receiver use one or both methods when a message is transmitted and received.

verbal:
spoken

nonverbal:
a form of communication that involves body language, tactile stimulation (touch), and facial expressions

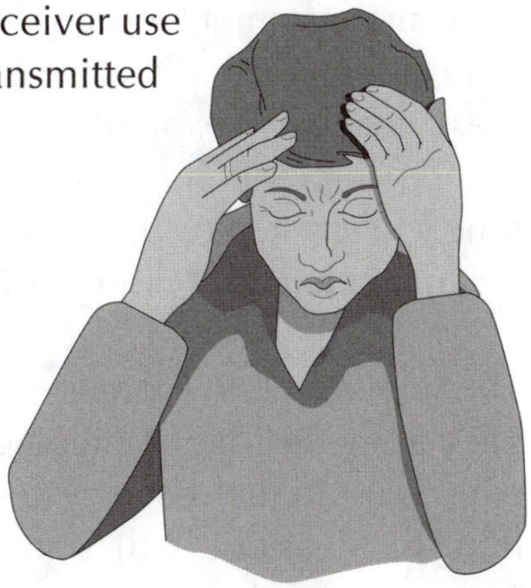

Figure 6-2: Some patients will provide nonverbal clues as to the nature of their complaint.

Transmitting the Intended Message

Although the process of communication may appear simple, several factors may interfere with the transmission and receipt of the intended message. Effective transmission of the message is the responsibility of the sender. The sender must deliver a message clearly and effectively. Clear messages are communicated in terms the receiver understands. Healthcare workers often communicate with each other using medical terminology, but patients and their significant others may not be educated in the meaning of medical terms. Therefore, the healthcare worker must translate medical terms into words the patient may understand. This will improve the communication.

For example, saying to the patient, "I am going to auscultate breath sounds," does not explain the procedure. However, saying, "I am now going to listen to your breathing," means the same thing and is easier for the patient to understand. Terminology may need to be simplified even more for children and individuals with limited education. Some words will need to be modified or substituted so the message may be clearly transmitted.

Besides using proper terminology, the verbal message must be transmitted using correct grammar and punctuation. It is very important to pronounce words properly. The use of slang words and vocabulary with more than one meaning, should be avoided. Terms such as *like, you know,* and *uh-huh* are meaningless and also should be avoided. Emphasis of a particular word and the way a statement is phrased can also affect the clarity of the message. The tone of the voice and pitch of the voice reveals the underlying meaning of the message. For example, practice saying, "I am having a really good time," several different times. Vary the phrasing, tone and pitch of your voice each time you say it. Now try saying it emphasizing different words. See how the meaning changes with the different speech patterns?

The speed at which someone speaks also affects how the receiver interprets the verbal message. A message transmitted at a rate of speed that is too fast may result in the receiver misinterpreting the message, (eg, *hearing* something that was not said). These factors must be applied to all types of verbal communication.

Not only must healthcare workers learn which questions to ask, but they must also learn how to phrase their questions. **Open-ended questions** generally provide more information because they permit the **receiver** to elaborate on the answer (eg, "Describe the pain to me."). **Closed-ended questions** only allow a short answer. Typically, only a "yes" or "no" response is required. "Does your head hurt?" is an example of a closed-ended question. Practice and experience will enhance your verbal communication skills.

Receiving the Message

The previous section focused on the responsibilities of the sender during the transmission of the message. However, the receiver also plays a very important role in effective communication. The receiver must be able to hear the message adequately. If the message is written, the person must be able to read and have an adequate vocabulary and understanding of the terminology used.

Several factors also may affect the receiver's interpretation of the message. Medication, age, level of education, and limited English all impact the interpretation of the information communicated. Patients who are under the influence of pain medication may have their **sensorium** altered. The sensorium refers to the part of the brain that receives and interprets sensory stimuli. It also refers to one's level of consciousness. Pain medication can affect the sensorium by impairing a patient's hearing or clouding his or her memory. These patients may nod their head as if they understand; but, it is advisable to relay the information to a significant other as well as the patient.

Those who are either elderly or very young may not fully comprehend the intent of the message. For example, young patients may not understand certain words you normally use. On the other hand, elderly patients may be insulted if overly simplified terminology is used. When an older person does not understand your message, it doesn't mean that they do not understand your terminology, it may mean they are hard of hearing! When you encounter a patient who has difficulty hearing, be sure to face the patient, speak clearly, and pronounce the words properly. Talk directly into the patient's ear if necessary, and repeat the message if needed; take your time with the hearing impaired. Use family members to help transmit the message. They understand the needs of the patient and can often communicate the message more effectively than the healthcare worker.

Visually impaired patients or those who are hearing impaired often have a communication system already intact. Ask them, or the significant other, about the most effective way they use to communicate their needs.

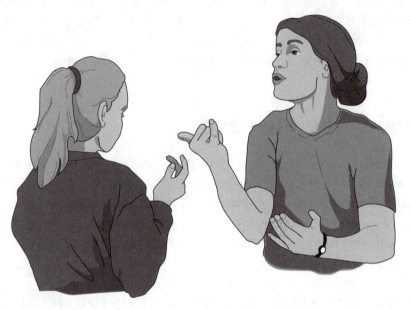

Figure 6-3: Some hearing impaired people use sign language as one of their communications systems.

People who are learning impaired may require special communication techniques. Patience and understanding are extremely important when rendering healthcare to this type of patient. Using the Social Services Department and the patient's significant other may help the communication.

The receiver will often hear the message, but may not understand it. Body language, facial expressions, and inappropriate responses may suggest lack of understanding by the patient. Rephrasing the message using terminology that is more familiar to the patient and using examples to illustrate what you mean may enhance the comprehension of the message. Learning to be sensitive to these signs is important. Many people hesitate to admit they do not understand a message because the sender may interpret the receiver as being dumb.

There are times when the receiver's attitude and prejudices may interfere with proper receipt of the message. For example, if the healthcare worker seems hurried or does not appear to be knowledgeable and informed during the transmission, the patient will not accept the information.

The receiver must have confidence and trust in the sender before the message is accepted and believed. Healthcare workers must be willing to say, "I do not know, but I will try to find out that information for you." Healthcare workers also must be aware of their own feelings of prejudice toward patients. For example, if you think that patients are lazy, ignorant, apathetic (uncaring, showing no emotion), or uncooperative, your actions may reveal and produce inappropriate reactions from the receiver.

Distractions and interruptions also interfere with effective communication. Loud noises, ringing phones, uncomfortable room temperatures or accommodations, and writing while speaking to someone can all alter the effectiveness of the intended message. An attempt to eliminate, or at least limit, the number of distractions will greatly enhance meaningful communication.

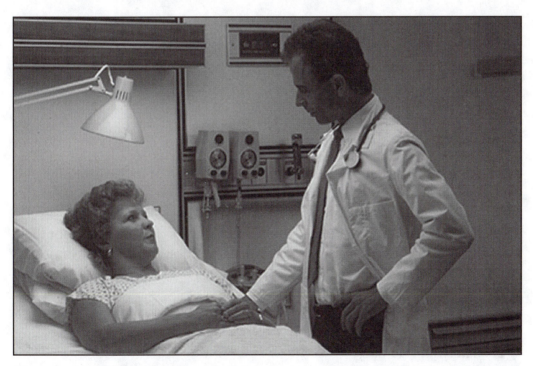

Figure 6-4: Looking directly at the patient as you speak or listen and ignoring or eliminating distractions will enhance the quality of your communication.

Active listening is an essential part of effective and meaningful communication. It requires a conscious effort from the receiver; the receiver must pay attention to exactly what the sender is communicating. The receiver must have a sincere interest and concern regarding the message the individual is sending. Eye contact, an open mind, and observation of the sender's nonverbal communication may help uncover hidden meanings to the message.

Reflective statements and **clarification** also aid the receiver's understanding of the message. Reflective statements tell the sender how the message was heard and received. Clarification allows the sender to explain any part of the message the receiver was unclear about. For example, a patient may say, "I feel awful today." As a healthcare worker, you should clarify what the sender means by "awful" by replying, "What do you mean by awful?" This is an open-ended question that will allow the sender to elaborate on the statement.

Written communication must be complete, clear, and legible. All words must be correctly spelled and the memorandum, message, or letter should contain correct grammar. The receiver of the message often considers the written form of communication to be a direct reflection of the sender.

need:
something (either physical or psychological) that is required by an organism

Mastery of the verbal and nonverbal communication skills requires constant practice. Breakdowns in communication will be prevented when both the sender and receiver use effective communication skills.

Abraham Maslow:
a psychologist who is credited with a theory of motivation that identified five levels of human needs in which the lower levels must be satisfied before attention is given to the higher levels

Human Needs

All humans have essential **needs** that must be met in order to live a fulfilling life. These needs motivate a person to act or behave in certain ways. A reputable psychologist, **Abraham Maslow**, identified five categories of human needs. Through his research and studies, he developed the order of priority for these needs known as **Maslow's Hierarchy of Needs**. Starting with the most important need, the five levels are as follows:

1. Physiological needs.

2. Safety and security.

Maslow's Hierarchy of Needs:
five categories of needs identified by psychologist Abraham Maslow, including physiological needs, safety and security, love and affection, esteem, and self-actualization

3. Affection and love.

4. Esteem.

5. Self-actualization.

Physiological needs include the physical, biological, or basic needs that are required by every human being in order to live. Examples include oxygen, food, water, elimination of waste products, protection from extreme temperatures, and sleep. If any of these needs remains unmet, death will occur. It is interesting that even in this category, priorities exist. For example, if a person is deprived of oxygen, death will occur sooner than if a person is deprived of food. This is an important concept to remember when taking care of patients. For example, a patient who is gasping for each breath will not be concerned with eating. Physiological needs also include sensory and motor stimulation.

Sensory stimulation refers to the senses, and includes touch, sight, taste, smell, and hearing. As these needs are fulfilled, the individual may respond to the environment. Deprivation of one or more of these needs may result in the loss of contact with reality. **Motor** stimulation involves muscle excitation. If a person's muscles are not stimulated, then **atrophy** (decrease in size) will occur.

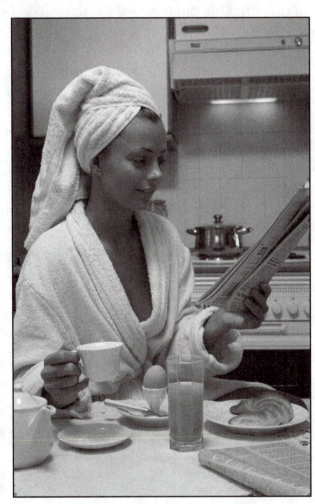

Figure 6-5: Nutritious food is one of our physiological needs.

The body automatically controls many physiological needs. For example, most people do not consciously think about the physical effort of breathing. Any loss of bodily function may affect the physiological needs of the patient. Be considerate of the patient. It is often embarrassing to ask for assistance. Remember to offer help to patients; this may prevent them from feeling humiliated.

Safety is the next level on the hierarchy of needs. Safety only becomes important after the physiological needs have been satisfied. This level includes the desire to feel secure in their environment and to be free from anxiety and fear. There are several methods by which a person strives to attain this level of safety. For example, the desire for order and routine often gives a person a sense of control and security. The loss of order and routine in his or her life often leaves the patient feeling out of control and results in insecurity and uncertainty.

People are comfortable with familiar faces, environments, and material things. Fear of the unknown often manifests itself as insecurity and fear. Explaining all procedures before the equipment is brought into the room may help alleviate this fear in the patient and may promote a sense of trust between the healthcare worker and the patient.

There are many factors that may affect an individual's sense of safety and security. For example, marital problems, financial struggles, and employment uncertainties may cause specific reactions from the patient. As the healthcare worker, it is important that you do not take the responses of the patient as a personal attack on you.

Love and affection is the next level on Maslow's Hierarchy of Needs. This includes the need for friendship, social acceptance, and love. The need to belong, relate to others, and receive social acceptance are the driving forces at this level. Attending social functions is usually important. Since the need for safety and security has been satisfied, it is easier to adapt to new environments, unfamiliar faces, and unknown routines.

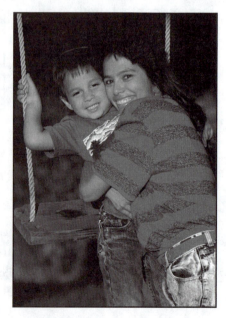

Sexuality is often included at this level as well as in the first level, physiological needs. Sexuality does not only include sexual relationships, but also considers a person's gender and the feelings, emotions, and needs associated with being either male or female. The way in which a person views his or her sexuality will often determine the ways in which his or her need for love and affection will be met.

Figure 6-6: Love and affection are basic human needs.

Feeling important and worthwhile is part of the fourth level, **esteem**. Receiving respect, approval and appreciation from others enhances one's self-esteem. Individuals often participate in activities that bring achievement, success, and recognition. These help create and maintain positive self-esteem in a person. When self-esteem is high, the fifth level, self-actualization, becomes possible for that person.

The last level is called **self-actualization**. When a person achieves this level, all other needs on the previous four levels have been satisfied. Self-actualization means that the individual is satisfied with the levels of growth and success he or she has achieved. Personal beliefs are strong, and ideas and beliefs are expressed with confidence. This does not mean that the person no longer has any goals, it simply means that the person's full potential has been explored and realized. This is the highest level in the Hierarchy. It cannot be attained unless the needs are met at all other levels.

Meeting Those Needs

As an individual identifies a need, he or she becomes motivated to act in a way that will attain that need. If the action is successful, the person will feel a sense of satisfaction, or fulfillment. However, if the action has failed to meet that need, tension or frustration may result. The desire for the fulfillment of more than one need at the same time may occur. At this point, the individual must set priorities and decide which need is the strongest. For example, a person may be both tired and hungry at the same time. In this case, the individual must decide whether to eat or take a nap.

As an individual grows, needs may be experienced at different levels of intensity. If the intensity is strong, the desire to satisfy that need also will be strong. As people experience new and different needs, they may try to fill that need through trial and error. As a person matures, satisfying those needs becomes easier.

There are two methods of fulfilling the hierarchy of needs. The first method is called *direct*. This technique uses realistic goals, hard work, and cooperation with others in order to meet the needs and obtain satisfaction. The second, and less preferred, method is *indirect*. This method usually relieves the tension and frustration created by the unmet need, or reduces the particular need. The need remains, but the intensity of the need may be reduced. The most common indirect methods are known as **defense mechanisms**. Defense mechanisms are used by everyone; they help people cope with stressful situations.

defense mechanisms: coping mechanisms; methods of unconscious behavior that assist people in coping and adapting to life

Defense Mechanisms

The coping mechanisms people use to meet a need or manage stress vary greatly from person to person. The term *defense mechanisms* covers a broad category of typical behavior patterns. It is believed that these mechanisms are used subconsciously, not intentionally. They provide a way for the individual to maintain his or her self-esteem and to relieve discomfort. If overused, defense mechanisms do not allow the person to cope realistically with specific needs and stressful situations. Several of the more commonly used defense mechanisms are rationalization, projection, compensation, and displacement.

Rationalization consists of using a logical reason or acceptable explanation for a particular behavior that makes the behavior seem appropriate. This type of behavior is often seen in patients who fear hospitalization. For example, a patient may be rude and abrupt with the healthcare staff. The patient rationalizes the behavior by thinking, "It's okay for me to act this way because I am sick."

Projection involves attributing one's own undesirable qualities to another person. In the example above, the patient may indicate that his rudeness stemmed from the "extreme rudeness and abruptness of the hospital staff."

Another defense mechanism is **compensation**. Physical and mental inferiorities may be the driving forces behind this type of coping mechanism. For example, a patient who is paralyzed below the waist may work very hard and diligently at strengthening the muscles of the upper body. This may mentally help the patient cope with the atrophy of the lower body. This is a healthy use of compensation. Healthy or unhealthy compensation methods are often a direct reflection of the physical, mental, and spiritual balance of a person's life. As mentioned earlier, if one of these aspects is not balanced with the others, a person may turn to unhealthy compensation methods (alcohol abuse, drugs, etc.) Redirecting goals may be another healthy method of compensation.

Displacement involves redirecting an emotion or behavior from the original person or object to another person or object. Displacement is often seen with anger. Sometimes people are angry with one person or a situation, but the anger may be displaced to other people if the original problem is not resolved.

It is important for healthcare workers to realize that the use of defense mechanisms is a normal part of everyday life. However, the healthcare worker must refrain from discussing his or her own problems with the patient and the patient's family. Healthcare workers who recognize the needs and coping mechanisms of others can provide better patient care.

Communication Devices

Today, there are many types of communication devices available for the consumer. Several devices that are frequently used by healthcare personnel will be discussed briefly in this section.

Perhaps the most common communication device is the telephone. This is a very important link between healthcare workers and the public. An impression is created by the receiver every time the telephone is used. Therefore, PROPER TELEPHONE ETIQUETTE (good manners) IS A MUST for healthcare workers.

Be sure to follow your organization's rules regarding telephone etiquette. Always remember the type of impression you wish to create when you are speaking to a caller. Avoid comments that might offend someone. Treat the caller as you would like to be treated; after all, you may be the caller someday! If you do not know the answer to a question that has been asked, try checking a manual. Operation and procedural manuals can be valuable sources of information when questions are asked by a caller, or when requests are made by other public agencies such as the Police Department, Fire Department, etc.

Practice the following guidelines until proper telephone etiquette becomes a habit.

1. Efficient management of the telephone requires the use of many different skills. Always have a pad of paper and pencil or pen in front of you before you answer the telephone. The impression you create can influence the caller greatly. Therefore, you must be professional at all times. This means you must use a combination of tact, friendliness, sincerity, and courteousness. You must also be able to be firm when discussing procedures, yet flexible enough to make the caller feel comfortable. It can be very challenging to incorporate all of these traits into one telephone conversation, yet sometimes it must be done. Above all, YOU MUST ACT RESPONSIBLY WHEN MAKING DECISIONS!

2. Your tone of voice must be pleasant. It will help if you answer the telephone with a smile on your face. Avoid using an indifferent tone, and keep your voice low pitched, clear, and distinct. DO NOT MUMBLE! Mumbling can be avoided if you hold your head up and do not lean the telephone receiver on your shoulder while speaking.

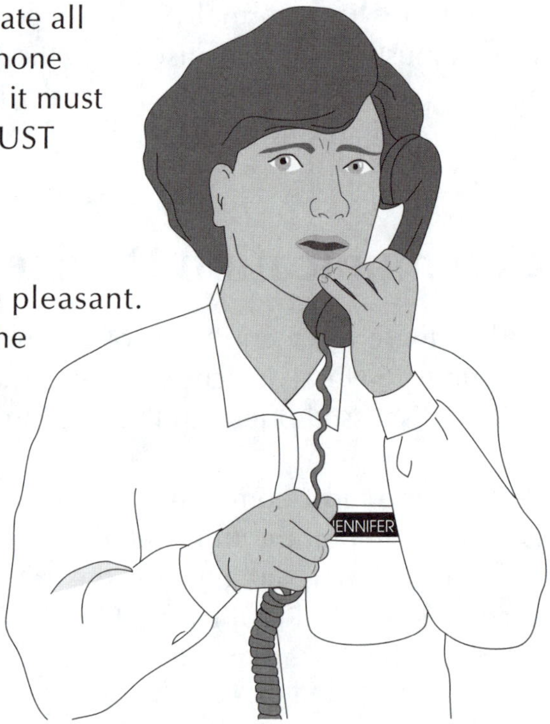

Figure 6-7: Proper use of the telephone requires etiquette.

3. Answer the telephone in three rings or less.

4. Identify the facility or department and yourself. Refrain from answering by just saying, "Laboratory." Use the phrase, "Laboratory, Debi speaking, may I help you?" This lets the person calling know what department they have contacted and to whom they are speaking.

5. Remember to use common courtesy and manners during the conversation. Do not forget to say "please" and "thank you." If someone says "Thank you," say "You're welcome," rather than "No problem," which is less courteous.

6. Always ask for the caller's name. Do not hesitate to ask for the correct spelling. Do not use statements such as "Who is this?" or "What is your name?" Instead, smile and ask, "May I please have your name?" or "May I say who is calling, please?"

7. Screening calls properly requires practice and experience. A few suggestions and guidelines will be provided here; but you should always refer to the agency's policy and procedure manual for their specific requirements:

    A. Determine the purpose of the call. This will help you decide if another person could assist the caller, or if a message needs to be taken and the call returned. Simply say to the caller, "I'm sorry, but the doctor is with a patient. May I take a message and have him return your call?"

    B. Learning to use discretion while screening calls takes practice. It is inappropriate to say to the caller, "The doctor is at lunch now," or, "The surgeon will be here in about two hours, she's playing golf." A more appropriate statement would be, "The doctor is not available now. I'll ask her to return your call as soon as possible." Or you could say "I expect the doctor at 7:00, may I take a message for her?"

8. Emergency calls are inevitable. Proper handling and referral of those calls to the appropriate person or department requires specific skills. It is important to remember that the general public may view an emergency situation differently than a healthcare worker would view it. View the emergency call from the perspective of the caller. Many of the calls will not seem overly serious to you; yet, to the medically uneducated public, certain situations warrant a call for assistance from a medically trained person. Be sure to refer the call to the appropriate person (ie, the nurse or doctor). Remember, giving medical advice over the phone can impose certain liability risks; therefore, be aware of your facility's policy concerning telephone medical advice.

9. Problem calls also will be encountered. Some people may not comply with your requests for their name or the purpose of their call. This must be dealt with in a firm, professional, and courteous manner. Remain calm and do not lose your temper! Politely explain to the caller that you cannot help him or her without knowing the nature of the call or who is calling. Handle the situation tactfully.

10. Placing callers on hold must be kept to a minimum. If you must place the caller on hold, politely ask, "Can you hold for a short time while I find out for you?" If there is an unanticipated delay, be sure to let the person who is holding know this. Offer to take the caller's name and number and return the call. Consideration is the key!

Some healthcare agencies prefer to use a telephone memo book. This is sometimes called a telephone log. The sole purpose of this log is to serve as a record of all calls received. Most memo books follow the same basic format. Record the information as follows:

1. Use the full, complete name of the caller—check for the correct spelling.

2. Indicate the date and time the call was received.

3. Briefly summarize the purpose of the call.

4. Record your response to the call (ie, if the caller was referred to another person or department, then document this).

5. Place your initials at the end of the message.

6. Indicate if the caller will call back or wishes to have the call returned.

Today's technology has made the cellular telephone both popular and affordable for many people. These phones allow verbal contact with someone almost anywhere. Many physicians have a telephone in their car and others have a cellular phone that is portable, or mobile. This means that it can be removed from the car, home, or office and physically carried by the person to another location (eg, hospital, golf course, another person's home, etc.). When communicating with someone via their cellular telephone, it is very important to speak clearly and listen carefully. The connection often is not as clear as it is when using a telephone via the cable line.

The telephone is a valuable communication tool. Learning to use it properly and practicing proper telephone etiquette greatly enhances the agency's relationships with the public and other professionals.

One of the most important communication devices is the computer. Computers are used in every department of the hospital. They are the communication link of the healthcare facility. Computers are used to generate patient records, and to transmit a physician's orders for patient care, including diagnostic testing, diet, medications, treatments, supplies, equipment, and so on to the various departments. Every healthcare worker should become familiar with the use of the facility's computer system and must understand the importance of maintaining patient confidentiality when using this important communication device.

Another useful communication device is a pager. A pager is a small device that may be carried in the pocket or on the belt. There are three types of pagers. The first is a *beeper*. This device is a simple pager in that it just beeps when the person has a call. When they receive a call, they contact a central number (their office) and ask why they were beeped. This type of pager is not used very often now that voice pagers and digital pagers are on the market.

The voice pager is accessed by dialing the pager number, waiting for three beeps, and then verbally relaying the message you want the person to receive. You must speak clearly because most of the time it is difficult for a clear message to be transmitted.

Although the voice pager is still used, the digital pager is gaining in popularity. One advantage of the digital pager is that messages cannot be misunderstood. Accessing a digital pager is similar to the voice pager. First, dial the pager number, and wait for three beeps, then dial the number you want the person to call, wait for the busy signal, and hang up. When you do this, the digits, or numbers, you dialed over the telephone for the person to call will appear on the pager's display area. When the person is able to get to a telephone, your call should be returned. As long as the person wearing the pager has it turned on, the message will be received. Allow the person approximately fifteen minutes to return your call before paging again. Sometimes it may take awhile for someone to respond to the page if he or she is not near a phone.

Recent advances have enabled companies to develop pagers that will allow the caller to enter letters and words as well as numbers. These are called alphanumeric pagers. Many hospitals and healthcare facilities have upgraded their communications systems to accommodate this new technology. Healthcare professionals can sit at a special keyboard and type their entire message onto a computer screen. Once the message is complete and correct, one additional key stroke will electronically send the message to the pager. This new technology saves time when updating physicians on a patient's condition or following up on lab results.

Intercoms are used in many healthcare facilities. They may be as simple as a telephone intercom or as complicated as the overhead system used in hospitals. Often the intercom system is located in each patient's room, the nursing station, and the staff lounge. It is easily accessed through specific buttons or switches or by dialing a specific code. Whenever a patient activates the intercom system, it should be answered promptly.

Due to advanced electronic technology, contact with anyone is available 24 hours a day. To have effective results, you must be skilled in the use of the telephone and the paging system. During orientation, ask questions and use the devices under supervision in case problems should arise. These are skills that should be polished through persistent and diligent practice.

Other methods of communication exist within all healthcare facilities, small businesses, and corporations. Department memorandums are an effective way of notifying personnel of changes and upcoming meetings, seminars, etc. These are called *memos* and are usually posted for everyone to read.

Department supervisors and committee members often attend meetings. Minutes are recorded and appropriate information from the meeting will be shared with other staff members in additional meetings and memos. Try to attend as many staff meetings as possible; this will keep you informed of any policy and procedure changes, new equipment, in-services, and other valuable information that is pertinent to the efficient operation of the department. Staff meetings are the most suitable time to share areas of concern dealing with policies and procedures of the department. These meetings should never be used as a time to gossip or complain.

Chapter Summary

Meaningful relationships are built through communication. Many factors influence the quality of a communication. The ability to identify those factors and learning how to prevent misunderstandings will greatly enhance your personal, and professional relationships.

Everyone has needs that must be satisfied. Circumstances, attitudes, emotions, feelings, and prejudices often affect when and how those needs are met. Sensitivity to those factors will open and enhance communication between you and the patient. As a healthcare worker, your job is to nurture patients to a state of wellness. This includes verbal and nonverbal communication with the patient, significant other, and family members.

Modern technology has introduced several different types of communication devices. Computers are the communication link of the healthcare facility, and cellular telephones, pagers, memos, and meetings are just a few additional means of communicating information and messages from one source to another in the work environment. Proper etiquette must be used with each of these devices in your place of employment!

Mastery of communication skills requires persistent practice. It is through valuable communication skills that meaningful and lasting relationships will be developed and nurtured.

Name _____

Date _____

Student Enrichment Activities

Complete the following statements.

1. The three parts of any communication are the _____, the _____, and the _____.

2. Body language and tactile stimulation are examples of _____ _____.

3. The effective sending of a message is enhanced when _____ and _____ are kept to a minimum.

4. Accurate information is best obtained by asking _____ questions.

5. _____ listening requires a conscious effort from the receiver.

6. Five categories of human needs were identified by _____ _____.

7. Two methods of satisfying human needs are _____ and _____.

8. A category of indirect methods of meeting human needs is called _____ _____.

9. When placing callers on hold, remember that _____ is the key.

10. Two examples of communication, other than the telephone, are

    _____ and _____.

11. Computers are the communication _____ of the
    healthcare facility.

Unscramble the following terms.

12. MARHABA SMOWAL   _____ _____

13. UNTIMAICOMCON   _____

14. SNEEFED SCHEMASMIN   _____ _____

15. CHRYARIEH   _____

16. CRIEVERE   _____

17. DRESEN   _____

18. BLAVER   _____

19. XYLASUITE   _____

Chapter Seven
The Safe Workplace

Objectives

After completing this chapter you should be able to
do the following:

1. Define and correctly spell each of the key terms.

2. Identify the three natural curves of the back.

3. Name at least four basic guidelines for proper body mechanics, and explain why using them is important.

4. List at least three rules for the use of siderails.

5. Identify three hazards that may result in falls.

6. Name at least two restrictions for patients who smoke.

7. List at least five ways to reduce the risk of electrical shock.

8. Identify at least three rules to follow for chemical safety.

9. Describe the steps that should be taken if a fire occurs.

10. Explain how to use a fire extinguisher.

Key Terms

- alignment
- body mechanics
- cardiopulmonary resuscitation
- hazard communication label

- Material Safety Data Sheet
- range of motion
- sudden death

Safety at Work

The term *safety* simply means keeping from harm. In the work environment, injuries sustained while working are called **industrial accidents**. The healthcare worker is at risk for several different types of injuries. Back injuries, puncture wounds from needles, electrical shock, and slip and fall injuries are all common among healthcare workers. Prevention of such injuries is the responsibility of both the employer and the employee. As a responsible employee, you MUST make an effort to communicate possible safety hazards and to exercise proper judgment while working.

Proper Body Mechanics

body mechanics: the efficient and safe use of the body during activity

You will face the possibility of injury to your back in every area of healthcare. All hospital personnel must understand and use proper **body mechanics** to preserve their physical health. If not done correctly, positioning, turning, and transferring patients or equipment can result in injury to you.

Using body mechanics means using all of your body parts efficiently in daily activities to prevent injury and correct problems related to posture and lifting. In caring for patients, healthcare workers often put a great deal of strain on their backs. In fact, studies have shown that clinical healthcare workers put as much strain on their back as a construction worker does! Because of this, low back pain is an occupational hazard for many who are in this type of profession. Back injuries cause more loss of time from the job than any other injury. Work-related back injuries are often costly for the employer and miserable for the injured worker. It is important to take care of your back! Understanding how your back works will keep your back healthy and help reduce the risk of injury.

The Anatomy of a Healthy Back

The back has three natural curves: the **cervical** curve of your neck; the **thoracic** curve of your middle back; and the **lumbar** curve of your lower back. By maintaining these three curves in proper **alignment**, your body weight is evenly distributed throughout the vertebrae and discs. Alignment refers to the proper positioning of parts in a line. When the back is properly aligned, the ears, shoulders, and hips form a straight line, resulting in correct posture. The spine is composed of thirty-three individual bones called **vertebrae**: seven cervical; twelve thoracic; five lumbar; five sacral, which actually fuse to form one bone; and four in the coccyx, which also fuse to form one bone. The vertebrae are separated by round-shaped cartilage called **discs**, which absorb shocks to the spine.

alignment: a physical position in which there is not stress or strain on any part of the body; the proper anatomical position; the positioning of parts in a straight line

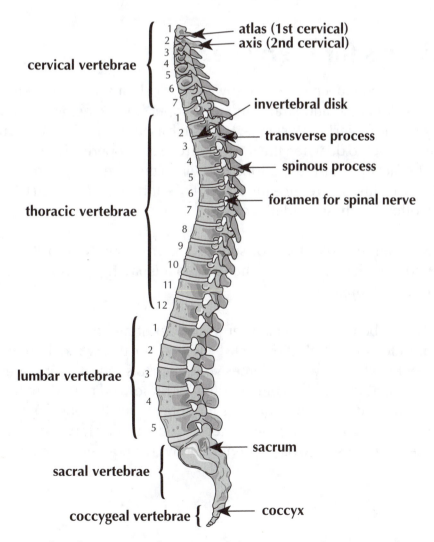

cervical vertebrae
1
2 — atlas (1st cervical)
— axis (2nd cervical)
3
4
5
6
7 — invertebral disk

thoracic vertebrae
1
2 — transverse process
3
4 — spinous process
5
6
7 — foramen for spinal nerve
8
9
10
11
12

lumbar vertebrae
1
2
3
4
5

sacral vertebrae — sacrum

coccygeal vertebrae — coccyx

Figure 7-1: The Three Natural Curves of the Spine and Associated Structures

Besides the vertebrae and discs, there are several groups of muscles that help support the spine. The muscles of the thighs, buttocks, abdomen, and back play a significant role in the prevention of serious injury to the back. These muscle groups support the three natural curves of the back and allow you to move freely. These muscles must be kept strong and flexible!

range of motion:
the extent to
which a joint
can move

The joints of the hips, knees, and ankles are essential in promoting a healthy back. Healthy and flexible joints give the entire body the full **range of motion**, or range of movement, that is needed to maintain the proper alignment of the three natural curves of the spine.

The back, or spine, is a marvelous machine; but it is not indestructible. Proper body mechanics are essential for a healthy back!

Back Tips for Everyone

Using good body mechanics will lower your risk of self-injury and greatly reduce back fatigue and strain. In fact, proper body mechanics can even make your job easier! For instance, tasks such as lifting, pulling, and pushing are much easier to do when the muscles are used properly. This is primarily due to the fact that muscles perform best when they are used correctly. Keep your back healthy and reduce the amount of effort that is required to do your job by following these guidelines.

1. Maintain a broad base of support, approximately 6 to 8 inches in width, with your feet. This helps keep the natural curves of your back in proper alignment.

2. Always bend your knees, keep your back straight, and use the largest muscles (the thighs, buttocks, etc.) to do the work. Bending and reaching from the waist forces your back to support your upper body as well as the load. Avoid bending for prolonged periods of time. For example, if your work involves mopping beneath beds, kneel on one knee and bend your hips and knees. When leaning forward, do not just use your arms—move your entire body. Do not bend from the waist!

3. Keep the load close to your body. This reduces the strain on your lower back and gives you the proper leverage. This tip keeps your back in proper alignment and distributes the weight evenly throughout your spine. Over time, poor body mechanics can lead to disc, muscle, and nerve damage. For example, a 2 lb load held close to the body exerts a 2 lb force on the lumbar spine; but A 2 LB LOAD HELD AWAY FROM THE BODY EXERTS A FORCE OF 200 LBS ON THE LUMBAR SPINE!

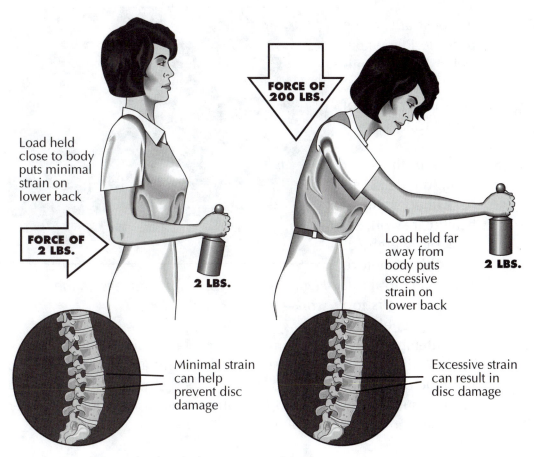

Figure 7-2: Keep the load close to your body.

4. Use your body weight to push or pull an object. Whenever possible, push or pull instead of lifting, and use patient transfer aids if they are available. Just make sure you have been taught how to use them properly. Injuries can occur from improper use of equipment as well as from improper performance of the task!

5. Instead of twisting and turning, turn your entire body while keeping your feet and hips pointed in the same direction. Position yourself so that you have the best advantage possible. Remember to let your **extremities** (arms and legs) do the work—not your back!

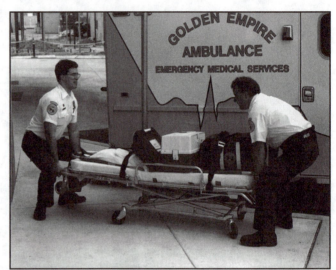

6. Lifting is the most common cause of back injuries among healthcare workers. Test the weight of the object before attempting to lift it. If the object is too heavy, get help be-

Figure 7-3: Let your arms and legs do the work—not your back!

fore attempting to lift it again. This applies to lifting patients too. Many patients will be too heavy for you to lift alone. Remember to keep the object or patient close to your body, maintaining a broad base of support. Don't bend from the waist. Push or pull whenever possible, and do not twist when lifting.

Using these guidelines, you will significantly lower your risk of back injury. Remember, you are the backbone of the healthcare facility! TAKE CARE OF YOUR BACK!

Needle Sticks

Although back injuries are the most common injuries among healthcare workers, there is always the risk of receiving a needle stick. Many clinical healthcare workers are at risk: laboratory assistants, radiology assistants, housekeeping and janitorial services, transportation personnel, nursing assistants, medical assistants, home health aides, physicians and nurses. Any healthcare worker who provides direct patient care is at risk of obtaining a needle stick from a dirty needle or other sharp object, such as a scalpel blade, that has been used on a patient. Needle sticks can expose healthcare workers to a number of diseases, such as hepatitis and acquired immune deficiency syndrome (AIDS). Specific guidelines concerning prevention of needle sticks and information about hepatitis and AIDS will be detailed in Chapter Nine.

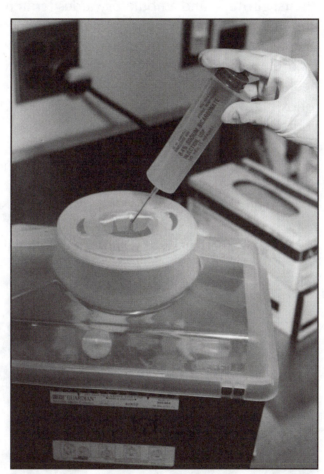

Figure 7-4: Sharps always must be handled with care to prevent injury and illness.

Patient Safety

Over the years, particularly in the past decade, there have been numerous lawsuits stemming from injuries received by patients from omissions concerning basic patient safety. The main responsibility for the safety of the patient falls on the healthcare worker. It is imperative that you, as a healthcare worker, take every precaution to ensure the safety of the patient.

Transfers

There will be many instances when transferring a patient from one area of the hospital to another will be necessary. This will involve using wheelchairs, **gurneys**, and ambulatory aides (crutches, walkers, canes, etc.). It is important to remember the guidelines discussed at the beginning of the chapter when transferring patients. In this instance, the patient will be the *load* or *object*. Some patients may be too ill to offer assistance to the healthcare worker during transfer from a hospital bed to a gurney. By following a few simple guidelines, you can help prevent injury to both yourself and the patient.

1. First you should get help from at least one other coworker. There will be times when the help of two or more additional workers will be needed. If in doubt, ASK FOR ASSISTANCE!

2. Tell the patient what will happen during the transfer and she should do.

3. Make sure the bed is locked and adjusted to the level of the gurney.

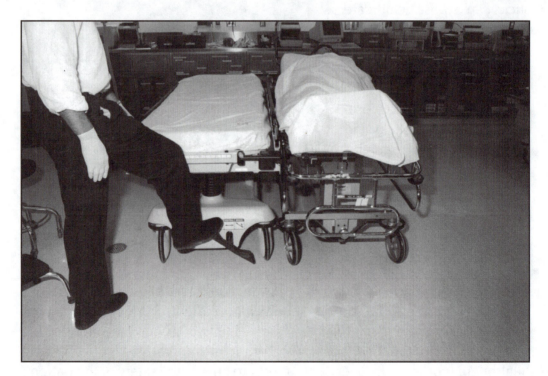

Figure 7-5: Lock the bed in place.

4. If a patient slide board is available, use it to make the move easier. If the unit does not have a slide board available, consider placing plastic bags under the patient or pull the sheet to make sliding easier.

5. Lock the gurney in place; make sure it is the same height as the bed.

6. Put one knee on the gurney for proper spinal alignment and balance. If possible have the patient move to the edge of the bed.

7. Make sure everyone is physically ready. Count to three aloud before moving the patient. For example, the person in charge should say, "Is everyone ready? We move on the count of three: one, two, and three."

8. If possible, have the patient clasp her hands or cross her arms across the chest in preparation for the transfer.

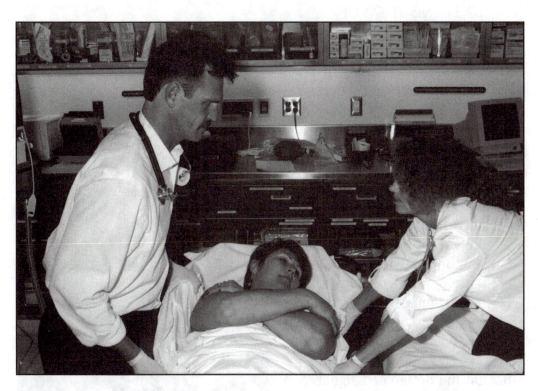

Figure 7-6: Have the patient clasp her hands or cross her arms across her chest.

9. Transfer the patient in two stages if possible; first to the edge of the bed and then to the middle of the gurney.

10. Be sure to let your legs, buttocks, and arms do the work—not your back!

Another common transfer will be moving the patient from the bed to a wheelchair. Unless the patient is paralyzed, the patient may be able to assist in this transfer. Once again, following a few simple guidelines will provide optimum safety to the patient and help prevent injury to you:

1. Lock the wheelchair in place close to the bed.

2. Adjust the height of the patient's bed to the height of the wheelchair's seat.

3. Thoroughly explain the procedure to the patient. Ask the patient how much he or she is able to help and verbally plan the transfer.

4. Help the patient sit on the edge of the bed. Allow the patient to rest there for a minute so that any dizziness or weakness can be assessed. Abrupt changes in position can cause dizziness or light-headedness. Be sure to specifically ask your patient if this is occurring BEFORE YOU ATTEMPT TO STAND THEM UP.

5. If the patient has a weak leg, support that extremity by placing it between your knees.

6. Tell the patient that on the count of "three" you will assist him or her to a standing position.

7. Have the patient place his or her arms around your waist or on your shoulders for added support if needed. Don't let the patient *hug* your neck; this places unnecessary stress on the cervical spine and may interfere with your balance.

8. On the designated signal, and with your knees bent and bending from the hips, assist the patient to a standing position. Using proper body mechanics will provide balance for both you and the patient.

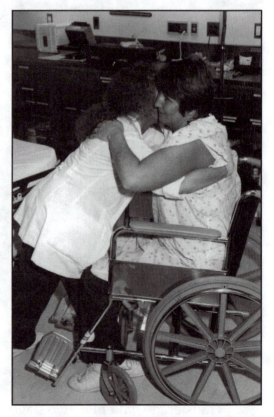

Figure 7-7: The patient should place her arms around your waist or on your shoulders for added support if needed.

9. If possible, instruct the patient to place his or her hands on the arm rests of the wheelchair.

10. Pivot and lower the patient into the wheelchair by bending your knees.

Whenever possible, use mechanical aids to help with patient transfers. Always practice good body mechanics to help PREVENT INJURY TO BOTH YOU AND THE PATIENT!

Preventing Injuries With Siderails

It is the responsibility of ALL healthcare personnel to make every effort to provide a safe environment for patients. Every hospital bed and gurney is equipped with **siderails** to keep patients from falling out of bed. Using these simple equipment items can help prevent unnecessary injuries to patients. The following guidelines will help you establish good habits for using siderails.

1. Explain the rationale for the siderails to all patients.

2. EVERY patient should have the siderails raised during the night. Only those who have signed the hospital's Siderail Release form may leave the siderails lowered.

3. Siderails may be left in the low position during the daytime unless the physician or nurse has specifically ordered that they be raised at all times, or if the patient experiences periods of confusion.

4. If the patient has been given medication to help him or her relax during a procedure, raise the siderail.

There have been numerous lawsuits stemming from the failure of healthcare workers to use the siderails. Patients sometimes fall out of bed when siderails are not raised, leading to injuries in the form of fractured arms, fractured hips, lacerations (cuts), and contusions (bruises). Hospitals and individual healthcare workers have lost thousands of dollars in lawsuits from failing to use the siderails. This is a simple piece of equipment; use common sense when patient safety is at issue. WHEN IN DOUBT, RAISE THOSE SIDERAILS!

Preventing Falls

Although many lawsuits have occurred from the failure to properly use siderails, lawsuits also have resulted from patients falling while under the care of a hospital. Some of the more common falls occur from wheelchairs, beds, gurneys, lack of assistance from the healthcare worker, and spilled liquid or dropped objects left on the floor. Lacerations, abrasions, and fractures often result from such falls. The following guidelines can help you prevent falls and avoid injury to your patients.

1. Know the physical abilities of your patient as well as your own physical limitations.

2. Obtain help if needed. Wait for help to arrive.

3. Explain all procedures to the patient as well as what assistance you expect from the patient.

4. Lock all pieces of equipment (beds, wheelchairs, bedside commodes, mechanical patient lifts, gurneys, etc.).

5. If necessary, secure the patient to the equipment with safety straps or belts according to the policy and procedure of your facility.

6. NEVER LEAVE A PATIENT UNSUPERVISED!

7. Immediately notify Housekeeping to clean up any spilled liquids.

8. Remove any small objects, such as needle caps that roll, needles, etc. from the path of traffic.

Following these guidelines will help you prevent falls and injuries to patients who expect healthcare workers to make every effort to provide for their safety. Reducing the risk of falls decreases the possibility of a liability lawsuit!

Patients Who Smoke

Although many diseases are aggravated or caused by smoking and more and more hospitals forbid it, you may at some point have to care for patients who smoke. As a healthcare worker, your top priority is to provide the patient with the highest level of care possible. Smoking is a sensitive issue with many people; therefore, use caution when discussing this topic with patients who insist on smoking. It may be difficult for healthcare personnel to understand why some patients continue to smoke—especially if the patients have a serious respiratory disease. However, you will find that many patients will insist on their right to do so. It is important for you to be aware of how YOU feel about this issue, because those feelings may inadvertently affect how you communicate with and treat the patient.

There are safety factors to consider when patients insist on smoking. As the healthcare worker, be aware of the smoking policy in the healthcare facility and be sure to adhere to it. Other safety guidelines follow.

1. PATIENTS MUST NEVER BE ALLOWED TO SMOKE IN PLACES WHERE OXYGEN IS NEARBY!
Even if the oxygen is in the *off* position, there is always the possibility of a small leak. Do not take any chances—there could be an explosion!

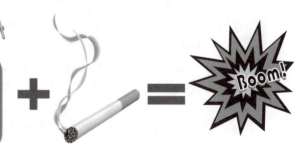

2. Do not allow any patient to smoke while in bed. If he or she falls asleep while smoking, the possibility for a fire greatly increases! Some patients have accidentally burned themselves, and others have inadvertently started a fire while smoking in bed.

3. All elderly patients should be watched by a responsible person while they are smoking.

4. Keep lighters and matches away from children and confused patients.

If the patient is uncooperative with the hospital's policy and the safety guidelines, report this to the unit supervisor. This can be a dangerous situation for everyone; the problem must not be allowed to continue.

Cardiopulmonary Resuscitation (CPR)

**cardiopulmonary
resuscitation
(CPR):**
the basic life-
saving procedure
of artificial
ventilation and
chest compres-
sions that is done
in the event of a
cardiac arrest

Cardiopulmonary resuscitation (CPR) is the administration of external cardiac compressions and rescue breathing to someone who is not breathing and who's heart may have stopped beating. **Cardio** refers to the heart and **pulmonary** refers to the lungs. **Resuscitate** means to revive, or to bring back to life. Cardiopulmonary resuscitation, in essence, means to bring life back to the heart and lungs. The startling effects of this lifesaving technique were first published in 1960. Now, because of this discovery, people who have been trained in the procedure often can reverse **sudden death**, an emergency that requires the prompt response of trained personnel.

sudden death:
the unexpected
and instanta-
neous cessation
of breathing
and the pulse, or
within 60 min-
utes of the onset
of symptoms in
patients without
known preexist-
ing heart disease

The purpose of CPR is to provide oxygen quickly to the brain, heart, and other vital organs until appropriate medical treatment can restore normal function to the heart and lungs. Due to the importance of this lifesaving procedure, all new employees in an acute care hospital should be trained in cardiopulmonary resuscitation. If you are not given the opportunity to become properly certified and trained in the procedure by your employer, contact the nearest branch of the American Heart Association or the American Red Cross for the next available Basic Life Support class. This class will instruct, test, and certify or recognize qualified participants in theory and technique of cardiopulmonary resuscitation and airway obstruction. Since you are providing care to the public, you MUST be certified or recognized in this procedure. (The terminology or the title varies depending upon the training agency.) This procedure is outlined in Chapter Eighteen: Basic First Aid.

The technique of cardiopulmonary resuscitation involves demonstration and hands-on practice. Patients expect healthcare workers to be skilled and current on this lifesaving maneuver. It is a simple procedure, and through diligent and precise practice, it can be mastered in as little as 8 HOURS! You owe it to the patients AND to yourself to become a certified or recognized provider of basic life support!

Equipment and Safety

Alerting supervisors and other workers to possible hazards in the work environment is the responsibility of every employee. Inspecting and certifying every piece of equipment in a hospital is the responsibility of the Engineering Department. However, if a safety hazard is discovered by someone other than an employee of the Engineering Department, the piece of equipment MUST be removed from use and the hazard reported to the appropriate person.

Electric Shock

One of the most common and serious accidents that can occur while using a piece of equipment is the possibility of **electric shock**. This type of shock occurs when an electric current passes through the body. It can cause injuries ranging from mild burns to complete destruction of the skin, unconsciousness, and even death. Observance of the following guidelines will help reduce the risk of electric shock.

1. Follow all safety standards established by the hospital. Review the safety manual at least once a year and participate in all mandatory safety drills.

2. Do not use any piece of equipment until you have been properly instructed and supervised in its correct use.

3. Read and follow all instructions before using any equipment. If clarification is needed, ask your supervisor for assistance.

4. Inspect the electrical cord on the piece of equipment. DO NOT USE IT OR PLUG IT IN IF THE CORD IS DAMAGED OR FRAYED!

5. All equipment used in the hospital is equipped with a three-prong plug. The third prong is used for grounding purposes. If the third prong has been removed, DO NOT USE IT!

6. Any damaged or malfunctioning piece of equipment must be reported to your supervisor and removed from the area. DO NOT ATTEMPT TO USE IT!

7. Avoid practical jokes when using equipment—these tend to cause accidents.

8. Always make sure your hands, the patient, and the floor are dry!

9. Follow every safety guideline and standard that is established by your facility.

Electric shock is a very serious and potentially life-threatening injury. Daily practice of the guidelines provided will reduce the risk of electric shock to both you and the patient.

Avoiding Chemical Injuries

Chemical injuries (**chemical burns**, inhalation of toxic fumes, or eye injuries) also are possible in healthcare facilities. Housekeeping, janitorial, laboratory, dietary, and pharmacy assistants are just a few of the employees that may be accidentally exposed to chemical injuries.

A chemical is an acid, alkaline, or other substance, capable of causing injury either through direct contact on the skin or by inhalation of the gaseous fumes. Examples of chemicals are oxygen, cleaning solution, baking soda, bleach, hydrochloric acid, and sodium bicarbonate. A chemical may induce injury by itself or when it is combined with another chemical. The most common type of chemical injury is a burn. Simple redness and a burning sensation may be the only result; however, if proper first aid treatment is delayed, the possibility of blisters and further tissue damage may result. Harmful gases also may be produced from various chemicals, causing burns to the respiratory tract (ie, the nose, throat, and lungs), shortness of breath, pneumonia, or critical respiratory distress. Following these simple guidelines will greatly reduce the risk of chemical injury to yourself and others:

1. Always WEAR GLOVES when using solutions. Cleaning solutions can also be very harsh to the skin.

2. ALWAYS READ THE LABEL ON THE CONTAINER AT LEAST THREE TIMES: (1) when you first pick up the container; (2) before you pour the solution or mix solutions; and (3) immediately after you have poured the chemical (before you put it away).

3. If the label is not readable or is missing from the container, DO NOT USE IT! Immediately remove the container from the supply area so that others will not use it either.

4. Always use chemicals in a well-ventilated area.

5. Immediately clean up any spills.

6. If a chemical touches your skin or eyes, immediately flush that area with water and report the incident to your supervisor. Seek medical attention if the burning continues or if it becomes difficult to breathe.

7. Follow your facility's reporting procedures.

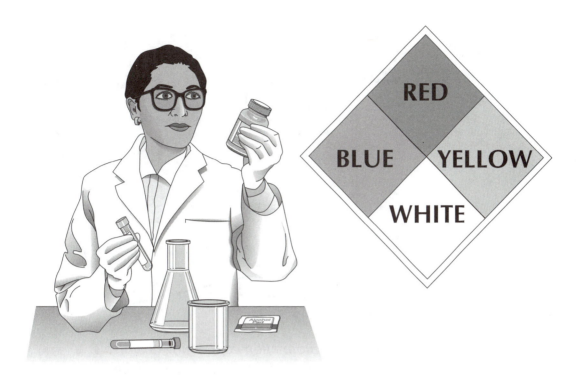

Figure 7-8: Safety precautions must be used when dealing with chemicals. Always read the hazard communication label on the container at least three times.

Every department in the hospital is provided with an information sheet on every chemical used in their department. This sheet contains information concerning the chemical makeup, possible hazards, first aid treatment, appropriate dilution and mixture concentration, and indications and uses. This information sheet is called the **Material Safety Data Sheet**. OSHA requires each chemical container to display a diamond-shaped, **hazard communication label** displaying the following information within four smaller, colored diamonds:

- the degree of health hazards (blue diamond).

- the degree of flammability hazards (red diamond).

- the degree of reactivity hazards (yellow diamond).

- the degree to which specific hazards exist (white diamond). (Specific hazards are defined as the part of the body that would be affected if contact with the chemical occurs.)

The hazard level for each category ranges from 0 to 4. A *0* means the substance is a minimal hazard, whereas a *4* indicates an extreme hazard. Rules and regulations may vary among states; so it is essential that you become familiar with your facility's policies and procedures.

Material Safety Data Sheet: an official, required document that identifies all the chemicals that are used in a specific department and that details important information regarding those chemicals

hazard communication label: a label (usually diamond-shaped) with four colored diamonds that each represent a specific aspect of the chemical's hazards

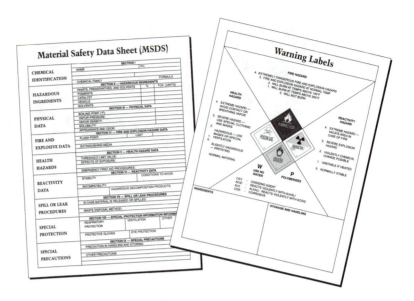

Figure 7-9: Information concerning chemicals is provided on the Material Safety Data Sheet.

Fire Safety

One of the most frightening events that can occur is a fire. A fire may occur at any time; therefore, the healthcare workers must be properly prepared to manage this type of emergency. All healthcare facilities are required by law to provide fire drills throughout the facility. The more drills you participate in, the more efficient you will become in the facility's fire procedure.

Fire prevention is one of the most important aspects of safety. All departments in an acute care hospital are provided with that facility's fire manual. It is your responsibility to become thoroughly familiar with the procedures that are outlined and explained for you in the fire manual.

Remember—RACE!

1. **R**ESCUE THE PATIENT.

2. **A**CTIVATE (SOUND) THE ALARM.

3. **C**ONTAIN THE FIRE.

4. **E**XTINGUISH THE FIRE.

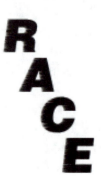

If a fire DOES occur, remember the following safety tips.

1. NEVER SHOUT, "FIRE!" Summon help when you discover a fire; but don't shout the word *fire*. It will cause panic.

2. Remain calm and do not panic. Portray an image of confidence and ultimate safety to the patients and visitors. Remember, patients and visitors rely on you for guidance, safety, and direction.

3. If patients or visitors are in immediate danger, move them to safety.

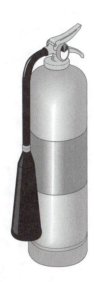

4. Turn off all oxygen.

5. Be familiar with the locations of the fire alarms and how to operate the fire extinguishers.

6. Notify the operator concerning the location of the fire.

7. Close all doors and windows. This reduces the spread of smoke and may reduce the amount of oxygen that is feeding the fire.

8. Do not enter an area if the door is closed and feels warm to the touch.

9. Use the fire-fighting equipment.

10. If the fire is not in your area of work, take the following precautions:

   A. Close all doors and windows. This decreases the draft.

   B. Do not use the telephone except for business calls.

   C. Follow instructions from the designated authority figure.

A fire is the result of a chemical reaction between three components: fuel, oxygen, and heat. When all three are present, a fire will result. It is important to remember that where there is smoke, there is fire. Follow the same procedure for smoke as you would a visible, flaming fire.

During orientation to the hospital, learn the location of all the exits, the proper evacuation routes, and how to operate the fire extinguishers. Fire extinguishers are usually classified according to the type of fire they can put out. Classification is universal; every facility uses the same letter classification system. For example, **Class A** extinguishers are for paper, wood, fabric, rubber, and certain plastic material fires; **Class B** extinguishers are for flammable liquids, oil, paint, fat, and gasoline fires; and **Class C** extinguishers are used to combat fires caused by energized electrical equipment such as motors, appliances, and switches. **Class D** extinguishers are for combustible metals such as sodium, magnesium, potassium, uranium, and powdered aluminum.

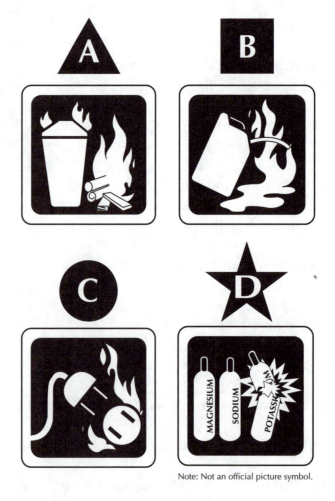

Note: Not an official picture symbol.

Figure 7-10: Classes of Fire Extinguishers

Fire extinguishers are easy to operate; but your confidence and skill during emergencies will increase if you become familiar with their use and operation in advance. Using a fire extinguisher is as easy as 1-2-3.

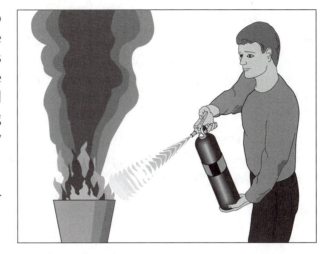

Figure 7-11: Make sure you are trained in the proper use of a fire extinguisher.

1. Hold the extinguisher upright.

2. Pull the pin.

3. Direct the spray at the base of the fire.

Taking the proper steps to prevent a fire from occurring, spreading, or causing injury is the responsibility of the healthcare facility's employees. Remember to make every attempt to provide the safest environment possible for the ones who depend on you the most—the patients!

Chapter Summary

Several aspects concerning employee and patient safety have been addressed in this chapter. The issue of professional liability lawsuits was discussed to point out the risks associated with the field of healthcare today. Chapter Four provides specific information regarding the components of a lawsuit and how these components affect a healthcare worker's job.

The proper use of body mechanics is essential to safe and injury-free patient care. The clinical healthcare worker must put forth a conscious effort in the use of proper body alignment.

Guidelines are provided for the clinical healthcare worker for various areas of safety. Transferring patients, using siderails, preventing patient falls, managing patients who smoke, preventing chemical injuries, understanding cardiopulmonary resuscitation and the clinical healthcare worker's responsibility, and equipment safety all require diligent and daily practice from the healthcare workers.

Safety drills should be conducted frequently in all healthcare facilities. For example, instruction concerning the use and proper handling of fire extinguishers is usually provided for employees. Requirements for participation in training sessions and drills will vary among healthcare facilities; however all training sessions are important—attend as many of them as you can!

The main responsibility of the healthcare worker is to provide the safest environment possible for the patients and their visitors. Remember, SAFETY BEGINS WITH YOU!

Name _____

Date _____

Student Enrichment Activities

Complete the following statements.

1. The three natural curves of the back are the _____, the _____, and the _____ curves.

2. The thirty-three bones of the spinal column are called _____.

3. The muscles of the _____, _____, _____, and _____ help support the spine. Keeping them strong and flexible can help prevent serious injury to the spine.

4. Self-injury is at its lowest risk when proper _____ _____ are used.

5. Two serious diseases capable of being transmitted to healthcare workers through dirty needles or sharp objects are _____ and _____.

6. During a patient transfer, the _____ is the *load* or *object*.

7. Many lawsuits stem from healthcare workers NOT using _____.

8. One of the keys to the prevention of falls is never leave the patient _____.

9. Patients must never be allowed to smoke when _____ is near.

10. All hospital personnel must complete a course in cardiopulmonary

    _____.

11. The possibility of _____ _____ always exists

    when using equipment.

12. The most common type of chemical injury is a _____.

13. Where there is _____, there is _____.

Unscramble the following terms.

14. TIMEGLANN   _____

15. OBYD SCHEMACIN   _____ _____

16. RICARDOPLAYONUM   _____

17. ISTARTSCIONUE   _____

18. DEDSUN HATED   _____ _____

19. ROCHATIC   _____

20. ICRAVECL   _____

Chapter Eight
Disasters: Preparedness, Hazards, and Prevention

Objectives

After completing this chapter you should be able to do the following:

1. Define and correctly spell each of the key terms.

2. List at least four guidelines for managing disasters.

3. Name two agencies involved with developing guidelines for safety in the workplace.

4. Identify the main difference between OSHA and NIOSH.

5. List the four parts of an effective hazard communication safety program.

6. Name at least three types of potential hazards in the hospital work environment.

7. List the three parts of an effective safety program.

Key Terms

- disaster
- Occupational Safety and Health Administration

- triage

Disasters: Expecting the Unexpected

disaster:
an unexpected event that causes great damage and depletes or exhausts currently available resources

The previous chapter provided you with some basic safety guidelines to follow on a daily basis. But unexpected events sometimes occur, which require healthcare workers to take additional steps to ensure the safety of their patients and themselves. In recent years, increased attention has been given to **disaster** preparedness and the preservation of human life. In this chapter you will learn how disasters can affect the healthcare system, and what healthcare workers can do to prepare for these emergencies.

Disasters can be caused by a number of different events, ranging from relatively minor electrical failures to catastrophic earthquakes, tornadoes, floods, and hurricanes. Many other occurrences can be classified as disasters too. These include severed water mains, gas leaks, multi-vehicle collisions, airplane accidents, bomb threats, hazardous waste accidents, etc. Clinical healthcare workers must be prepared to function in ANY type of disaster.

Disaster Triage

triage:
to sort or prioritize care for a group of patients

Effective management of a disaster depends on a quick and accurate **triage** system. *Triage* is a French word that means, to choose, pick, sort, or select. It is a valuable tool that is used often in pre-hospital care as well as the hospital environment. When a disaster occurs, one or more people will be responsible for assessing patients according to the seriousness of their condition. Triage involves the use of specific guidelines for categorizing patients, so it is very important for you, as a clinical allied healthcare worker, to cooperate with the person in charge of this very important process.

In a disaster, triage relies heavily on objective assessment. An **assessment** is an evaluation of the patient. The word **objective** refers to the information obtained from observing the patient. Therefore, the person performing triage must be skilled in assessing the condition of patients on the basis of both verbal information received, if any, and direct patient observation. Physicians and nurses are trained in triage, which includes observing the patient's general appearance, obtaining the vital signs, and performing a physical examination.

Sometimes patients can provide healthcare workers with information about their condition. This type of information is called **subjective** data because it is provided by the patient. A clinical decision concerning the urgency of treatment is based on a combination of subjective and objective information.

All clinical healthcare workers use triage in their work. For example, deciding which patients need to have blood drawn first and determining which patients should be seen by the nurse are forms of triage. Nurses and physicians are highly skilled at this because of their experience and broad base of medical knowledge.

During a disaster, cooperating with the other members of the medical team is extremely important. Learn to be both a follower and a leader. These two skills are very valuable in the field of healthcare. Learn to TAKE DIRECTIONS as well as HOW TO DIRECT.

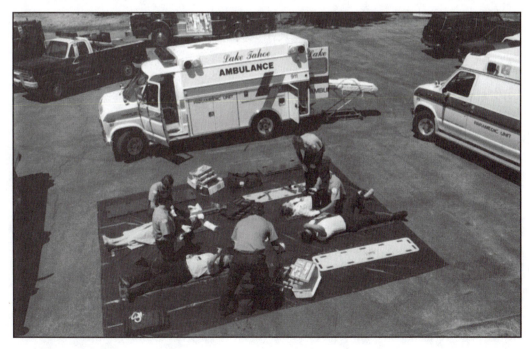

Figure 8-1: Disaster Triage

Chaos is common during emergencies; but PROMPT AND EFFICIENT PATIENT CARE IS THE GOAL! Remember, the primary responsibility for triage rests on the shoulders of the nurses and the physicians.

Disaster Preparedness

Disaster preparedness has become a recognized specialty of Emergency Medical Services (EMS), healthcare facilities, public safety agencies, communities, counties, and states. Although everyone is responsible for their own preparedness, successful response to a disaster in the healthcare environment requires the cooperation of many people and agencies.

Proper disaster preparation takes foresight, thought, and planning. Experience is one of the greatest teachers, but not everyone involved with disaster preparedness has had actual disaster experience. Some people specialize in helping other people prepare for disasters by studying disasters that have already occurred. These specialists visit the location of the disaster and observe different aspects of disaster preparedness. For example, a specialist might ask whether the members of the community were educated in basic first aid procedures. Were the community's hospitals well-versed in their disaster response protocols? Were all aspects of the EMS communication system adequate? Who was in charge at the time of the disaster? What areas were identified as weaknesses (ie, routes to the nearest healthcare facility, communication system failures, etc.)?

As a result of the work of disaster preparedness specialists, simple guidelines and suggestions have led to the formation of formal disaster plans by businesses and healthcare institutions. In the acute care hospital, every department should possess a copy of that facility's disaster manual. It is your responsibility to become thoroughly acquainted with the policies and procedures contained in the manual.

Preparing for a disaster involves participating in disaster drills conducted by a public service agency. The fire department, Emergency Medical Services Agency, or a local healthcare facility often manages these disaster drills. Several agencies such as the Highway Patrol, local police department, fire department, and local hospitals participate in these unannounced drills. Furthermore, these drills involve all departments in the hospital; therefore, it is vital that every employee possess a working knowledge of disaster procedures.

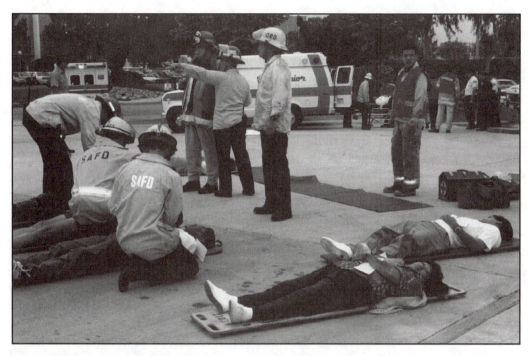

Figure 8-2: A Disaster Drill

The following are basic guidelines for action in a disaster:

1. REMAIN CALM! Remember, patients depend on you for guidance and safety.

2. Know who the designated person-in-charge is and promptly report your availability to him or her.

3. If the telephones are still functional, do not use them for personal business. KEEP THE TELEPHONE LINES CLEAR FOR OFFICIAL BUSINESS!

4. Communicate and cooperate with other workers.

5. If in doubt, ASK!

6. Report to the person in charge frequently. This will permit efficient changes in assignments, if needed.

7. Always speak in a firm, caring voice to the patients. The firmness suggests control of the situation and a caring tone shows compassion.

True disasters are frightening experiences for everyone. Read the disaster manual and participate in disaster training regularly! Being prepared for a disaster means being ready for the sudden and unexpected event BEFORE it happens, not during it! Imagine yourself in the following situation...

You are working in the Emergency Department when a moderate-sized earthquake occurs. When the shaking stops, you attempt to assess the situation. You note that some of the patients are screaming in panic. There is no power, and none of the communication systems, telephones, or elevators are working. Broken glass, spilled liquids, and fallen supplies lie on the floor in various places. It is unclear whether any of the patients received additional injuries during the quake. You also know that aftershocks may occur.

Because you have attended the hospital's disaster drills, you know that the evacuation plan must be put into action. A temporary communication system must be established, and a central reporting area must be set up as well. Patients and family members must be kept from panicking. Extra patient care supplies such as bandages, cold packs, gurneys, and stretchers must be obtained and placed in a central location. Patients must be evacuated from the hospital and placed in a central area for care. Above all, YOU must remain calm and be in control of the situation. Everyone is depending on your expertise!

Can you imagine a situation such as this? It is important for all personnel to participate in the facility's disaster drills on a regular basis. Disaster preparedness begins with you! Don't become part of the disaster; frequent participation in drills will build your confidence and skills. Always be prepared!

Occupational Safety and Hazards

Failing to follow safety guidelines can result in different types of disasters. One of the more common accidents in the hospital environment involves the mishandling of infectious and hazardous waste products. Because of the increasing numbers of healthcare personnel contracting illnesses from infectious and hazardous waste, agencies have been formed to develop guidelines to protect employees in the work environment.

Development and enforcement of job safety and health regulations are the main responsibilities of the **Occupational Safety and Health Administration (OSHA)**. The United States Department of Labor directs this agency, which keeps employers informed about industrial hazards through educational programs.

OSHA's regulations cover a variety of subjects including fire prevention, personal protection equipment (PPE), railings, and other safety items. They also establish maximum levels of exposure to many hazardous materials such as lead and asbestos. OSHA provides inspectors who check healthcare facilities and other buildings for violations. Employers who fail to meet the standards established by OSHA must pay a fine. This agency has encouraged states to develop their own rules and regulations according to federal guidelines.

Another agency concerned with the safety of workers is the **National Institute for Occupational Safety and Health (NIOSH)**. This agency is under the direction of the United States Department of Health and Human Services. The main purpose of NIOSH is to investigate requests submitted by employers or employees concerning working conditions and how they relate to illnesses contracted by employees. Once the investigation is completed, standards and guidelines are recommended to the Occupational Safety and Health Administration, which then enforces them. NIOSH conducts studies that examine the effects on workers of exposure to excessive noise, hazardous chemicals or radiation, and other questionable conditions on the job. Assuring quality in the work environment is this agency's primary responsibility.

> **Occupational Safety and Health Administration (OSHA):** a government agency that develops safety standards and establishes maximum levels of exposure to many hazardous materials

Other Hazards and Potential Disasters

Being aware of potential hazards in the work environment will help you prevent accidents. PREVENTION IS THE KEY TO SAFETY IN THE WORKPLACE. There are a variety of hazardous gases used in the hospital setting. Surgery and the Post Anesthesia Care Unit contain gases used for **anesthesia** (loss of sensation and/ or consciousness caused by the administration of drugs). If, for example, a gas leak occurs, the danger of explosion exists. Furthermore, inhalation of these gases can cause serious health problems. In addition, Central Supply, the department responsible for sterilizing hospital equipment and instruments, uses a gas that can damage the skin as well as the respiratory and nervous systems. It is essential that only properly trained personnel use the gases. Be sure to wear the recommended protective items!

Chemotherapy agents are very **toxic** (poisonous) drugs used in the treatment of cancer. They not only destroy cancer cells, they also kill normal, healthy cells. Improper handling of these drugs can expose the healthcare worker to cancer and birth defects. Mixing the chemotherapy agents is usually done in a special area of the pharmacy by the pharmacist. Pharmacy assistants may be accidentally exposed if care is not used. Follow all guidelines when handling and disposing of these chemicals or transporting them to the proper nursing area of the hospital, using leakproof containers and wearing the recommended attire.

The Radiology Department exposes the clinical healthcare worker to waves and particles of radiation. If safety guidelines are not followed, the employee becomes a high risk for developing tissue damage, becoming **sterile** (not able to produce children), developing birth defects, or contracting cancer. Radiology assistants and technicians wear film badges that safely monitor the level of radiation exposure of that employee. Safety guidelines are developed for the protection of everyone in that hospital. Choosing to follow them is the choice of a responsible employee!

Asbestos is a mineral formerly used in construction and for fireproofing. If it is disturbed or becomes old, it breaks into tiny fibers that are small enough to be inhaled into the lungs. Studies have shown that these fibers can lead to respiratory diseases and possibly lung cancer. This mineral is no longer used for construction and facilities are required to take protective measures for the employees wherever asbestos is used in the building. Warning signs should be posted wherever it is located. If you discover asbestos in the workplace, notify the appropriate supervisor. This should not occur unless the hospital was constructed before the 1970s.

In addition to the risks of infectious waste, medical gases, chemotherapy, and radiation, there are hundreds of different chemicals used in the hospital environment. The Material Safety Data Sheets in each department are for the protection and education of all employees. Chemicals that are handled incorrectly can cause burns, explosions, and other serious hazards. ALWAYS READ THE LABEL AND MIXING INSTRUCTIONS BEFORE USING ANY CHEMICAL! Wear the protective gear that is recommended for each chemical you use, and report any accidents and necessary cleanup to the appropriate supervisor!

Safety = Accident Prevention

The safety guidelines contained in the hospital's safety manual were designed to protect employees from the dangers of chemicals and medical gases. They are part of the safety program known as the **Hazard Communication Program**. It is commonly called HazCom. This program consists of four parts: employee training, the written program, Material Safety Data Sheets, and warning labels.

Safety guidelines are not designed to make your job difficult. They are created to protect employees, visitors, and patients. Employees have a right to work in a healthy and safe work environment. Following a few general guidelines will help promote a safe workplace for you and your coworkers.

1. KNOW THE HAZARDS! Infectious diseases and common hospital materials put the clinical healthcare worker at risk for contracting potentially life-threatening ailments. Learn to recognize the hazards!

2. PROTECT YOURSELF! Use the personal protective equipment provided by the hospital (required by OSHA), follow safe working practices, and stay alert to potential hazards!

3. WORK AS A TEAM! Get involved with the hospital's safety committee—WORK WITH your employer, NOT AGAINST IT!

An effective HazCom program includes a written program, which consists of various manuals for safety, fire, and disasters. Every department in the hospital should have each of these manuals. Review them during orientation and ask any questions that you have.

Ongoing training is also part of the safety program. Participation in periodic fire drills and knowledge of fire extinguisher operation is required by all employees. Frequent **in-services** also should be provided to inform all staff members of changes in legislation, policies, or procedures. Remember, AN INFORMED EMPLOYEE IS A PREPARED EMPLOYEE!

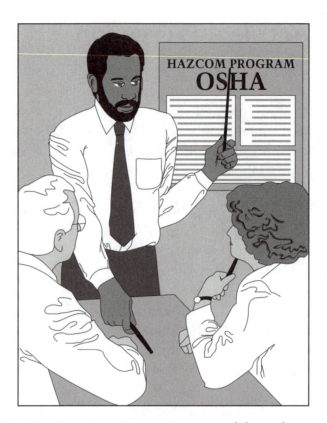

Figure 8-3: HazCom is an important part of the safety program.

Various warning labels and Material Safety Data Sheets are also a part of an effective safety program. Read and follow the instructions provided by these sources. They are for your safety as well as for the safety of the patient!

Chapter Summary

Disasters occur in various forms. Participation in the community's and hospital's disaster drills will help you develop competence in various skills needed during a disaster. Disasters are frightening for everyone; however, the patients expect the healthcare workers to know what to do! Review the safety manuals periodically and become involved with the hospital's safety committee to help you learn the hospital's policies and procedures for disasters.

Working in the healthcare profession can expose clinical healthcare workers to serious health risks. Knowing those risks and taking extra precautions will minimize the healthcare worker's possibility of developing a potentially serious, even fatal, disease.

Name _____

Date _____

Student Enrichment Activities

Complete the following statements.

1. An unexpected event that causes great damage or exhausts currently available resources is called a _____.

2. A recognized specialty in many departments and agencies concerned with public safety is _____ _____.

3. One of the more common disasters in a hospital occurs from the mishandling of _____ and _____ waste.

4. _____ is responsible for the development and enforcement of job safety and health regulations.

5. Requests submitted by employers or employees concerning working conditions and how they relate to illnesses and diseases contracted by employees are investigated by _____.

6. The key to safety in the workplace is _____.

7. The four parts of the HazCom program are: employee _____, the _____ program, _____ _____ Data Sheets, and _____ _____.

8. An _____ employee is a _____ employee.

Unscramble the following terms.

9. STARSIDE _____

10. IGREAT _____

11. STABESOS _____

12. UNTALCOPAOCI FEYATS _____ _____

13. ONITALAN ISNUTETIT _____ _____

Chapter Nine
Infection Control

Objectives

After completing this chapter you should be able to
do the following:

1. Define and correctly spell each of the key terms.

2. Describe the six components of the infection cycle, and
    the methods of interrupting each.

3. Thoroughly explain the meaning of the phrase
    sterile technique.

4. List the precautions for preventing puncture wounds from
    needles and other sharp objects.

5. Explain and demonstrate the proper procedure for
    donning sterile gloves.

6. Name three serious illnesses clinical health personnel may
    contract from patients.

7. Describe the main difference between viruses
    and bacteria.

8. Explain the procedure for proper handwashing.

9. Identify body secretions for which Standard Precautions or
    Airborne, Droplet, or Contact Precautions must be used.

10. Name the recommended cleaning solution for use
    in hospitals.

Key Terms

- AIDS
- airborne transmission
- aseptic
- asymptomatic
- bacteria
- Centers for Disease Control and Prevention
- clean technique
- contact transmission
- droplet transmission
- hepatitis A

- hepatitis B
- hepatitis C
- infection cycle
- nosocomial infection
- pathogen
- reverse isolation
- Standard Precautions
- sterile technique
- Transmission-based Precautions
- virus

AIDS: acquired immune deficiency syndrome; a viral disease caused by the human immunodeficiency virus (HIV), which damages the immune system leaving the patient susceptible to other infections. It is contracted through infected blood and other body fluids and sexual contact

pathogen: a disease-causing microorganism

Centers for Disease Control and Prevention (CDC): the government agency responsible for protecting public health through the prevention and control of disease

Invisible Enemies

Previous chapters have provided you with information concerning disasters and safety in the workplace. This chapter will focus on another aspect of safety—infection control. Since the early 1980s, infection control has become an increasingly important aspect of quality patient care. The **AIDS** epidemic has emphasized the need for precise and consistent steps to ensure the safety of the healthcare workers and their patients.

Though germs are too small to see with the naked eye, their presence can be detected in many ways. For example, when introduced into the human body, they can result in numerous infections—some of them life-threatening. Infectious diseases were once the major cause of illness and death throughout the world, and although medical science has made great strides in the fight against these pathogen-induced illnesses, the invisible enemies that cause them still remain. Thus, the best way to control these diseases is to keep the **pathogens** from spreading.

This chapter will provide you with information concerning occupational hazards, risks, and safety guidelines associated with infection control. The importance of strict adherence to the recommended guidelines of the hospital and the **Centers for Disease Control and Prevention** cannot be overemphasized. YOU are responsible for your safety as well as the safety of the patient.

Centers for Disease Control and Prevention

The government agency that assists in formulating safety guidelines regarding infectious diseases is the Centers for Disease Control and Prevention (CDC). This agency is part of the Public Health Service as well as part of the United States Department of Health and Human Services. The main responsibility of this agency is to protect public health through the prevention and control of disease. By studying the causes and distribution of diseases, employees of this agency are able to provide the general public and healthcare workers with valuable information concerning the prevention and control of various diseases.

As a result of this agency's work, it now is the employers' responsibility to provide a safe working environment for the employees. Standards and guidelines established by the CDC and other agencies require all employers to provide continuous training for their employees concerning the management of infectious and hazardous waste products.

The Infection Control Department

The Infection Control Department of the hospital is responsible for writing and implementing hospital policies and procedures designed to reduce the risk of **industrial illnesses** (illnesses received from infections contracted at work) for the employee, and **nosocomial infections** for the patient.

nosocomial infection: an infection that is acquired during a stay at a hospital

The hospital is required by law to protect all employees from infectious and hazardous waste products. The employee is responsible for knowing and understanding the policies and procedures established by the healthcare facility. There are many diseases that can be contracted by an employee in the hospital environment. Two of the more common, and serious, diseases will be discussed briefly in this chapter.

How the Infection Cycle Starts

Our environment is filled with microorganisms. Although many microorganisms are helpful, some are capable of causing disease. Since both types of microorganisms exist in the hospital environment, it is important for you to understand the various ways infection can be transmitted as well as the methods by which the **infection cycle** can be broken.

infection cycle: a pattern that describes the origin and transmission of a disease or illness

The cycle of infection can be thought of as a chain of events that is given the opportunity to take place when a pathogen, or infectious agent, is present. There are six components to the infection cycle.

1. **Infectious Agent:** any disease-causing microorganism (pathogen).

2. **Reservoir Host:** the individual in which the infectious microorganisms reside. Examples include animals, water, air, soil, and human beings. Humans or animals who do not show any outward signs or symptoms of a disease but are still capable of transmitting the disease are known as **carriers**.

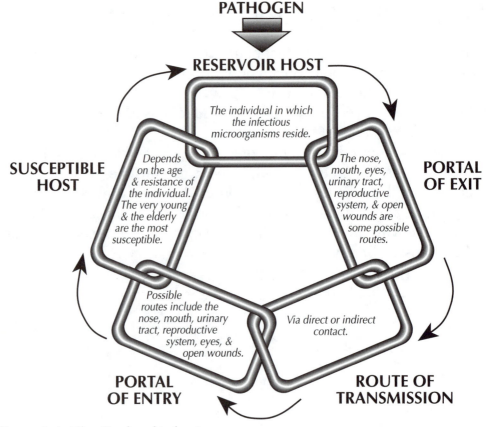

Figure 9-1: The Cycle of Infection

3. **Portal of Exit:** the route by which a pathogen leaves the body. Examples of portals of exit are breaks in the skin, respiratory secretions, reproductive secretions, and blood.

4. **Route of Transmission:** the method by which the pathogen gets from the reservoir to the new host. Transmission may occur through direct contact, air, insects, etc.

5. **Portal of Entry:** the route through which the pathogen enters it's new host. The respiratory, gastrointestinal, urinary, and reproductive tracts, and breaks in the protective skin barrier are common points of entry.

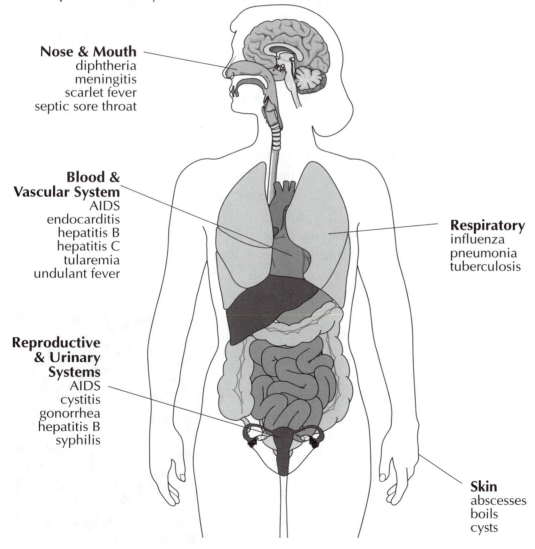

Nose & Mouth
diphtheria
meningitis
scarlet fever
septic sore throat

**Blood &
Vascular System**
AIDS
endocarditis
hepatitis B
hepatitis C
tularemia
undulant fever

Respiratory
influenza
pneumonia
tuberculosis

**Reproductive
& Urinary
Systems**
AIDS
cystitis
gonorrhea
hepatitis B
syphilis

Skin
abscesses
boils
cysts

Figure 9-2: Possible Portals of Entry and Potential Illnesses

6. **Susceptible Host:** a person capable of being affected or infected by invading microorganisms, depending on the degree of that person's **resistance**. Some examples of susceptible hosts are people who are malnourished, people who have suppressed immune systems, or others who are in poor health.

As a healthcare worker, it is important for you to be able to identify the various parts of the infection cycle and take appropriate measures to interrupt it. This is an essential part of patient care and self-protection.

How to Interrupt the Infection Cycle

For each component of the infection cycle there is a specific method that may be used to prevent or interrupt that aspect of the cycle. These methods follow.

1. **Infectious Agent:** the infectious agent (pathogen) must be rapidly identified by the physician and appropriate treatment promptly started.

2. **Reservoir Host:** the employee must maintain proper personal hygiene and **asepsis**. The working environment must be disinfected and sanitized.

3. **Portal of Exit:** the employee must wear the proper attire (a uniform); take Standard or Transmission-based Precautions; control body secretions (eg, use kleenex when sneezing, etc.); and wash hands according to protocol.

4. **Route of Transmission:** the employee must practice good handwashing, disinfection, and sterilization techniques; properly dispose of all potentially infected materials; isolate infected patients from others; and REFRAIN FROM WORKING IF YOU ARE INFECTIOUS!

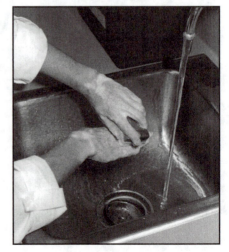

Figure 9-3: Proper handwashing can interrupt the infection cycle.

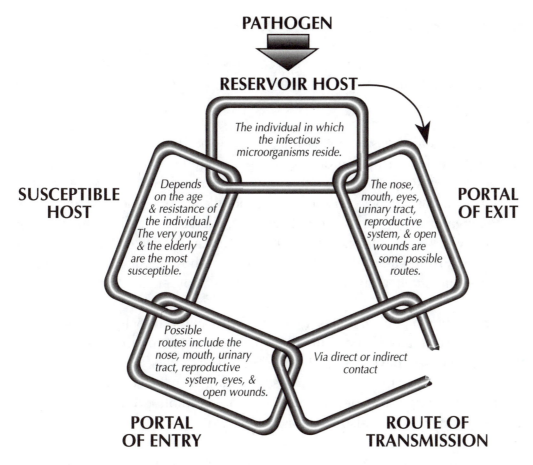

Figure 9-4: Breaking the Cycle of Infection

5. **Portal of Entry:** employees must practice good asepsis, disinfection, and sterilization.

6. **Susceptible Host:** employees must recognize and identify high-risk patients and take appropriate action to avoid unnecessary exposure.

The Infection Control Department is responsible for investigating reports of potentially infectious patients and staff members. You are responsible for knowing the policies and procedures for infectious disease control in the hospital setting. Remember—quality patient care is YOUR responsibility and every step should be taken to ensure the wellness of the patient.

Microorganisms and Disease

An **organism** is any living thing that is composed of one cell, such as bacteria, or many cells, such as man. A **microorganism** is an organism that is not visible with the naked eye.

A pathogen is a disease causing microorganism. There are several types of pathogens, including fungi, protozoa, viruses, bacteria, and rickettsia. **Fungi** are a large group of simple plants. Of this group, only **molds** and **yeasts** are capable of causing disease. Fungi-caused diseases include athlete's foot and ringworm. Some fungal diseases can be very dangerous, such as coccidioidomycosis, or Valley Fever. These yeast (mold) based diseases can lead to chronic, recurrent infections. **Protozoa** are the only group of microbes classified as an animal. They are single-celled and cause diseases such as dysentery and malaria.

virus:
a microscopic parasitic organism capable of causing an infectious disease

A **virus** is a tiny organism that is not visible with an ordinary light microscope. Viruses are so small they can only be seen with an electron microscope. More than 300 viruses have been identified by researchers. Some seem to be harmless; however, many cause illnesses ranging from the common cold or flu to life-threatening forms of pneumonia. Certain childhood diseases, such as chickenpox and croup, also are caused by a virus.

Because viruses are simple in their makeup and organization, they multiply easily as long as they have access to food. They get their food and nutrients from the cell in which they are living. Viruses are not affected by **antibiotics**; antibiotics can destroy bacteria, but not viruses.

bacteria:
the plural of bacterium; single-celled microorganisms in the class Schizomycetes

Bacteria are single-celled microorganisms first observed under the microscope in 1693 by the Dutch naturalist, Antoni van Leeuwenhoek. About 1600 species have been identified; but only a small percentage of these are known to cause disease in man. Normal flora, which are naturally occurring bacteria on and in the body, live on the skin and in the mouth. For example, everyone has bacteria on the surface of their skin known as **Staphylococcus**, or **Staph**. These bacteria help defend the skin against disease; however, if they enter into the body through a break in the skin, they become harmful. Normal flora help fight off infection when they stay where they belong.

Bacteria can grow with or without oxygen. This means they can live and multiply outside the body as well as inside the body. The bacteria that need oxygen to grow are referred to as **aerobic**; those that do not require oxygen are called **anaerobic**.

Bacteria have many shapes: round ones are called **cocci**, rods are called **bacilli**, and those shaped like spirals are called **spirilla**. Round bacteria in grape-like clusters are called **Staphylococci**, those arranged in chains are called **streptococci**, and those in pairs are **diplococci**. Staining is a procedure used by trained personnel in the laboratory. This procedure helps identify specific kinds of bacteria. Gram-staining is a particular procedure named for Hans C. J. Gram. Gram negative bacteria stain red and gram positive bacteria stain violet. Some bacteria can encase themselves in a cellular shell to protect themselves from destruction; these are known as *spores*. Steam under pressure, or heat above a certain temperature, will kill all bacteria and their spores.

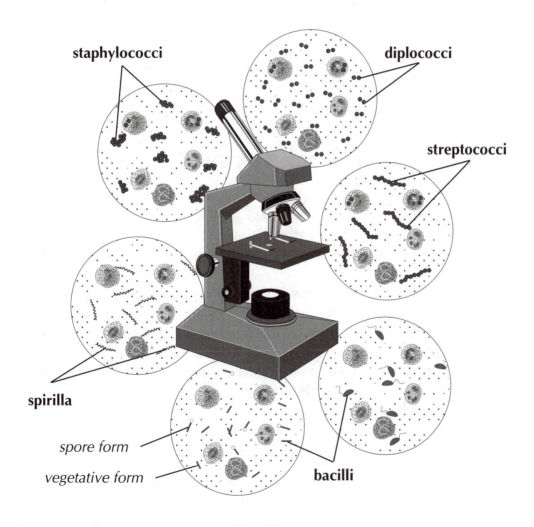

Figure 9-5: Types of Bacteria and Their Shapes

Staphylococci are capable of causing boils, impetigo, and osteomyelitis. Streptococci can cause diseases like rheumatic fever, streptococcal pneumonia, and scarlet fever. Gonorrhea and meningitis are caused by diplococci; tetanus and tuberculosis are induced by bacilli; and a type of spirilla can cause a form of rat bite fever. Almost all bacteria can be destroyed with antibiotics, which are a special classification of medication capable of destroying microorganisms by inhibiting their growth. However, several types of bacteria recently have been identified which are unaffected by antibiotics.

Rickettsiae are smaller than bacteria. They are barely visible under a light microscope. Rickettsiae are members of the plant family. They are responsible for causing such diseases as typhus and Rocky Mountain spotted fever.

Viruses, bacteria, fungi, protozoa, and rickettsiae are pathogens capable of producing life-threatening diseases in humans. The most effective way to fight the transmission of disease is through consistent and thorough handwashing!

Medical and Surgical Asepsis

aseptic:
sterile; preventing infection

It is vital that healthcare workers understand the importance of maintaining a clean, or **aseptic**, environment. Pathogens are everywhere, but they can be controlled or eliminated for a period of time by following certain procedures. Preventing the spread of pathogens is part of every healthcare worker's job.

clean technique:
the removal or destruction of infected material or organisms; medical asepsis

Medical asepsis, also known as **clean technique**, refers to practices and procedures that are designed to ensure a clean environment by removing or destroying disease causing microorganisms. The Housekeeping Department, or Environmental Services Department, is vitally important in maintaining a clean hospital environment; but clinical allied healthcare workers are involved in providing direct patient care. Therefore, the first step in medical asepsis is proper and adequate handwashing on the part of these workers. Other aseptic practices include wearing a clean uniform, not touching your hair or your face with your hands, and holding contaminated items away from you.

sterile technique:
the procedure used by healthcare workers when performing or assisting with a sterile procedure; surgical asepsis

The highest level of protection for patients is **surgical asepsis**. Surgical asepsis, or **sterile technique**, is used whenever the skin is broken open, as in surgery or from a traumatic injury; when a normally sterile body cavity is entered, such as during urinary catheterization; during the treatment of open wounds (ie, dressing changes); and to decontaminate items between patients. Sterile instruments and supplies are completely free from all microorganisms; therefore, all instruments used for putting in stitches or performing an operation are sterile.

The CDC has established guidelines which, if followed, will minimize the risk of introducing disease causing organisms to both the healthcare worker and the patient. These specific guidelines will be described later in this chapter.

Handwashing—The Key to Medical Asepsis

Now that you are familiar with disease-causing microorganisms, it will be easy to understand how clinical healthcare workers and patients contract illnesses in the hospital environment. Staphylococci occur naturally on the skin; so, of course, they reside on your hands. Research has shown the most effective method to reduce the risk of industrial illnesses and nosocomial infections is by frequent and correct handwashing. Therefore, clinical healthcare workers are responsible for giving care to each patient with CLEAN hands! This means that all patient contact must be preceded and followed by thorough handwashing. The procedure on the next page is the accepted method of handwashing to protect clinical healthcare workers and patients from the spread of disease.

Proper handwashing will minimize the risk of spreading infection from one patient to another, from the clinical healthcare worker to patients, and from patients to the clinical healthcare worker. Handwashing must be done at the following times:

- when first arriving to work.
- before performing each procedure on a patient.
- during a procedure if your hands become contaminated.
- between each patient for whom you provide care.
- after using the restroom.
- after removing gloves from your hands.
- before eating.

Remember, medical asepsis is clean technique. Handwashing is the key to successful medical asepsis.

Handwashing Technique

Materials needed:
- ✓ liquid soap
- ✓ dry paper towels

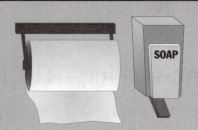

1. Procedural Step: Turn on the faucet. Adjust the temperature of the water to warm—don't burn yourself! *Reason: Warmer water helps remove pathogens.*

2. Procedural Step: Always wet your hands with the fingertips pointing down into, but not touching, the sink. *Reason: Keeping your hands down keeps your forearms dry and prevents contaminated water on your forearms from running over your clean hands. (In most cases, your hands will be dirtier than your arms anyway, so concentrate on getting your hands clean.)*

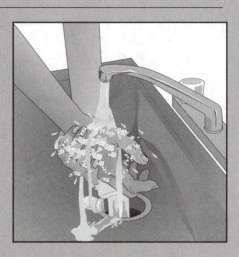

3. Procedural Step: Use a liberal amount of soap and rub the palms of your hands together several times. *Reason: This friction will create a lather and help remove any unwanted viruses or bacteria from the skin surface.*

4. Procedural Step: Put the palm of one hand over the back of the other hand and briskly rub them together. *Reason: All parts of the hands are capable of carrying germs.*

5. Procedural Step: Repeat step #4 using the opposite hands. *Reason: To clean the other hand.*

6. Procedural Step: Interlock the fingers of both hands and vigorously rub them together. You should scrub your hands for a total of two minutes. *Reason: To remove harmful germs.*

7. Procedural Step: Use an orange (cuticle) stick to clean under each nail. If a cuticle stick is not available, use a sterile brush. *Reason: To remove germs from under the nails.*

8. Procedural Step: Rinse all soapy lather from the wrists and hands, continuing to point the hands downward. *Reason: To prevent contaminated water on your forearms from running over your clean hands.*

Handwashing Technique (Cont.)

9. <u>Procedural Step:</u> Leave the water running and dry all areas of the hands using a paper towel.
   <u>Reason:</u> *Paper towels are disposable and prevent the spread of germs.*

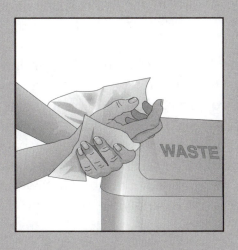

10. <u>Procedural Step:</u> Dispose of the wet paper towel. Obtain another paper towel and, placing the paper towel on the faucet handles, turn off the water. Make sure the towel is dry.
    <u>Reason:</u> *A wet paper towel allows microorganisms to pass through the towel and back onto your clean hands. The dry paper towel will shield your hands from germs on the faucet. THE FAUCET AND SINK ALWAYS ARE CONSIDERED TO BE CONTAMINATED.*

11. <u>Procedural Step:</u> Discard all debris and leave the sink and surrounding area clean, taking care not to recontaminate your hands.
    <u>Reason:</u> *The area must be ready for the next person who wants to wash.*

Disinfection

The most common method of maintaining an environment free from many pathogens is **disinfection**. The hospital uses many different kinds of disinfectants, but the one most recommended is 10% bleach solution. Household bleach kills all pathogens. However, it is very strong, and bleach fumes can harm the respiratory tract. Before using any disinfectant, READ THE LABEL CAREFULLY AND FOLLOW THE DIRECTIONS AS SPECIFIED! Each disinfectant and germicide is used for a particular purpose. For example, alcohol and iodine are commonly used on the skin surface, whereas 10% bleach solution is used on objects contaminated with body secretions. **Contamination** means not pure or unclean, and usually indicates the presence of pathogens. When using any disinfectant or chemical, be sure to review the Material Safety Data Sheet for pertinent information.

Sterilization

A sterilized item is free from all microorganisms. An **autoclave** is an effective means of **sterilization** that uses heat and steam under pressure to produce a sterile product. The autoclave may be large, like the ones in a hospital, or small enough to fit in a private physician's or dentist's office. Autoclaving is the preferred method of sterilization because it destroys all pathogens including viruses and spores. Gas sterilization also is used in hospitals on items that can be damaged by autoclaving. The Central Supply Department is responsible for sterilizing many nondisposable items for use in the various departments throughout the hospital.

All items must be prepared for the autoclave before putting them in it. This includes removing secretions and debris from the surface so those substances do not interfere with sterilization and become baked on during autoclaving. In Central Supply, ultrasound often is used to do this. Linens and other supplies will then be combined with certain instruments to form a pack. Each pack is prepared and labeled for a specific procedure (eg, suturing, burn care, minor surgical procedures, etc.). These packs are wrapped in disposable towels and then secured in a tough plastic wrap. Prior to applying the plastic wrap, indicator strips are placed on the outside of the disposable towels. These indicator strips turn a different color when the sterilization process is completed. In addition, autoclave tape is applied to the outside of the package. This tape will display black lines when the package has gone through the autoclave. Central Supply personnel place expiration dates on all items that have been sterilized. The expiration dates vary according to the items sterilized. For example, a pack may expire within a month, or it may be good for up to a year. Always check the date prior to opening the package! DO NOT SELECT A PACKAGE FOR THE NURSE OR DOCTOR IF THE DATE HAS PASSED!

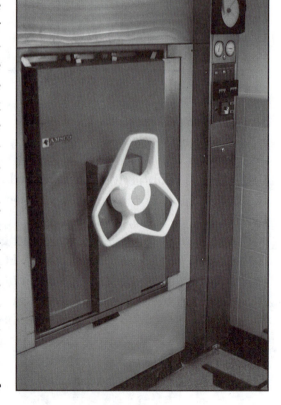

Figure 9-6: An Autoclave

Sterile Technique

Once the instruments or items have been sterilized they must be handled very carefully, using **sterile technique** (surgical asepsis). Sterile technique is the specific procedure used by healthcare workers who are performing a sterile procedure or assisting with one. Part of this procedure involves an awareness of the **sterile field**. The sterile field includes the area and supplies that are sterilized. The healthcare worker must follow these guidelines concerning sterile fields and sterile technique.

1. Wash your hands.

2. Assemble all the equipment that will be needed for the procedure BEFORE PUTTING ON STERILE GLOVES.

3. Open all packages. Be careful not to contaminate the sterile contents with your clean hands.

4. Consider 1 to 1½ inches around the edge of the field to be contaminated. DO NOT TOUCH ANYTHING STERILE IN THAT AREA!

5. NEVER reach across the sterile field.

6. Hold sterile items above waist level.

7. Pour all liquids into sterile containers without touching the rim of the container of liquid with the sterile container. BE CAREFUL NOT TO SPLATTER THE LIQUID! Do not extend the liquid's container over the sterile field. If you do this you risk the chance of contaminants falling from your hands or arms.

8. Put on sterile gloves without contaminating them using the procedure on page 9-17.

    Remember:

    sterile to sterile = STERILE;

    sterile to unsterile = UNSTERILE;

    sterile to unsure = CONTAMINATED.

9. Do not cough, sneeze, or talk over the sterile field!

10. TRY TO NEVER LEAVE A STERILE FIELD UNSUPERVISED. Do not take your eyes off of it if there is not another healthcare worker to watch it. If you must leave the sterile field unsupervised, BE SURE TO COVER IT WITH A STERILE TOWEL. Remember, sterile technique is a precise skill. Although you may never perform a sterile procedure, you may be asked to assist. Responsible healthcare personnel carefully monitor their own techniques and do not hesitate to recognize when they, or others, have broken that technique. To knowingly contaminate an item, or be aware of a contaminated item's existence and NOT CORRECT the error, is NOT ACCEPTABLE. It could cause further injury to the patient.

11. BE AWARE OF ALL NEEDLES AND OTHER SHARP OBJECTS USED DURING THE PROCEDURE. Make a mental note of their location before reaching for items from the procedure tray and surrounding area.

12. Wear gloves when you are cleaning up after the procedure is completed. This prevents accidental contamination from blood or other body fluids that may be present on the instruments or in solutions. Dispose of all needles and sharps in the appropriate container.

13. At the completion of the procedure, carefully remove your gloves in a manner that will not risk self-contamination; this must be done without any part of your bare hands coming in contact with the contaminated gloves.

Sterile technique is used in many healthcare settings. It must be practiced in order to prevent accidental contamination of the sterile field. Competency in this procedure cannot be overemphasized!

Donning Sterile Gloves

Materials needed:

✓ 1 pair sterile gloves

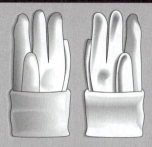

1. Procedure: Obtain a pair of sterile gloves in your hand size.
   Reason: For proper fit.

2. Procedure: Inspect the glove package for signs of contamination: water spots, moisture, tears, or rips.
   Reason: The gloves must be sterile.

3. Procedure: Remove all jewelry and scrub your hands.
   Reason: Standard Precaution. This reduces the number of normal bacteria on the skin.

4. Procedure: Dry your hands well.
   Reason: Moisture increases bacterial growth.

5. Procedure: Peel open the sterile package and lay the inner package on a flat, clean, dry surface so the end nearest you shows the word "cuff."
   Reason: This will allow you to don them properly.

6. Procedure: Open the inner wrapper like a book with right glove on the right, touching only the folded edge of the wrapper.
   Reason: A 1 to 1¹/₂ inch border around the wrapper of the inner package is considered to be contaminated. The inside of the package is sterile.

7. Procedure: With the non-dominant hand pick up the glove touching only the inside of the cuff. (You will glove your dominant hand first.)
   Reason: The inside of the glove will be next to the skin. This area is not sterile.

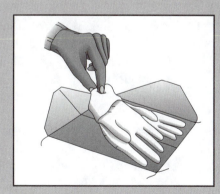

Donning Sterile Gloves (Cont.)

8. <u>Procedure:</u> Keeping your hands above your waist, step back from the table or tray. Hold your hands away from your body and slide your dominant hand into the sterile glove. Leave the cuff folded for now.
   Reason: To avoid contamination.

9. <u>Procedure:</u> Pick up the second glove with the gloved hand by slipping the fingers of the gloved hand under the cuff.
   Reason: Sterile surfaces can only touch other sterile areas.

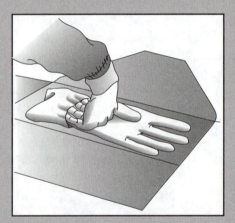

10. <u>Procedure:</u> Slide your second hand into the glove, keeping the gloved thumb extended (like a hitchhiker) to avoid touching your skin. Avoid touching anything else while you do this.
    <u>Reason:</u> *To avoid contamination.*

11. <u>Procedure:</u> Move the glove up the hand and slide the fingers into position.
    <u>Reason:</u> *To secure the glove properly.*

12. <u>Procedure:</u> Unroll the cuff of the first glove, touching only the outside of the glove. Do not touch your bare arm with the sterile fingers of the glove.
    Reason: To avoid contamination.

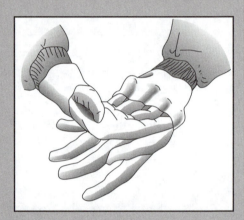

13. <u>Procedure:</u> Unroll the cuff of the second glove, touching only the outside of the glove. Do not touch your bare arm with the sterile fingers of the glove.
    <u>Reason:</u> *To avoid contamination.*

14. <u>Procedure:</u> Interlock your fingers to adjust the gloves, but do not adjust the gloves below the heels of your hands.
    <u>Reason:</u> *To obtain a snug fit and to avoid contamination.*

15. <u>Procedure:</u> Keep your hands above your waist and do not touch anything outside the sterile field. Ask for assistance if needed.
    <u>Reason:</u> *To avoid contamination.*

Disposable Supplies and Infection Control

Because of the time involved in hospital **sterilization** procedures today, many patient care items now are disposable. These commercially sterilized products are designed to be used once, and then discarded. Always check the expiration date on disposable supplies, and never use the item if it has been dropped on the floor. Packages that have been dropped may have holes in them that are too small to be seen by the human eye, yet large enough to result in contamination.

Avoiding Contaminated Sharps

A serious risk associated with providing clinical patient care is the possibility of receiving a puncture wound from a needle or other sharp object. In today's healthcare field, there is a significant risk of contracting either hepatitis B, C, or acquired immune deficiency syndrome (AIDS) from contaminated body fluid and blood.

All needles, scalpel blades, and other sharp objects should be disposed of in the proper puncture-resistant container. During your orientation, try to learn the locations of all the **sharps containers**. Although the colors of these containers may vary, most of them will be either red or beige. Follow the manufacturer's instructions for the proper filling, sealing, and disposal of this container.

The following guidelines are suggested for reducing the risk of a puncture wound from a contaminated needle or other sharp object.

1. Never recap, bend, or manually remove a dirty needle.

2. Always deposit the entire syringe and needle or sharp object in the puncture-resistant container.

3. Immediately clean any puncture wound with alcohol and betadine and cover the wound. Report the incident to your supervisor or instructor.

4. Never carry needles or sharps from one location to another with the tips pointing toward other people or yourself. POINT THEM TOWARD THE FLOOR.

Removing Contaminated Gloves

Materials needed:

✔ a trash can lined with a red biohazard bag

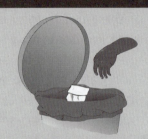

1. <u>Procedure:</u> Hold your gloved hands over a trash can.
   <u>Reason:</u> *You will throw away your used gloves.*

2. <u>Procedure:</u> Without touching the bare skin of your forearm, grasp the contaminated (or outside) area of the dominant glove cuff (approximately 1 to 2 inches from the top) with your gloved nondominant hand.
   <u>Reason:</u> *To avoid contamination.*

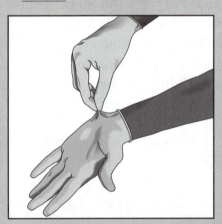

3. <u>Procedure:</u> Pull the glove off. It will now be inside out. Do not snap gloves when removing them.
   <u>Reason:</u> *Microorganisms on the gloves could become airborne.*

4. <u>Procedure:</u> Discard the glove directly into the trash container lined with a red biohazard bag.

<u>Reason:</u> *Gloves cannot be reused. They are considered hazardous waste, and therefore, must be disposed of in the proper manner.*

5. <u>Procedure:</u> Place the bare fingertips of the dominant hand inside the other glove and grasp it near the top. Don't let your bare hand touch the contaminated portion of the glove.
   <u>Reason:</u> *To avoid contamination.*

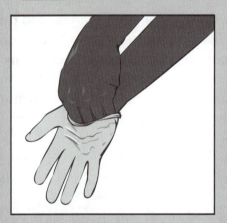

6. <u>Procedure:</u> Pull the second glove off. It also will be inside out. Discard it in the trash can lined with a red biohazard bag.
   <u>Reason:</u> *Gloves cannot be reused.*

7. <u>Procedure:</u> Wash your hands thoroughly before touching anything.
   <u>Reason:</u> *Standard Precaution.*

Most needle sticks occur because of carelessness. Always be aware of their location as well as the location of surrounding people. Wear gloves and other protective wear. TAKE ALL PRECAUTIONS, and do not allow yourself, the patient, or a fellow worker to become a victim of a needle stick!

The Risks—Hepatitis and AIDS

There are several risks to the healthcare worker while providing care to patients. Using aseptic technique and making a conscious effort to reduce the risk of contamination for both the employee and the patient will help reduce the chances of contracting a very serious illness.

Two important diseases that can pose a significant risk to the employee are **hepatitis** and acquired immune deficiency syndrome, or AIDS. Hepatitis is a disease that results in inflammation of the liver. **Hepat-** means pertaining to the liver, **-itis** means inflammation of.

Many different agents can cause hepatitis. This disease may be caused by a virus, bacteria, or a variety of physical or chemical agents. There are several types of hepatitis, but the three most common types that can be contracted from patients and **transmitted** (transferred) to another, are hepatitis A, hepatitis B, and hepatitis C. **Hepatitis A** is caused by a virus. It is the most common form of the disease occurring in children and young adults. Spread of the illness occurs through the fecal-oral route by failing to wash the hands after using the restroom. This is important to the clinical healthcare worker providing direct patient care. Diligent and thorough handwashing CAN protect the healthcare worker. **Hepatitis B** and **C** are caused by viruses too; however, these forms of the disease are spread through blood products and infected body fluids. Clinical healthcare workers in contact with blood MUST wear gloves and practice careful and frequent handwashing! Cover any breaks in the skin with a dressing BEFORE any patient contact occurs. If the dressing becomes contaminated or soiled, remove the dressing, wash your hands, and apply a new dressing. Hepatitis can become a chronic, and sometimes fatal, illness.

Acquired immune deficiency syndrome, or AIDS, is a fatal disease that only has been identified within the past decade, and for which there is no cure. This is a disease that is transmitted through blood and sexual contact. The illness is caused by a virus that attacks the **immune system** (blood cells that work together to fight off infections and disease). An immune system that

hepatitis A: inflammation of the liver that is caused by the hepatitis A virus and spread by the fecal-oral route either from poor handwashing or contaminated food

hepatitis B: inflammation of the liver that is caused by the hepatitis B virus and spread through contact with blood products or infected body fluids (It is the most common form contracted by healthcare workers)

hepatitis C: inflammation of the liver caused by the hepatitis C virus and spread through contact with infected blood or body fluids

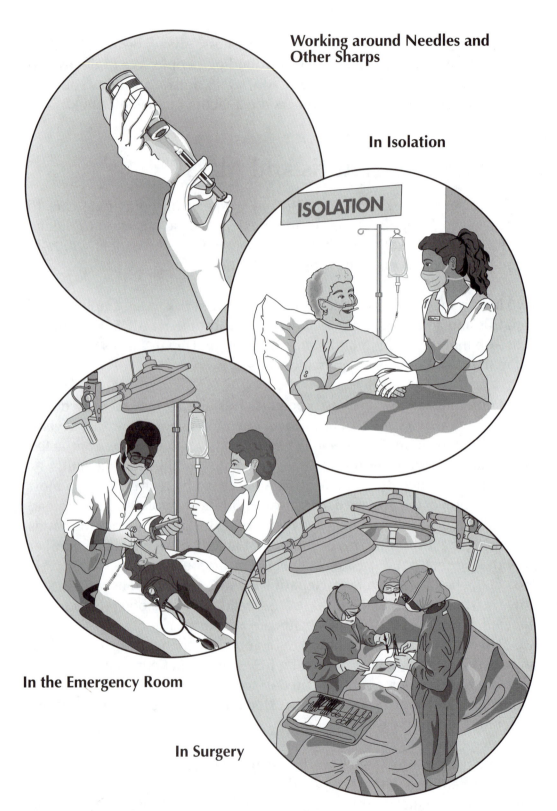

Working around Needles and Other Sharps

In Isolation

ISOLATION

In the Emergency Room

In Surgery

Figure 9-7: Wear the appropriate personal protection equipment during patient care.

does not function properly makes a person susceptible to many different kinds of infections, called **opportunistic infections**. Certain types of cancer and pneumonia are two of the most common disease processes that can be caused by opportunistic infections. AIDS damages the immune system and leaves the patient susceptible to other infections. NO ONE IS COMPLETELY PROTECTED FROM THE VIRUS! You should be aware that according to current laws, it may NOT be mandatory to inform healthcare workers if a patient is infected with the AIDS virus. Currently, there is PROPOSED federal legislation that would require disclosure of testing and counseling data regarding HIV status to healthcare workers who come in physical contact with infected body fluids. Be sure and check your state law regarding disclosure of this information.

AIDS is recognized as a worldwide disease and people from all ages and racial backgrounds can be infected. According to statistics provided by the Centers for Disease Control and Prevention, as of June 1997 more than half a million (612,078) AIDS cases have been reported in the United States since 1981, and approximately 380,000 (1 in 300) Americans have died of AIDS. Furthermore, the World Health Organization estimates that 30.6 million people are living with the AIDS virus (HIV) worldwide.[1] Of these, 29.5 million are adults and 1.1 million are children younger than 15. During 1997 HIV-associated illnesses caused the deaths of an estimated 2.3 million people, including 460,000 children younger than 15. According to the Global AIDS Policy Coalition, if current trends continue, by the end of the year 2000, between 60 and 70 million adults will be infected with HIV.

You must take every precaution available in order to protect yourself from infection, and to keep from transmitting the illness to patients or other healthcare workers. People who are positively infected with the virus may remain **asymptomatic** for many years. However, despite the fact that no symptoms are present, it is still possible for them to transmit the virus. For additional information about AIDS and HIV you may contact the Centers for Disease Control and Prevention's National AIDS Clearing House Services at 1 (800) 342-AIDS. These services are designed to facilitate the sharing of information about HIV, AIDS and other sexually transmitted diseases. They can be found on the internet at http://www.cdcnac.org.

asymptomatic: not showing any signs of disease

---

1. *Statistical Information on HIV/AIDS Cases*, National AIDS Clearinghouse, Centers for Disease Control and Prevention, http://www.cdcnac.org (27 Feb. 1998).

Keeping Pathogens in Their Place With Isolation

The healthcare worker may be exposed to many types of infections while working in the hospital. Transmission of diseases occurs quickly and can easily spread to other people. Asepsis is one method of greatly reducing the spread of communicable diseases. The other method that is common in the hospital is known as isolation.

In the isolation process, pathogens are isolated to the patient care unit. Transmission-based Precautions protect the healthcare worker from contact with ALL body secretions and includes the utilization of Standard Precautions. A special sign on the outside of the patient care unit door will notify all hospital employees and visitors that special procedures must be done both before and after entering the patient care unit.

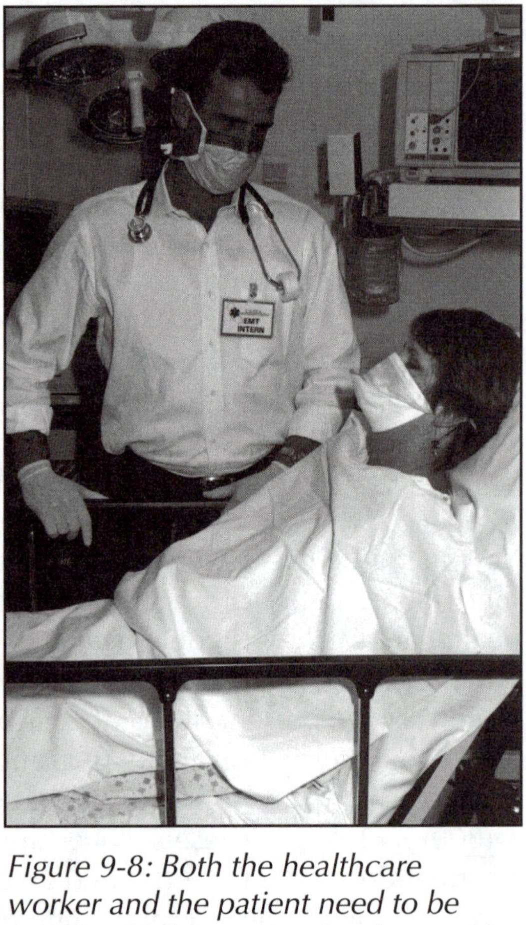

Because some patients' immune systems are so suppressed, they are very susceptible to acquiring many different types of infections and illnesses. It is imperative to pay careful attention to following the type of precautions that may be indicated on the patient care unit door or the patient care plan. This procedure is known as **reverse isolation**, meaning the healthcare worker must protect the patient from exposure to any pathogen which the worker may be able to transmit to the patient. Strict adherence to the procedure protects the patient from pathogens the healthcare worker, or visitors, may be harboring.

reverse isolation: a method of protecting a patient with a suppressed immune system from pathogens that might be transmitted by the staff, other patients or visitors, or through the air

Figure 9-8: Both the healthcare worker and the patient need to be protected when caring for those with a communicable disease.

Standard and Transmission-based Precautions

For your own protection, the CDC has developed guidelines, known as **Standard Precautions**, WHICH ARE TO BE USED EXACTLY AS RECOMMENDED DURING THE PROVISION OF CARE TO EVERY PATIENT. In addition to Standard Precautions, there is a second tier of precautions, known as **Transmission-based Precautions**, that are to be used IN ADDITION to Standard Precautions for patients strongly suspected of having an illness that can be transmitted by droplets, in the air (airborne), or through direct or indirect contact. All hospitals have identified what those illnesses are and have devised a specific infection control plan which, when adhered to by healthcare workers, patients, and visitors, can greatly reduce the risk of nosocomial infections and cross-contamination. Usually hospital personnel post the type of precaution that must be followed on the patient's care plan and on the door to their room.

Transmission-based Precautions and isolation procedures are based upon the following information recently released by the CDC.

1. **Contact transmission** is the most frequent route of transmitting pathogens, especially for nosocomial infections. There are two types of contact transmission: direct and indirect. Patient care activities that could potentially expose the healthcare worker to an infectious disease include turning a patient, bathing a patient, providing oral care, etc. Each of these represents a form of **direct contact** transmission. Gloves, gowns, and possibly eye and mucous membrane protection may be required when providing direct patient care. **Indirect contact** transmission can occur when a susceptible host comes in contact with a contaminated, inanimate object. This type of exposure for the healthcare worker often occurs when changing a patient's bed or gown, cleaning up the bedside (eg, tissues, emesis basins, dressings and bandages, etc.), not cleaning a stethoscope or pen after use, not changing gloves and washing hands, etc. Once again, gloves, gowns and other personal protective equipment may need to be donned prior to performing those various tasks. Examples of illnesses that may be transmitted through either direct or indirect contact are certain forms of hepatitis, AIDS, staphylococcus infections, varicella (chicken pox), herpes zoster, shigella, scabies, pediculosis (lice), and impetigo.

Standard Precautions: guidelines developed by the Centers for Disease Control and Prevention for protecting healthcare workers from exposure to blood-borne pathogens in body secretions

Transmission-based Precautions: guidelines developed by the Centers for Disease Control and Prevention to help prevent transmission of specific infectious and communicable diseases of patients either suspected of having, or confirmed to have, a certain pathogen

contact transmission: direct and indirect transmission of pathogenic microorganisms

droplet transmission: a method of transmitting pathogens when a susceptible host becomes exposed or infected through the droplets emitted during coughing, sneezing, talking, singing, or while performing ventilations

2. **Droplet transmission** occurs when a susceptible host is exposed through contact with droplets emitted during talking, sneezing, coughing, whispering, singing, etc. Healthcare workers may also incur exposure when performing such patient care activities as assisting with a bronchoscopy, suctioning, performing ventilations during cardiopulmonary resuscitation, etc. The actual infected droplets are propelled through the air for approximately three feet. The infected particles are considered to be large in size (greater than 5 microns) and are usually deposited on the mucous membranes or conjuctiva of the susceptible host. Usually gloves, gown, eye and mucous membrane personal protective equipment must be donned. Examples of illnesses transmitted through droplets are streptococcal pharyngitis, pneumonia, scarlet fever, influenza, rubella, mumps, and pertussis (whooping cough).

airborne transmission: a method of transmitting pathogens when a susceptible host is exposed or infected by the nuclei of evaporated, infected droplets

3. **Airborne transmission** occurs when a susceptible host is exposed to the nuclei of evaporated, infected droplets. The nuclei are considered to be small in size (5 microns or smaller). As with droplet transmission, these particles are also emitted during talking, sneezing, coughing, whispering, singing, etc. Unlike droplets, these particles remain suspended in the air for long periods of time and are capable of being emitted farther distances. Because of those two characteristics, special handling of the patient is required. These patients must be admitted to a patient care unit that has special ventilation techniques and air pressure requirements. Healthcare workers must don gloves, gowns, eye protection, and a special mask (a tuberculosis respirator, N95) that must be specially fitted for the healthcare worker. Examples of illnesses transmitted through the air are measles, tuberculosis, and varicella (chicken pox).

It is important to remember that frequent, thorough handwashing remains the most efficient method for reducing the healthcare worker's exposure to communicable and infectious diseases. Gloves are to be changed between patient contacts and, if necessary, during multiple dressing changes on the same patient in order to prevent cross-contamination of wounds. For your own protection, use the following Standard and Transmission-based Precautions as recommended.

1. WEAR GLOVES whenever contact with any body secretion may occur. Do not re-use gloves!

2. COVER CUTS AND OTHER LESIONS with a plastic bandage.

3. WEAR PROTECTIVE EYE WEAR AND A MASK during any procedures that may expose you to splattering blood or other body fluids.

4. WEAR DISPOSABLE GOWNS if blood or body fluids may splatter.

5. Thoroughly wash your hands and other skin surfaces immediately following contamination.

6. Carefully and properly dispose of all sharp objects (needles, scalpel blades, etc.) in appropriate puncture-resistant sharps containers. DO NOT RECAP, BEND, BREAK, OR MANUALLY REMOVE NEEDLES! If you get stuck by a used needle, clean the area with Betadine, fill out the necessary forms to notify supervisors of the needle stick and get a blood test for hepatitis and AIDS. If you know on which patient the needle was used, hospital policy usually requires the patient's blood to be tested for hepatitis B; however, the patient must sign an HIV Test Release Form first.

7. AVOID GIVING MOUTH-TO-MOUTH RESUSCITATION. Instead, use the mouth-to-mask method, resuscitator bags, and other available equipment.

8. AVOID DIRECT PATIENT CONTACT if you have open wounds or other skin conditions.

9. WASH YOUR HANDS after each patient contact and after removing gloves.

10. Use a 10% bleach solution to clean your pen and stethoscope should they become contaminated.

The Centers for Disease Control and Prevention have recommended these Standard Precautions to protect both healthcare workers and patients from contracting hepatitis B, C, or AIDS. These guidelines and recommendations are not intended to make patient care time consuming or difficult. They are intended to provide a safe, healthy environment for everyone concerned.

Body secretions for which Standard Precautions are appropriate include: tears, saliva, urine, sputum, fecal material, wound drainage, semen, vaginal secretions, tissues, **synovial fluid** (fluid around a joint), **cerebrospinal fluid** (fluid around the brain and spinal cord), **pleural fluid** (fluid in and around the lungs), **peritoneal fluid** (fluid from the abdominal cavity), **pericardial fluid** (fluid from around the heart), and **amniotic fluid** (fluid from the sac containing the growing fetus in the uterus). The CDC maintains that the risk of healthcare workers contracting the hepatitis B virus or the AIDS virus from these secretions is not as high as from blood and sexual secretions; however, it does exist! Recognizing common health hazards and infectious diseases can be difficult—especially since viruses and bacteria cannot be seen with the naked eye. Being aware of the potential hazards and risks, and following the Standard and Transmission-based Precautions established by the CDC as well as the recommendations of your hospital, can greatly reduce your exposure to potentially fatal diseases.

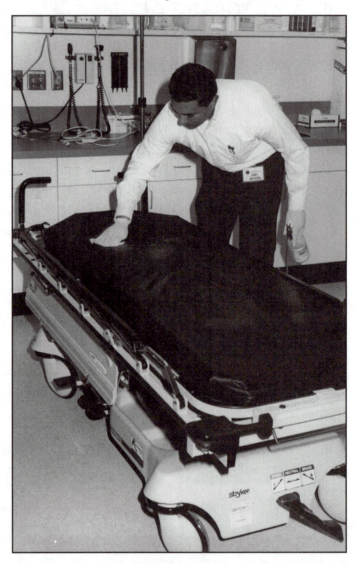

Figure 9-9: Treat blood and other body fluids as potentially infectious.

Chapter Summary

Since the recognition of AIDS in the 1980s, the healthcare industry has put more emphasis on infection control than ever before. In the hospital environment, it is especially important for healthcare workers to understand the significance of the infection cycle. It is their responsibility to be familiar with the methods for interrupting the infection cycle.

Advances in technology and research have made it possible for hospitals to sterilize and disinfect instruments, equipment, linen, floors, and counter tops to reduce the chances of infection. Pathogens occur everywhere, and the healthcare worker must provide an optimal healing environment for the patient. Standard Precautions, Transmission-based Precautions, and isolation techniques have been recommended by the CDC for everyone's protection. Diligent use of these precautions will help ensure minimal transmission of infectious diseases.

Although safety in the workplace is of prime importance, DO NOT FORGET THE PATIENT IS A PERSON! It is the blood and body secretions that can be infectious, not the patient. You must treat the patient with respect and care. Be sympathetic and sensitive to the various needs of the patient, significant other, and family members. A simple explanation concerning the personal protection equipment will help calm any fears the patient or relatives may have. Remember, entering an ill patient's room wearing gloves, gown, mask, and protective eye wear, may indicate to the patient that his illness is more serious than he originally was told. Try to calm the fears and misunderstandings that can be created by your personal protection equipment. Don't forget, YOU are responsible for the safety and protection of the patient, your coworkers, and yourself!

Name _____

Date _____

Student Enrichment Activities

Complete the following statements.

1. The _____ _____ _____ _____ _____
    _____ is the government agency responsible for protecting the public
    health through the prevention and control of disease.

2. Label the six parts of the infection cycle.

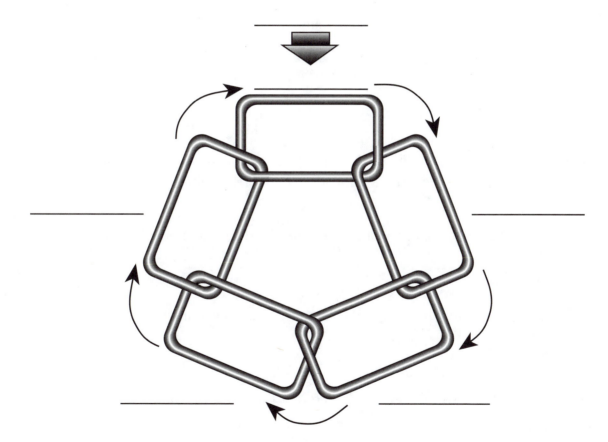

3. Bacteria that need oxygen to grow and reproduce are called _____.

4. *Staph* is an abbreviation for _____.

5. The first step in asepsis is proper and thorough _____.

6. List six times at which handwashing is a MUST. _____

    _____

    _____

7. The preferred method of sterilization is to use an _____ because
    it destroys all _____.

8. Round bacteria are called _____.

9. Organisms that cause disease are called _____.

10. Bacteria that naturally occurs on various parts of the body are called

    _____.

11. Sterile technique is a precise skill used by _____ _____
    who are performing a sterile procedure or assisting with one.

12. The puncture resistant container used for the disposal of needles is called a

    _____ _____.

13. Two diseases that healthcare workers are at risk of contracting are

    _____ and _____.

14. Patients with AIDS are susceptible to _____

    _____.

15. The Centers for Disease Control and Prevention recommend healthcare workers
    practice the use of _____ _____ if they
    may be exposed to body fluids.

Name _____

Date _____

16. In hospitals, the recommended cleaning solution is _____ _____

    _____.

17. Containment of pathogens to the patient care unit is called _____.

Unscramble the following terms.

18. SAID   _____

19. TRACIBEA   _____

20. COMSONLOIA   _____

21. SETIERL CHQTIENUE   _____ _____

22. SPASISE   _____

23. IENFITCON CEYLC   _____ _____

24. GRAMOCIRMSION   _____

25. SIRVU   _____

26. SPEITHIAT   _____

27. ATROOPZO   _____

Chapter Ten
Fundamental Skills

Objectives

After completing this chapter you should be able to
do the following:

1. Define and correctly spell each of the key terms.

2. List the four basic vital signs.

3. Explain three methods of heat loss.

4. Describe the two different temperature scales.

5. Explain the term *core temperature*.

6. Explain the differences between an oral glass thermometer
   and a rectal glass thermometer.

7. Name the normal numeric value for oral, rectal, and
   axillary temperatures.

8. Identify five locations on the body where a pulse can be felt.

9. Describe the normal resting heart rate for an adult.

10. Identify at least three conditions that can change a heart rate.

11. Describe the respiratory cycle.

12. Explain the term *blood pressure*.

Key Terms

- artery
- blood pressure
- bradycardia
- Celsius
- central circulation
- core temperature
- diaphragm
- diastolic
- Fahrenheit
- homeostasis
- hypertension

- hypothalamus
- peripheral circulation
- PMI
- pulse
- respiration
- systolic
- tachycardia
- trauma
- vein
- vital signs

The Importance of Skillfulness

As a clinical healthcare worker, a thorough understanding of fundamental skills and procedures will be helpful to you in many ways. The ability to perform certain skills efficiently and accurately makes the job interesting, exciting, and fun. Furthermore, technical ability increases your self-confidence and boosts the confidence your patients have in you!

> **Note:** During routine care, gloves are not usually worn unless there is potential for exposure to blood or other body fluids, or to non-intact skin, including open lesions. When in doubt, put on appropriate protective wear.

Vital Signs

vital signs:
assessments of temperature, pulse, respirations, and blood pressure; body functions essential to life

The phrase **vital signs** is commonly used in direct patient care. The meaning and value of vital signs often are underestimated. **Vital** means essential to life; indispensable. A *sign* is an obvious, objective finding or evidence of an illness or bodily malfunction. Therefore, *vital signs* provide essential information concerning the condition of the body. There are four basic vital signs: temperature (T), pulse (P), respirations (R), and blood pressure (B/P). They should be recorded on the patient's chart using these abbreviations in the following order: T, P, R, and BP. Recording vital signs in this manner will prevent misunderstandings and false interpretations of the patient's condition.

Homeostasis and Methods of Heat Loss

Heat is an important by-product of the chemical activities that constantly occur inside the body. While heat is being produced, the body is losing heat in a variety of ways. The ability to maintain a constant body temperature despite external and internal influences is one mechanism of **homeostasis**. Homeostasis is a state of equilibrium within the body that is maintained by compensating for changes in the environment or bodily function. Each of the vital signs represents a different mechanism in the process of homeostasis.

The heat-regulating center of the body, known as the **hypothalamus**, lies within the brain. By monitoring nerve impulses from temperature receptors in the skin, and the flow of blood to the brain, the hypothalamus tracks and controls the amount of body heat that is lost. In many ways, it does the same thing for the body that a thermostat does when it controls the temperature in a room.

Approximately 80% of total heat loss occurs through the skin. When the blood temperature rises, the hypothalamus sends signals via nerve impulses to dilate (expand) the blood vessels in the skin. This increases the amount of heat lost through **convection** (the transfer or loss of heat due to the circulation or replacement of a surrounding liquid or gas) and **radiation** (the transfer or loss of heat from or by its source to the surrounding environment in the form of heat waves or rays). The hypothalamus also sends nerve impulses to the sweat glands to stimulate perspiration, which leads to heat loss through **evaporation** (the conversion of a liquid or solid to a gas.) Evaporation cools the body by eliminating body heat whenever the air temperature equals or exceeds the body's temperature.

homeostasis: a state of equilibrium within the body maintained through the adaptation of body systems to changes in either the internal or external environment

hypothalamus: the portion of the brain that controls the temperature of the body

Oral and Rectal Temperatures

Obtaining and recording an accurate body temperature provides the primary healthcare provider with important information concerning the general condition of the patient. It may be your responsibility to take a patient's temperature and communicate the findings to the patient's primary care giver.

The most common methods of obtaining a patient's temperature are **oral** and **rectal**, but sometimes **axillary** or **tympanic** temperatures are taken. The oral and rectal methods are the most desirable ways of measuring the patient's **core temperature**. Generally, the rectal temperature will be approximately one degree higher than the oral reading.

core temperature: the internal body temperature

Fahrenheit:
a temperature scale used in medicine that uses 212° as the boiling point of water and 32° as the freezing point of water

Celsius:
a temperature scale used in medicine that uses 100° as the boiling point of water and 0° as the freezing point of water

There are two temperature scales used to identify a patient's temperature: **Fahrenheit** and **Celsius**. Glass thermometers use the Fahrenheit scale, but digital electronic thermometers can display the temperature in either Fahrenheit or Celsius. The Fahrenheit scale, named after the German physicist who developed it, is the most commonly used scale. This scale uses 32° as the freezing point of water and 212° as the boiling point. It is denoted by placing an *F* after the numerical reading of the temperature.

The Celsius, or Centigrade, scale also is used in the medical field to indicate body temperature. This scale was discovered by a Swedish astronomer named Anders Celsius, and uses a thermometer divided into 100 increments. On this scale, the boiling point of water is 100° and the freezing point of water is 0°. To convert from one scale to the other use the following formulas:

1. To convert from Fahrenheit to Celsius, subtract 32 from the Fahrenheit value and multiply by $5/9$ (or .555). Round off your answer to the nearest tenth degree.

    $5/9$ (F - 32) = Celsius
    .555 (98.6 - 32) = Celsius
    .555 (66.6) = Celsius
    36.96 = Celsius
    37° = Celsius

2. To convert from Celsius to Fahrenheit, multiply the Celsius value by $9/5$ (or 1.8) and add 32. Round off your answer to the nearest tenth.

    (C x $9/5$) + 32 = Fahrenheit
    (37 x 1.8) + 32 = Fahrenheit
    66.6 + 32 = Fahrenheit
    98.6° = Fahrenheit

Proper measurement of the body's **core temperature** is essential to determine both subtle and drastic changes in a patient's condition. The following pages include the procedures for taking patients' temperatures using glass, electronic, and tympanic thermometers.

Note: Remember when performing the following procedures to always raise the siderails on the bed and to return the bedside table to its proper position before leaving the patient.

Measuring an Oral Temperature Using an Electronic Thermometer

Materials needed:
✓ an electronic oral thermometer
✓ a disposable thermometer cover
✓ gloves (if blood or other body fluids are present)

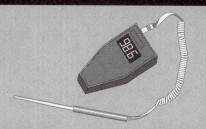

1. Procedural Step: Wash your hands.
   Reason: Standard Precaution.

2. Procedural Step: Put on gloves if blood or other body fluids are present.
   Reason: Standard Precaution.

3. Procedural Step: Identify the patient by his or her identification bracelet.
   Reason: To make sure you are working with the correct patient.

4. Procedural Step: Explain the procedure to the patient using terms he or she can understand.
   Reason: This keeps the patient calm and provides information the patient needs to give informed consent.

5. Procedural Step: Remove the thermometer from the charging unit or unplug the machine.
   Reason: The unit is charged when not in use.

6. Procedural Step: Remove the temperature probe from the storage compartment and place a disposable cover over the probe.
   Reason: To avoid contamination.

7. Procedural Step: Have the patient discard any chewing tobacco or gum.
   Reason: It may affect the temperature reading.

8. Procedural Step: Ask the patient if he or she has had anything by mouth within the last 15 minutes. Wait 15 minutes if he or she has had anything to eat, drink, chew, or smoke.
   Reason: It may affect the temperature reading.

9. Procedural Step: Wait for the *ready* signal to be displayed.
   Reason: This means the thermometer is ready for use.

10. Procedural Step: Place the probe in the patient's mouth under the tongue. Have the patient close his or her lips.
    Reason: This area is close to a rich blood supply.

Measuring an Oral Temperature
Using an Electronic Thermometer (Cont.)

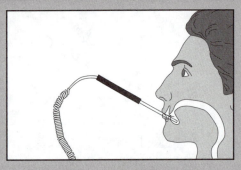

11. Procedural Step: At the sound or flashing light, remove the probe from the patient's mouth.
Reason: The signal indicates the thermometer is ready to read.

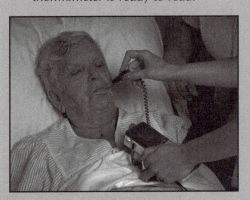

12. Procedural Step: Press the probe cover release and dispose of the cover. Do not insert the probe into the body of the thermometer until you have recorded the temperature.
Reason: This allows removal of the probe cover without touching it and prevents alteration of the thermometer reading.

13. Procedural Step: Remove your gloves if it was necessary to put them on.
Reason: The gloves are now contaminated and must be removed before touching anything or another patient.

14. Procedural Step: Wash your hands.
Reason: Standard Precaution.

15. Procedural Step: Read the display. Record the temperature on the patient's chart.
Reason: To provide documentation.

16. Procedural Step: Return the thermometer to the charging unit.
Reason: The equipment will be ready for the next patient.

17. Procedural Step: Report any abnormal readings to the primary healthcare provider and your supervisor immediately.
Reason: This may indicate a health problem. A normal oral temperature is 98.6° F.

Chart it like this: **T=99⁶** or **T 99.6**.

Measuring a Rectal Temperature Using an Electronic Rectal Thermometer

Materials needed:
✓ an electronic rectal thermometer (red-tipped probe)
✓ a disposable probe cover
✓ lubricating jelly
✓ gloves

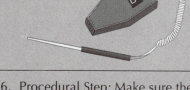

1. Procedural Step: Rectal temperatures are taken on children under age 5, unconscious patients, and patients who cannot tolerate an oral thermometer.
   Reason: It provides more accurate measurement on a patient who is unable to follow safety directions regarding oral thermometers.

2. Procedural Step: Wash your hands.
   Reason: Standard Precaution.

   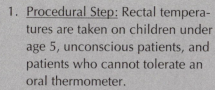

3. Procedural Step: Wear gloves.
   Reason: Standard Precaution.

4. Procedural Step: Identify the patient by his or her identification bracelet.
   Reason: To ensure you are working with the correct patient.

5. Procedural Step: Explain the procedure to the patient using terms he or she can understand.
   Reason: This keeps the patient calm and provides the information the patient needs to give informed consent.

6. Procedural Step: Make sure the thermometer has a red-tipped end.
   Reason: This means it is a rectal thermometer.

7. Procedural Step: Place a protective probe cover over the thermometer.
   Reason: The disposable cover prevents contamination.

8. Procedural Step: Lubricate the probe cover with **KY Jelly** or **Lubifax**.
   Reason: For ease of insertion.

9. Procedural Step: Provide privacy for the patient by drawing the curtain completely around the patient's bed or closing the door to the patient's unit.
   Reason: This makes the procedure less embarrassing for the patient.

10. Procedural Step: Position the patient on his or her side with the top thigh and knee pulled toward the chest. Have the patient lean forward slightly. Turn back the sheets to expose the anus.
    Reason: This allows easy access to the rectum.

Measuring a Rectal Temperature Using an Electronic Rectal Thermometer (Cont.)

11. <u>Procedural Step:</u> Insert the thermometer into the anus 1 to 1½ inches in an adult, 1-inch in a child, and ½ inch in an infant. If the thermometer does not advance easily, remove the probe and report this to the primary care provider. NEVER FORCE THE RECTAL PROBE!
    <u>Reason:</u> This is the proper position for an accurate reading. Forcing the probe could injure the patient.

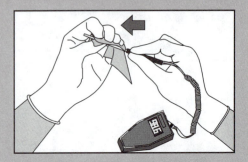

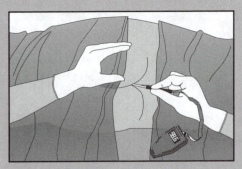

12. <u>Procedural Step:</u> Hold the thermometer in place until you hear the sound or see a flashing light.
    <u>Reason:</u> Prevents injury in case the patient moves and ensures an accurate reading.

13. <u>Procedural Step:</u> Carefully remove the thermometer. Wipe any excess lubricant from the rectal area and cover your patient.
    <u>Reason:</u> The thermometer is ready to read. To make the patient as comfortable as possible.

14. <u>Procedural Step:</u> Remove the protective probe cover and discard. Wipe the thermometer from stem toward bulb end and discard tissue.

<u>Reason:</u> The probe cover and tissue are contaminated.

15. <u>Procedural Step:</u> Remove your gloves.
    <u>Reason:</u> Standard Precaution.

16. <u>Procedural Step:</u> Wash your hands.
    <u>Reason:</u> Standard Precaution.

17. <u>Procedural Step:</u> Read the thermometer and record the temperature on the patient's chart using the proper abbreviation, *R*, to indicate that it is a rectal temperature.
    <u>Reason:</u> Normal rectal temperature is 99.8° F.

18. <u>Procedural Step:</u> Reposition the patient comfortably.
    <u>Reason:</u> To make the patient as comfortable as possible.

Measuring a Rectal Temperature Using an Electronic Rectal Thermometer (Cont.)

19. Procedural Step: Clean and disinfect the thermometer according to facility policy. Open the curtain surrounding the patient and return the equipment to its proper place.
    Reason: Aseptic technique. The equipment will be ready for the next patient. Standard Precaution.

20. Procedural Step: Report any abnormal findings to the appropriate healthcare provider and your supervisor immediately.
    Reason: Abnormal findings may indicate a health problem.

21. Procedural Step: Wash your hands again before providing care to another patient.
    Reason: Standard Precaution.

Chart it like this: T=102⁴Ⓡ or T 102.4Ⓡ

The procedures outlined above are for electronic digital thermometers. Almost all facilities use this type of thermometer exclusively. However, there will be a few occasions, such as when a patient is in isolation, or a digital thermometer is being repaired, in which a glass thermometer will be used.

It is very important to use the correct thermometer to take a temperature. A patient's temperature can reveal an early infection or disease process that may not be apparent to the patient. The oral glass thermometer usually has a longer bulb and is colored blue at the stem end. The glass rectal thermometer has a short, stubby bulb and is colored red at the stem end. The entire bulb may be a specific color, or there may be an area near the bulb with the appropriate color.

The procedures for using electronic thermometers and glass thermometers are essentially the same, however, there are a few important differences. Glass thermometers contain liquid mercury, which is toxic if swallowed. When using the glass thermometer, caution the patient about the hazards of biting the glass. If the glass is broken, the patient may cut his or her mouth and swallow the mercury. The procedures for using glass thermometers follow.

Measuring an Oral Temperature Using a Glass Thermometer

Materials needed:
- ✓ a glass oral thermometer
- ✓ a thermometer cover
- ✓ a clock or watch
- ✓ gloves (if blood or other body fluids are present)

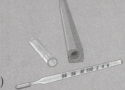

1. <u>Procedural Step:</u> Wash your hands. *Reason: Standard Precaution.*

2. <u>Procedural Step:</u> Put on gloves if blood or other body fluids are present. *Reason: Standard Precaution.*

3. <u>Procedural Step:</u> Identify the patient by his or her identification bracelet. *Reason: To make sure you are working with the correct patient.*

4. <u>Procedural Step:</u> Explain the procedure to the patient using terms he or she can understand. *Reason: This keeps the patient calm and provides information the patient needs to give informed consent.*

5. <u>Procedural Step:</u> Remove the thermometer from the package or cleaning solution. Clinics may put them in a cleaning solution, whereas hospitals have them individually wrapped. *Reason: To prevent contamination.*

6. <u>Procedural Step:</u> Hold the thermometer at eye level and rotate it until the column of silver-colored mercury can be seen. Check for cracks, breaks, or chips in the glass. *Reason: A cracked or chipped thermometer can injure the patient.*

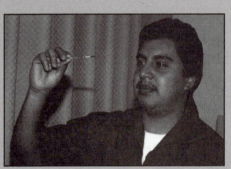

7. <u>Procedural Step:</u> Grasp the thermometer with your thumb and forefinger. With a sharp, snapping motion of the wrist, shake it until the mercury line falls below 96° F. DO NOT DROP THE THERMOMETER OR HIT IT AGAINST ANY OBJECT! Read it by holding it horizontally at eye level and rotating it between your fingers until the mercury line can be seen easily. Each long line on the thermometer designates 1 degree, and each short line designates 0.2 of a degree (2 tenths, 4 tenths, etc.). A longer line usually designates 98.6° F (ideal body temperature). *Reason: For accurate interpretation of the temperature reading, the thermometer must be below 96° F at the time the procedure is begun.*

Measuring an Oral Temperature Using a Glass Thermometer (Cont.)

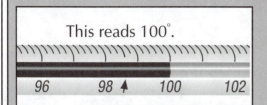

This reads 100°.

96   98 ↑   100   102

8. Procedural Step: Place a disposable cover over the thermometer if one is to be used.
Reason: Standard Precaution.

9. Procedural Step: Warn the patient about the hazards of biting the glass.
Reason: If the glass is broken, the patient may cut his or her mouth and swallow the mercury.

10. Procedural Step: Place the bulb of the thermometer in the patient's mouth under the tongue. Have the patient close his or her lips.
Reason: This area is close to a rich blood supply.

11. Procedural Step: Wait at least 3 minutes before removing the thermometer.
Reason: Non-electronic oral temperatures take at least 3 minutes to register.

12. Procedural Step: Remove the thermometer and the protective cover and read the thermometer to the nearest tenth degree.
Reason: The temperature is recorded to the nearest tenth degree.

13. Procedural Step: Shake the mercury below 96° F, wash it in cold water, and dry it with a paper towel.

Reason: Washing in cold water removes secretions so the disinfectant will be effective (See step #15), and prevents the mercury from rising. Items must be dried before being disinfected to prevent the solution from becoming diluted by the water.

14. Procedural Step: Place the thermometer in disinfecting solution for at least 15 minutes or according to the manufacturer's directions. Continue to wear your gloves until the thermometer is submerged in the solution.
Reason: Aseptic technique and Standard Precautions.

15. Procedural Step: Remove and discard your gloves if it was necessary to put them on.
Reason: Standard Precaution.

16. Procedural Step: Wash your hands before caring for another patient.
Reason: Standard Precaution.

17. Procedural Step: Record your findings on the patient's chart.
Reason: To provide documentation.

18. Procedural Step: Report any abnormalities to your supervisor and the primary healthcare provider.
Reason: An abnormality may indicate a health problem.

Chart it like this: T=98⁶ or T 98.6.

Measuring a Rectal Temperature Using a Glass Rectal Thermometer

Materials needed:
✓ a glass rectal thermometer (red-tipped)
✓ a prelubricated disposable thermometer cover
✓ gloves

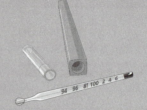

1. _Procedural Step:_ Rectal temperatures are taken on children under age 5, unconscious patients, and patients who cannot tolerate an oral thermometer.
   Reason: To provide more accurate measurement on a patient who is unable to follow safety directions regarding glass thermometers.

2. _Procedural Step:_ Wash your hands.
   Reason: Standard Precaution.

3. _Procedural Step:_ Wear gloves.
   Reason: Standard Precaution.

4. _Procedural Step:_ Identify the patient by his or her identification bracelet.
   Reason: To ensure you are working with the correct patient.

5. _Procedural Step:_ Explain the procedure to the patient using terms he or she can understand.
   Reason: Keeps the patient calm and provides information necessary for the patient to give informed consent.

6. _Procedural Step:_ Make sure the thermometer has a red-tipped end and a short bulb.
   Reason: This means it is a rectal thermometer.

7. _Procedural Step:_ Read the thermometer.
   Reason: To make sure it is below 96° F for an accurate reading.

8. _Procedural Step:_ If it is not there already, shake down the mercury column in thermometer below 96° F.
   Reason: To make the mercury level drop.

9. _Procedural Step:_ Place a prelubricated disposable cover over the thermometer.
   Reason: Disposable covers prevent contamination.

10. _Procedural Step:_ Provide privacy for the patient and position the patient on his or her side. Turn back the sheets to expose the anus.
    Reason: It may be more comfortable for the patient to lie on his side with one knee bent.

Measuring a Rectal Temperature
Using a Glass Rectal Thermometer (Cont.)

11. Procedural Step: Insert the thermometer into the anus 1 to 1¹/2 inches in an adult, 1 inch in a child, and ¹/2 inch in an infant.
Reason: This is the proper position for an accurate reading.

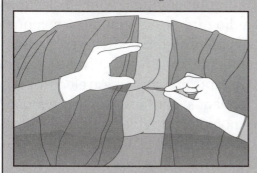

12. Procedural Step: Hold the thermometer in place for 3 to 5 minutes.
Reason: To prevent injury in case the patient moves.

13. Procedural Step: Carefully remove the thermometer. Wipe any excess lubricant from the rectal area and cover your patient.
Reason: The thermometer is ready to read. To make the patient as comfortable as possible.

14. Procedural Step: Remove the protective cover and discard. Wipe the thermometer from stem toward bulb end and discard the tissue.
Reason: The sheath and tissue are contaminated.

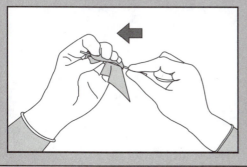

15. Procedural Step: Remove your gloves.
Reason: Standard Precaution.

16. Procedural Step: Wash your hands.
Reason: Standard Precaution.

17. Procedural Step: Read the thermometer and record the temperature on the patient's chart using the abbreviation, R, to indicate that it is a rectal temperature.
Reason: The normal rectal temperature is 99.8° F.

18. Procedural Step: Cover and reposition your patient comfortably.
Reason: To make the patient as comfortable as possible.

19. Procedural Step: Disinfect the thermometer according to facility policy. Open the curtain.
Reason: Standard Precaution.

20. Procedural Step: Report any abnormal findings immediately, and wash your hands again before providing care to another patient.
Reason: Abnormal findings may indicate a health problem. Standard Precaution.

Chart it like this: T=101⁴Ⓡ or T 101.4Ⓡ.

Axillary and Tympanic Temperatures

Oral and rectal temperature readings are the preferred methods for obtaining a patient's temperature. However, there will be instances when, due to the patient's condition, neither one of these methods is possible. For those patients, the temperature may need to be taken in the armpit (the axilla) or against the tympanic membrane in the ear.

The newest method of obtaining the body temperature is with an electronic thermometer designed to obtain a reading from the tympanic membrane (covering over the eardrum). The tympanic membrane shares the same blood supply as the hypothalamus. This temperature is actually the temperature of the blood flowing through the tympanic membrane. An electric probe (or **speculum**) is inserted into the patient's ear next to the tympanic membrane. Within seconds, the thermometer provides a readout of the patient's temperature. BE CAREFUL NOT TO INSERT THE PROBE TOO FAR—THIS CAN INJURE THE TYMPANIC MEMBRANE!

Measuring a Tympanic Temperature Using a Tympanic Thermometer

Materials needed:
- ✓ a tympanic thermometer (electronic)
- ✓ a disposable thermometer cover
- ✓ gloves (if blood or other body fluids are present)

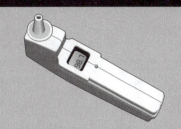

1. Procedural Step: Wash your hands.
   Reason: Standard Precaution.

2. Procedural Step: Put on gloves if any blood or other body fluid is present.
   Reason: Standard Precaution.

3. Procedural Step: Identify the patient by his or her identification bracelet.
   Reason: To make sure you are working with the correct patient.

4. Procedural Step: Explain the procedure using terms the patient can understand.
   Reason: This reassures the patient and provides information necessary for the patient to give informed consent.

5. Procedural Step: Remove the electronic device from the charging unit.
   Reason: The device is portable.

6. Procedural Step: Place the disposable cover over the ear speculum.
   Reason: Aseptic technique.

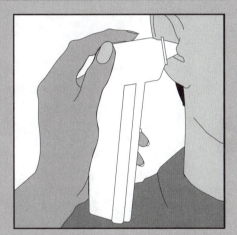

7. Procedural Step: Have the patient turn his or her head to one side. If the patient is a child, gently turn his or her head to one side and hold it in place.
   Reason: This makes the ear easily accessible.

8. Procedural Step: Place the speculum in either ear canal for 5 seconds. It only has to cover the opening!
   Reason: This measures the temperature of the tympanic membrane.

9. Procedural Step: Press the scan button, and release it when the temperature is flashing on the display screen.
   Reason: The signal indicates the thermometer is ready to be read. It usually takes about 2 seconds.

Measuring a Tympanic Temperature Using a Tympanic Thermometer (Cont.)

10. Procedural Step: Remove the thermometer from the patient's ear.
Reason: The temperature has been obtained.

11. Procedural Step: Read the thermometer and discard the disposable cover.
Reason: 98.6° F is normal.

12. Procedural Step: Remove and discard your gloves if it was necessary to wear them.
Reason: Standard Precaution.

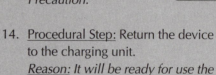

13. Procedural Step: Wash your hands.
Reason: Standard Precaution.

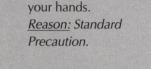

14. Procedural Step: Return the device to the charging unit.
Reason: It will be ready for use the next time.

15. Procedural Step: Chart the temperature using a T to show that it was a tympanic reading.
Reason: To provide documentation.

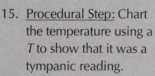

Chart it like this: **T=98⁴ Ⓣ** or **T 98.4 Ⓣ**.

An axillary temperature is taken on people who must breathe through the mouth, or who cannot be moved from side to side. It is obtained by placing the thermometer in the axilla (armpit) of the patient. This method may frequently be used for children; however, if the technique is incorrect, an invalid measurement will be obtained. Generally, the axillary temperature will be approximately 1 degree lower than the oral reading. Use the following procedure to ensure an accurate axillary temperature.

Measuring an Axillary Temperature

Materials needed:

✓ an oral (glass or electronic) thermometer
✓ gloves (if blood or other body fluids are present)
✓ thermometer cover

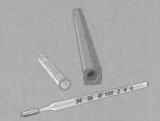

1. <u>Procedural Step:</u> Wash your hands.
   <u>Reason:</u> *Standard Precaution.*

2. <u>Procedural Step:</u> Put on gloves if there is any blood or other body fluid present.
   <u>Reason:</u> *Standard Precaution.*

3. <u>Procedural Step:</u> Identify the patient by his or her identification bracelet.
   <u>Reason:</u> *To ensure you are working with the correct patient.*

4. <u>Procedural Step:</u> Explain the procedure to the patient using terms he or she will understand.

   <u>Reason:</u> *This keeps the patient calm and provides the information necessary for the patient to give informed consent.*

5. <u>Procedural Step:</u> Remove the patient's top piece of clothing.
   <u>Reason:</u> *To gain access to the axilla.*

6. <u>Procedural Step:</u> If there is moisture in the axilla, gently pat the area dry.
   <u>Reason:</u> *Both moisture and intense rubbing can affect the temperature reading.*

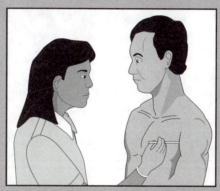

7. <u>Procedural Step:</u> Place the thermometer in the armpit, and bring the patient's arm close to the chest.
   <u>Reason:</u> *To get an accurate reading.*

8. <u>Procedural Step:</u> If using an electronic thermometer, wait for the signal indicating the reading is complete. If using a glass thermometer, hold it in place for at least 10 minutes.
   <u>Reason:</u> *This is necessary for an accurate reading.*

9. <u>Procedural Step:</u> Remove the thermometer and remove the protective cover.
   <u>Reason:</u> *It is ready to read.*

10. <u>Procedural Step:</u> Remove and discard your gloves.
    <u>Reason:</u> *Standard Precaution.*

Measuring an Axillary Temperature (Cont.)

11. **Procedural Step:** Wash your hands.
    Reason: Standard Precaution.

12. **Procedural Step:** Read the thermometer and record the temperature on the patient's chart. Be sure to use the abbreviation *Ax* to indicate axillary temperature.
    Reason: A normal axillary temperature is 97.8° F. (About 1° lower than an oral temperature.)

13. **Procedural Step:** Help the patient dress again if necessary.
    Reason: To assist the patient.

14. **Procedural Step:** Report any abnormalities to your supervisor and the primary healthcare provider immediately.
    Reason: An abnormality may indicate a health problem.

Chart it like this: T=102.4 (Ax) or T 102.4 (Ax).

Note: On a child, a thermometer patch can be placed on the forehead to obtain the skin temperature. The temperature is determined by color changes on the paper patch.

As a healthcare worker, you should be aware of some factors that may affect the core temperature:

- head injuries
- cerebrovascular accidents (CVAs), also known as strokes
- extreme environmental temperatures
- the amount of body fat present (fat is a natural insulator)
- the time of day (temperatures are usually lower early in the morning and higher toward evening)
- disease processes such as infection
- brain tumors or surgery

Practice is essential in order to perform these procedures confidently, accurately, and safely. Learning to recognize abnormal temperatures and reporting them immediately to the proper person will promote efficient patient care.

The Pulse

The **pulse** is another important vital sign that gives the clinical healthcare worker significant information concerning the health status of the patient. It is a rhythmical throbbing caused by the contraction and expansion of an artery as a wave of blood passes through the vessel. An **artery** transports blood away from the heart to the body, whereas a **vein** carries blood from the body back to the heart. Pulses are felt only in arteries.

The pulse provides valuable data on a patient's circulation and cardiac function. The normal range of the resting heart rate for an adult is 60-100 beats per minute. The pulse is recorded on the patient's chart as the number of beats per minute. This means that if a patient has a pulse rate of 72, the heart is beating 72 times in 1 minute. In the average size adult male, there are 5 liters of blood. The blood travels through the body at a rate of about 1 foot per second, with a complete circulation time of about 20 seconds.

Many circumstances can affect the heart rate. For example, a heart rate over 100 may be caused by medication, excitement, anxiety, heart problems, elevated temperature (hyperpyrexia), or many other factors. A rate lower than 60 may also be caused from a temperature below 97° F (**hypothermia**), medication, or heart abnormalities. A person's age and general physical condition can also influence the heart rate.

There are different locations on the body where a pulse can be felt. All pulses are easily felt in arteries close to the surface of the skin by pressing the artery against the underlying bone. The words *central* and *peripheral* are used to classify pulses and their relationship to circulation. **Central circulation** refers to the blood flow supplied to the internal, vital organs such as the brain, heart, and kidneys. The pulse sites used to assess this blood flow are the carotid and the femoral pulses. The **carotid** pulse is located on both sides of the neck, next to the **trachea** (windpipe). The **femoral** pulse is located in the **groin** area at the top of the thigh, near the trunk of the body. With adequate blood flow, a femoral pulse should be palpated, or felt, on both sides of the groin.

Figure 10-1: Pulse Sites

pulse:
a vital sign; a quantitative measurement of the heartbeat using the fingers to palpate an artery or a stethoscope to listen to the heartbeat

artery:
a blood vessel that carries highly oxygenated blood away from the heart to the tissues

vein:
a blood vessel that carries low-oxygenated blood to the heart

central circulation:
refers to the flow of blood to the internal organs

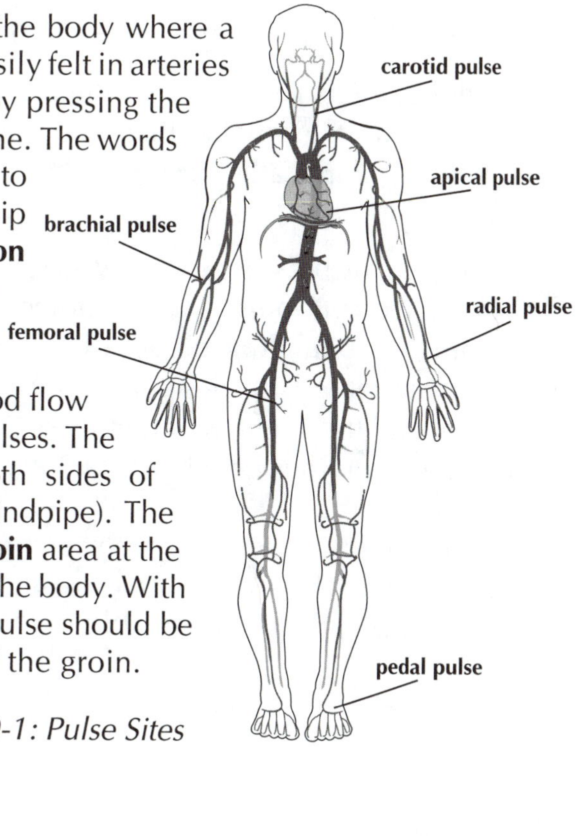

carotid pulse

apical pulse

brachial pulse

radial pulse

femoral pulse

pedal pulse

peripheral circulation: blood flow to the surface of the skin, extremities, ears, nose, and face

Peripheral circulation refers to all other circulation (ie, blood flow to the surface of the skin, arms, legs, ears, nose, and face). Pulse sites most commonly used to assess peripheral circulation include those found in the arms. The **brachial** pulse is located on the inside of the arm. It is easily palpated (felt) near the bend of the arm. The **radial** pulse is felt near the wrist area, extending up the arm from the thumb. One of the pulses located on the top of the foot also may be used to assess circulation to the foot. This pulse is known as the **pedal** pulse.

If there are any abnormalities, the pulse should be taken by placing a stethoscope directly over the heart at the apex, located at the bottom of the heart behind the left nipple. This is known as an **apical** pulse and should be indicated as such on the patient's chart. For example, if the patient's heart rate is 74, it should be recorded as *74Ap*.

Taking the pulse of a patient requires accurate counting and sensitivity to irregular rhythms and quality. The pulse rate varies with the size of the patient, overall physical condition, and age. General guidelines for determining normal resting heart rates are listed below.

- infants (under 1 year of age): 90 to 140 beats per minute.

- children (1 to 7 years old): 80 to 120 beats per minute.

- children (over 7 years old): 72 to 90 beats per minute.

- adults: 60 to 100 beats per minute, with average heart rate being 70 to 80. Rates higher than 100 are known as **tachycardia**; rates below 60 are called **bradycardia**.

tachycardia: a pulse rate above 100 beats per minute

bradycardia: a pulse rate below 60 beats per minute

The rhythm of the pulse is described as *regular* or *irregular*. Quality indicates the strength of the pulse, and is noted as weak, strong, **thready** (weak and rapid), or **bounding** (unusually strong). When noting the pulse on the medical record or designated form, be sure to indicate the rate, regularity, and the strength or quality of the rhythm. Follow the procedural requirements for your healthcare facility.

You must be familiar with the age-specific pulse rates in order to recognize abnormalities. To be an asset to the healthcare team, you must be accurate in obtaining vital signs and be able to recognize atypical values.

Measuring a Radial Pulse

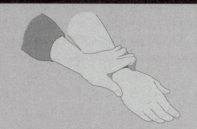

Materials needed:

✓ a watch with a second hand
✓ gloves (if blood or other body fluids are present)

1. Procedural Step: Wash your hands.
   Reason: Standard Precaution.

2. Procedural Step: Put on gloves if there is any blood or other body fluid present.
   Reason: Standard Precaution.

3. Procedural Step: Identify the patient by his or her identification bracelet.
   Reason: To make sure you are working with the correct patient.

4. Procedural Step: Have the patient sit, stand, or lie down, according to his or her medical condition. If he or she has recently changed position, wait a few minutes before taking the pulse.
   Reason: This allows the heart rate to adjust to the patient's shift in position.

5. Procedural Step: Tell the patient what you are going to do using terms he or she will understand.
   Reason: This keeps the patient calm and provides the patient with necessary information to give informed consent.

6. Procedural Step: Place the palm of the hand downward. If the patient is lying down, rest his or her forearm across the chest.
   Reason: This position will help you count the patient's respirations.

7. Procedural Step: Place the pads of your first two fingers directly over the **radial artery**. Apply slight pressure.
   Reason: The fingertips are sensitive and can feel the pulse, located on the inside of the wrist on the thumb side.

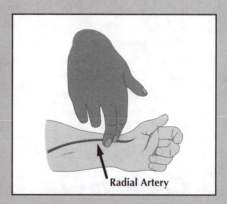

Radial Artery

8. Procedural Step: Feel for the pulsations as the heart beats. Don't push too hard.
   Reason: You could stop the blood flow and stop the pulse.

Measuring a Radial Pulse (Cont.)

9. Procedural Step: Look at the second hand on your watch and begin counting. Ideally, the pulse should be counted for 1 full minute; however, if the pulse is regular it is acceptable to count for 30 seconds and multiply the number by 2.
Reason: This will give you the rate per minute quickly. The pulse rate is charted as the rate per minute.

10. Procedural Step: If the rhythm is irregular, then count it for a full minute.
Reason: It is possible to miss some heartbeats by not counting an irregular pulse for a full minute.

11. Procedural Step: When measuring a pulse rate, note the RHYTHM and QUALITY of the beat as well.
Reason: Rhythm refers to whether the pulse is regular (doesn't change) or irregular (speeds up and/or slows down). Quality refers to the strength of the pulse. A weak, thready pulse may indicate **shock***, while a full bounding (strong) pulse could indicate high blood pressure.*

12. Procedural Step: Remove and discard your gloves.
Reason: Standard Precaution.

13. Procedural Step: Wash your hands before providing care to another patient.
Reason: Standard Precaution.

14. Procedural Step: Record the rate, rhythm, and quality of the pulse in the designated place on the proper form.
Reason: To provide documentation.

15. Procedural Step: Immediately report any abnormalities to your supervisor.
Reason: An abnormality may indicate a health problem.

Chart it like this: **P=80, R/S** (regular & strong)

or **P=116, irreg/thready** (irregular, thready)

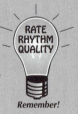

Note: Although the radial artery is the most common place for measuring the pulse rate, a pulse can be measured anywhere the pulsations of an artery can be felt.

Measuring an Apical Pulse

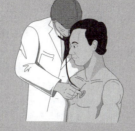

Materials needed:
- ✓ a stethoscope
- ✓ a watch with a second hand
- ✓ gloves (if blood or other body fluids are present)
- ✓ alcohol sponges

1. Procedural Step: Wash your hands.
   Reason: Standard Precaution.

2. Procedural Step: Clean the earpieces of the stethoscope with an alcohol sponge before using it.
   Reason: To protect against possible infection.

3. Procedural Step: Put on gloves if there is any blood or other body fluid present.
   Reason: Standard Precaution.

4. Procedural Step: Identify the patient by his or her identification bracelet.
   Reason: To ensure you are working with the correct patient.

5. Procedural Step: Tell the patient what you are going to do using terms he or she will under-stand. (ie, "I am going to listen to your heart," tells the patient exactly what is going to happen.)
   Reason: This keeps the patient calm and provides the information necessary for the patient to give informed consent.

6. Procedural Step: Close the curtains around the bed or close the door to the patient unit.
   Reason: To protect the patient's privacy.

7. Procedural Step: Carefully expose the left breast of the patient. Be careful not to expose more of the patient's chest than necessary.
   Reason: To protect the patient's privacy.

8. Procedural Step: The **apical** pulse can be heard with a stethoscope placed over the **apex** of the heart. It is located at the left fifth intercostal space, mid-clavicular line.
   Reason: This is the best location to hear the heartbeat.

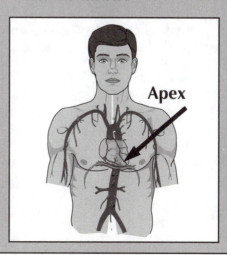

Apex

Measuring an Apical Pulse (Cont.)

diaphragm:
the portion of the stethoscope that is used for picking up sound

9. <u>Procedural Step:</u> Place the tips of the stethoscope in your ears with the tips pointing slightly forward, and place the **diaphragm** of the stethoscope directly below the left nipple or, if the patient is a woman, under the left breast (apex of the heart).
<u>Reason:</u> *The forward position of the earpieces will make it easier to hear because they will be following the direction of the ear canal. The tubes should be hanging freely so extraneous sounds won't be heard. This is where the apical pulse is located.*

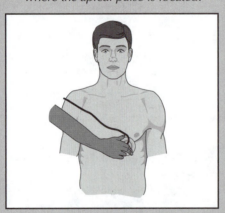

10. <u>Procedural Step:</u> Move the diaphragm until you hear the loudest heart sounds or **PMI** (point of maximal impulse). Listen for the sound of the heartbeat, *lubb-dubb*. Count each lubb-dubb as one beat. Count the apical pulse for a full minute.
<u>Reason:</u> *The apical pulse is measured when it is difficult to feel a pulse, when there is an irregular pulse, when the patient has a heart condition, or when it's ordered by the physician.*

PMI:
the abbreviation for point of maximal impulse

11. <u>Procedural Step:</u> Clean the earpieces and the diaphragm of the stethoscope with an alcohol sponge.
<u>Reason:</u> *The equipment will be ready for the next time.*

12. <u>Procedural Step:</u> After covering your patient, open the patient unit.
<u>Reason:</u> *You have obtained the pulse rate.*

13. <u>Procedural Step:</u> Remove and discard your gloves.
<u>Reason:</u> *Standard Precaution.*

14. <u>Procedural Step:</u> Wash your hands before providing care to another patient.
<u>Reason:</u> *Standard Precaution.*

15. <u>Procedural Step:</u> Record the rate, rhythm, and quality of the pulse in the designated place on the proper form.
<u>Reason:</u> *To provide documentation.*

16. <u>Procedural Step:</u> Immediately report any abnormalities to your supervisor.
<u>Reason:</u> *An abnormality may indicate a health problem.*

Chart it like this: **P=88** (AP) **R/S** (regular and strong).

Respiration

The respiratory rate provides valuable information that cannot be obtained from the temperature and pulse rates. The actual act of **respiration**, or breathing, occurs **spontaneously**, or without assistance. The breathing process begins when the level of carbon dioxide in the blood becomes higher than normal. This sends a signal to the respiratory center in the brain stem for inspiration to occur. **Inspiration** is the act of breathing in oxygen. There are two phases of respiration: internal and external. External respiration refers to the exchange of carbon dioxide and oxygen between the atmospheric air and that of the pulmonary capillaries (tiny vessels in the lungs). This is known as the **gas exchange**. Internal respiration refers to the exchange of oxygen and carbon dioxide between the peripheral capillaries and tissue cells. This is how the body's cells, tissues, and organs receive oxygen and eliminate carbon dioxide. The body eliminates carbon dioxide, a waste product, during **expiration**. Inspiration is an active motion, in which the diaphragm flattens and the intercostal muscles (those between the ribs) contract, raising the ribs. Expiration is a passive motion in which the diaphragm relaxes (returns to its original dome shape) as do the intercostal muscles, thereby decreasing the size of and amount of air in the lungs. One inspiration and one expiration forms one complete **respiratory cycle**. A respiratory cycle counts as one complete respiration, or one breath.

respiration: breathing; the process of bringing oxygen into the body and expelling carbon dioxide from the body

The rate of a patient's respirations provides the primary caregiver with vital information. The rate and depth of the respirations is centrally controlled in the brain and from voluntary and involuntary muscles. This is important to remember when counting respirations. Use the following general guidelines for the normal resting rates of respiration.

- premature infants (babies born before being carried in the uterus for 40 weeks): 40 to 90 breaths per minute.

- newborn infants (babies less than 4 weeks old): 30 to 50 breaths per minute.

- 4 weeks to 12 months old: 20 to 40 breaths per minute.

- 2 to 5 years old: 20 to 30 breaths per minute.

- 5 to 15 years old: 20 to 25 breaths per minute.

- 15 years and older: 15 to 20 breaths per minute.

The more you practice measuring respiratory rates, the more confident and accurate you will become. Practice will provide you with more experience in recognizing abnormal rates.

When measuring a patient's respirations, observing the pattern of the respirations must become routine. Some respiratory patterns are listed below.

- **abdominal:** respirations using primarily the abdominal muscles while the chest is mostly still.

- **apnea:** the temporary cessation of breathing.

- **bradypnea:** breathing that is abnormally slow.

- **Cheyne-Stokes respiration:** a grossly irregular breathing pattern composed of a period of apnea lasting from 10-60 seconds followed by respirations that gradually increase in frequency and depth.

- **decreased:** very little air movement in the lungs.

- **dyspnea:** difficult or painful breathing; shortness of breath.

- **hyperpnea:** breathing that is faster or deeper than that which is produced during normal activity.

- **Kussmaul's breathing:** deep, gasping respirations; *air hunger.* (Seen in serious diabetic acidosis and in comatose patients.)

- **labored breathing:** difficult breathing that uses shoulder muscles, neck muscles, and abdominal muscles (accessory muscles).

- **stertorous:** labored breathing in which snoring, rattling and/or bubbling sounds are heard.

- **tachypnea:** abnormally rapid breathing.

There are many types of medical conditions that will affect respiratory patterns. Different disease processes (eg, diabetes, kidney abnormalities, and lung diseases), cerebrovascular accidents (strokes), and emotions such as anxiety and fear can alter respirations. **Trauma** incidents such as head injuries, gunshot wounds, traffic accidents, diving accidents, or drownings also may affect the respiratory center in the brain.

trauma:
physical or psychological injury caused by an accident, violence, or a poisonous substance

The patient should not know that you are counting his or her respiratory rate. Although the breathing process is mostly spontaneous, people also use voluntary muscles to breathe. If the patient is aware that his or her respiratory rate is being calculated, self-consciousness may alter the true rate. Do not tell the patient when you will be monitoring the respiratory rate. You can do this procedure without the patient's knowledge by observing and counting the patient's respirations after you have completed taking the pulse.

Measuring Respiration

Materials needed:

✓ a watch with a second hand
✓ a stethoscope (if done following measurement of the apical pulse)
✓ gloves (if blood or other body fluids are present)

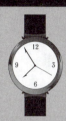

1. Procedural Step: Measure the respiration after obtaining the patient's pulse.
   Reason: To prevent the patient from knowing when his or her breathing is being counted.

2. Procedural Step: Wash your hands.
   Reason: Standard Precaution.

3. Procedural Step: Wear gloves if any blood or other body fluid is present.
   Reason: Standard Precaution.

4. Procedural Step: Identify the patient by his or her identification bracelet.
   Reason: To make sure you are working with the correct patient.
   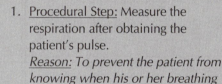

5. Procedural Step: Do not tell the patient when you will be monitoring the respiratory rate.
   Reason: This could alter the results.

6. Procedural Step: If you measured the radial pulse, keep the patient's arm across the chest and count one inspiration and one expiration as one breath. Breathe with the patient.

Reason: Having the patient's arm in this position will make it easier to detect the rise and fall of the patient's chest. Breathing with the patient helps you concentrate on the rise and fall of the chest.

7. Procedural Step: Count the rate for 30 seconds and multiply that number by two. This final value will be the number of breaths per minute (ie, if you count eight full respirations in 30 seconds, multiply 8 x 2 = 16 breaths per minute).
   Reason: Respiration is documented as the rate per minute.

8. Procedural Step: Remove your gloves.
   Reason: Standard Precaution.

9. Procedural Step: Wash your hands.
   Reason: Standard Precaution.

10. Procedural Step: Record the results on the patient's chart.
    Reason: To provide documentation.

11. Procedural Step: If you detect any difficulty in breathing, note it on the patient's chart after the rate, and report it to your supervisor.
    Reason: Difficulty in breathing indicates a health problem.

Measuring Respiration (Cont.)

Chart it like this:

R=16, labored

Note: If you are taking an apical pulse, keep the stethoscope in place on the chest and observe the rise and fall of the chest. Count the respirations in the manner described above.

A patient whose breathing is labored usually will sit up and lean forward in an effort to breathe easier. The first signs of oxygen deprivation are mental confusion, restlessness, and anxiety. A person who is experiencing dyspnea must be seen immediately by the physician.

Normal breathing should be quiet and effortless. Noisy respirations indicate an obstruction in the respiratory tract. Snoring sounds signal an upper airway obstruction and the position of the airway should be checked. If the patient has a lot of secretions, immediate suctioning may be needed. **Crackles** or **gurgling** may indicate fluid in the air passages. **Stridor** is a high-pitched noise, like a squeak, and occurs from upper airway obstruction, usually laryngeal edema. Narrowing of the airways also can produce a **wheeze** such as that heard in patients with asthma. To listen for sounds within the lungs, use the following procedure.

Listening for Lung Sounds

Materials needed:

✓ a stethoscope
✓ gloves (if blood or other body fluids are present)
✓ alcohol sponges

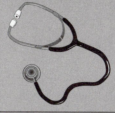

1. Procedural Step: Wash your hands.
   Reason: Standard Precaution.

2. Procedural Step: Clean the earpieces of the stethoscope with an alcohol sponge before using it.
   Reason: To protect against possible infection.

3. Procedural Step: Put on gloves if any blood or other body fluid is present.
   Reason: Standard Precaution.

4. Procedural Step: Identify the patient by his or her identification bracelet.
   Reason: To make sure you are working with the correct patient.

5. Procedural Step: Tell the patient what to expect using terms he or she can understand.
   Reason: This keeps the patient calm and provides information necessary for the patient to give consent.

6. Procedural Step: Place the earpieces of the stethoscope in your ears with the tips pointing slightly forward. Avoid letting the tubes rub together.

Reason: The forward position of the earpieces will make it easier to hear because they will be following the direction of the ear canal. The tubes should be hanging freely so extraneous sounds won't be heard.

7. Procedural Step: Place the stethoscope over the patient's chest. (See illustration for positions.) Move from points 1 through 5 on the anterior chest and repeat on the posterior chest.
   Reason: To listen for lung sounds.

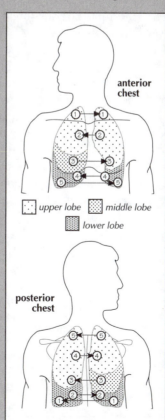

anterior chest

:::: upper lobe   ▨ middle lobe

▉ lower lobe

posterior chest

Listening for Lung Sounds (Cont.)

8. Procedural Step: Listen for air entering the lungs and for abnormal sounds.
   Reason: Normal breathing is quiet.

9. Procedural Step: Ask the patient to breathe deeply through the mouth while you listen to the chest.
   Reason: It amplifies the chest sounds.

10. Procedural Step: Listen for abnormal sounds. Crackles sound similar to the sounds made by rolling a few strands of hair next to your ear.
    Reason: Crackles indicate fluid in the **alveoli** of the lungs. If the lungs are full of fluid, as in **pulmonary edema**, the sounds can be heard without a stethoscope.

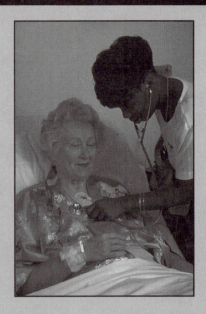

11. Procedural Step: Always compare the right and left sides of the chest as well as the front and back sounds.
    Reason: To detect differences in the sounds that are being made.

12. Procedural Step: Identify the area from which the sounds are coming.
    Reason: To help locate the problem.

13. Procedural Step: Count the number of breaths for 1 full minute.
    Reason: Respirations are recorded by the number of breaths per minute.

14. Procedural Step: Clean the earpieces and the diaphragm of the stethoscope with an alcohol sponge.
    Reason: The equipment will be ready for use the next time.

15. Procedural Step: Remove your gloves.
    Reason: Standard Precaution.

16. Procedural Step: Wash your hands.
    Reason: Standard Precaution.

17. Procedural Step: Record your findings on the patient's chart.
    Reason: To provide documentation.

Chart it like this:

Lungs clear, bilateral or, **Wheezes, left anterior lower lobe**

Blood Pressure

Blood pressure, like the previous vital signs, is a source of important information for the primary healthcare provider. **Blood pressure** is a measurement of the pressure of the blood exerted against the walls of the arteries. The measurement consists of two numbers; for example, 120/80. The top number is known as the **systolic** reading and refers to the contraction of the heart. The bottom number is the **diastolic** reading and refers to the relaxation of the heart.

Obtaining an accurate blood pressure is dependent on several factors: proper size of the blood pressure cuff (**sphygmomanometer**); movement and cooperation of the patient; lack of excessive noise and distractions; the emotional state of the patient; disease processes; trauma; and a properly working sphygmomanometer and stethoscope.

To get a proper reading, the width of the blood pressure cuff should cover approximately ³/₄ the size of the patient's upper arm. A false high reading can be obtained if the cuff is too narrow, and a false low reading can be obtained if the cuff is too wide. Pediatric and infant cuffs are available for children and infants.

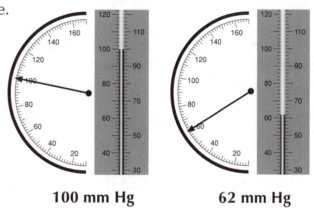

100 mm Hg   **62 mm Hg**

Figure 10-2: Examples of Sphygmomanometer Readings

There are many factors that may affect a patient's blood pressure. For example, **hypertension** (**HTN**) is a common disease. It is known as *the silent killer* because people often do not have any symptoms of the disease, and therefore, do not know they have it. Hypertension often manifests itself in the form of headaches, excessive fatigue, general weakness, visual disturbances such as double or blurred vision, dizziness, or cerebrovascular accidents. The diagnosis of hypertension is often made after at least three separate blood pressure measurements obtained at different times of the day indicate systolic readings of 140 or greater, and diastolic readings of 90 or greater. NEVER TELL THE PATIENT HE OR SHE HAS HYPERTENSION! Instead, ask the patient what his or her normal blood pressure is. Telling a patient he or she has hypertension can increase the blood pressure. If you obtain an abnormal reading, wait 1 to 2 minutes and retake the blood pressure. It also should be measured in the other arm. Notify your supervisor of any abnormally high or low measurements.

blood pressure: the pressure of the blood exerted against the arteries

systolic: the top number in a blood pressure reading; refers to the time between the first and second heart sounds in which the heart contracts

diastolic: the bottom number in a blood pressure reading; refers to the period of time between heart contractions in which the heart relaxes

hypertension (HTN): high blood pressure that has been diagnosed on the basis of several random readings of 140/90 or higher; known as *the silent killer*

Accurate measurement of a blood pressure requires practice. The values are measured in millimeters of mercury, abbreviated as *mm Hg*. There are three main types of blood pressure sphygmomanometers. The mercury sphygmomanometer contains a large column of mercury (Hg). Each separate mark on the gauge, or manometer, represents 2 mm Hg. The aneroid sphygmomanometer does not contain a mercury column; it involves only a needle dial in which each line represents 2 mm Hg pressure. The third type is an electronic cuff. The cuff is placed on the patient's extremity; and an electronic machine (computer) will calculate the blood pressure. Make sure you are familiar with the proper operation of the machine before attempting to use it. All of the above methods are termed **noninvasive blood pressure** (**NIBP**). This means it is an external procedure. The Emergency Department and the Critical Care Units frequently insert special devices that obtain blood pressure readings inside the blood vessels. These measurements are **invasive blood pressure** (**IBP**) readings.

Noninvasive blood pressure measurement is recommended for obtaining a blood pressure reading on children and adults. Blood pressure readings for newborns and infants require special instruction; therefore, do not attempt to obtain a blood pressure on an infant without proper training.

There are many different factors that can affect blood pressure measurements:

- emotions (anger, fear)
- medications (prescribed or illegal)
- diet and weight
- stress (hospitalization, death, divorce, etc.)
- the patient's position

Documenting the position of the patient while taking the blood pressure provides the nurse and physician with important information about the patient's health status. Normal blood pressure measurements are expected to be the lowest when in the lying (supine) position. In that position, the blood vessels are relaxed and **vasodilated**, and the heart and blood flow are not working against gravity. The next highest reading would occur while the patient is sitting, because the heart has to work harder to compensate for areas of the body in which the blood is flowing against gravity. Similarly, due to the affect of gravity on the flow of blood, the highest number occurs when the patient is standing. A ten point change in the reading between the different positions in a healthy patient is the normal variant.

Learning the normal limits of blood pressure will take time, but the ability to recognize changes in your patient's blood pressure values is an important part of your patient assessment skills.

Taking a Palpated Systolic Blood Pressure

Materials needed:

✓ a sphygmomanometer (in the proper size for the patient)

✓ gloves (if blood or other body fluids are present)

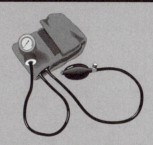

1. <u>Procedural Step:</u> Wash your hands and assemble the equipment. *Reason: Standard Precaution.*

2. <u>Procedural Step:</u> Put on gloves if there is any blood or other body fluid present. *Reason: Standard Precaution.*

3. <u>Procedural Step:</u> Identify the patient. *Reason: This confirms that you are assessing the correct patient.*

4. <u>Procedural Step:</u> Explain the procedure to the patient using terms he or she will understand. *Reason: This keeps the patient calm and provides the information necessary for the patient to give informed consent.*

5. <u>Procedural Step:</u> Have the patient sit or lie down. Roll the patient's sleeve about 6 inches above the elbow. If the sleeve is too tight, remove the arm from the sleeve. Extend the arm, palm up, at heart level.

Reason: A sleeve that is too tight may compress the brachial artery and distort the results. If the arm is above heart level the reading may be incorrectly low.

6. <u>Procedural Step:</u> Palpate the brachial artery, located on the inner aspect of the elbow on the patient's little finger side. Then place the blood pressure cuff smoothly and securely around the patient's arm about 2 inches above the bend in the elbow. Be sure the middle of the cloth-enclosed cuff is directly over the brachial artery. If the cuff has an arrow to indicate right or left arm, the arrow should be placed over the brachial artery.

Reason: The cuff should be tight enough to stay on, but not so tight as to be constricting. It should be high enough so that you can easily palpate the brachial artery, and if you will be auscultating the blood pressure after palpating it, the stethoscope will not touch the cuff and cause extraneous sounds. By placing the center of the bladder of the cuff over the brachial artery you assure that the pressure is applied equally over the artery.

Taking a Palpated Systolic Blood Pressure (Cont.)

7. Procedural Step: Place two fingers of your nondominant hand over the patient's radial artery, which is located on the inside of the wrist on the thumb side. Do not use your own thumb to feel for the pulse.
Reason: The thumb has a pulse of its own that could be mistaken for the patient's pulse.

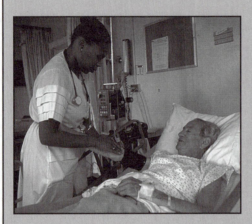

8. Procedural Step: Hold the rubber bulb of the blood pressure cuff in your dominant hand with your palm upward and the knob of the control valve pointing toward your thumb. Continue to palpate the radial pulse while you turn the control valve away from you using your thumb.
Reason: This will close the valve.

9. Procedural Step: Rapidly squeeze the bulb to pump air into the blood pressure cuff. Note on the calibrated scale of the sphygmomanometer the point at which the radial pulse cannot be felt.

10. Procedural Step: Do not pause. Continue to pump air into the blood pressure cuff to a level of 20 to 30 mm Hg above the point where the radial pulse disappeared.

11. Procedural Step: Immediately begin to release the air in the cuff by slowly and steadily turning the knob of the control valve toward you with your thumb.

12. Procedural Step: Note the point on the calibrated scale when you once again feel the pulse.
Reason: This is the palpated systolic pressure.

13. Procedural Step: Now you may rapidly deflate the cuff. Remember, you cannot obtain a diastolic blood pressure using the palpation method.
Reason: The diastolic blood pressure cannot be felt.

14. Procedural Step: If you are now going to take an auscultated blood pressure, wait at least 1 minute before inflating the cuff again.
Reason: To reduce the congestion of the blood vessels which can result in incorrect results.

15. Procedural Step: If you are not going to take an auscultated blood pressure, remove the cuff and proceed to steps 16, 17, and 18.

Taking a Palpated Systolic Blood Pressure (Cont.)

16. Procedural Step: Remove your gloves if it was necessary to put them on. *Reason: Standard Precaution.*

18. Procedural Step: Record the results on the patient's chart. *Reason: To provide documentation.*

17. Procedural Step: Wash your hands before providing care to another patient. *Reason: Standard Precaution.*

Chart it like this, indicating which arm was used and whether the patient was sitting or lying down: **BP=70/ palpated RA, sitting** meaning the blood pressure was taken on the right arm, and a systolic blood pressure of 70 was palpated.

After **palpating** the systolic pressure, you are ready to take an **auscultated** blood pressure. Both a systolic blood pressure reading and a diastolic blood pressure reading can be obtained by the auscultation method. To do this, use the procedure on the next page.

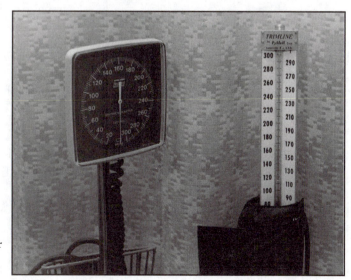

Figure 10-3: Types of Sphygmomanometers

Auscultating a Blood Pressure

Materials needed:
✓ a stethoscope
✓ a sphygmomanometer (in the proper size for the patient)
✓ alcohol sponges
✓ gloves (if blood or other body fluids are present)

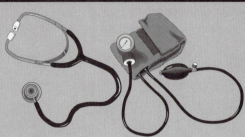

1. Procedural Step: Wash your hands and assemble the equipment.
   Reason: Standard Precaution.

2. Procedural Step: Clean the earpieces of the stethoscope with an alcohol sponge before using it.
   Reason: To protect against possible infection.

3. Procedural Step: Put on gloves if there is any blood or other body fluid present.
   Reason: Standard Precaution.

4. Procedural Step: Identify the patient.
   Reason: This confirms that you are assessing the correct patient.

5. Procedural Step: Explain the procedure to the patient using terms he or she will understand.
   Reason: This keeps the patient calm and provides the information necessary for the patient to give informed consent.

6. Procedural Step: Wait 1 minute after taking a palpated blood pressure before inflating the cuff again.
   Reason: To reduce the congestion of the blood vessels which can result in incorrect results.

7. Procedural Step: Place the earpieces of the stethoscope in your ears with the tips pointing slightly forward. Avoid letting the tubes rub together.
   Reason: The forward position of the earpieces will make it easier to hear because they will be following the direction of the ear canal. The tubes should be hanging freely so extraneous sounds won't be heard.

8. Procedural Step: Palpate the pulse at the brachial artery. Place the diaphragm of the stethoscope firmly over the point of maximal impulse (PMI).
   Reason: Proper placement of the diaphragm will help you hear the sounds of the blood pressure.

9. Procedural Step: Hold the diaphragm in place with your nondominant hand, close the control valve and quickly squeeze the bulb with your dominant hand to a level of 20 or 30 mm Hg above the point at which you palpated the systolic blood pressure.
   Reason: The range of 20 to 30 mm Hg is sufficient to be sure you have pumped the cuff high enough to accurately hear the systolic pressure. Inflating the rubber bladder in the cuff stops the flow of blood in the artery. The cuff is inflated quickly and smoothly to avoid congestion in the blood vessels.

Auscultating a Blood Pressure (Cont.)

10. Procedural Step: Slowly and steadily open the control valve at a rate of approximately 2 to 3 mm Hg per heartbeat. This will release the air in the cuff. Listen for the first clear, tapping sound. This is the systolic pressure. Notice the reading on the calibrated scale.
Reason: The systolic blood pressure represents the pressure against the walls of the arteries when the ventricles of the heart contract and blood surges through the aorta and pulmonary arteries.

11. Procedural Step: Continue to steadily deflate the cuff until the last sound is heard. This is the diastolic pressure.
Reason: The diastolic pressure refers to the point at which there is the least pressure in the arteries and occurs when the heart relaxes (diastole) before the next contraction (systole).

12. Procedural Step: Quickly release the rest of the air from the cuff and remove the cuff from the patient's arm. (Or leave the deflated cuff in place if frequent blood pressure readings are to be done.)
Reason: If left inflated, it will prevent circulation to the hand and arm.

13. Procedural Step: Immediately record the measurements obtained as a fraction, noting the time, arm used (right or left), and the patient's position (lying, sitting, or standing).
Reason: Charting immediately will ensure accuracy.

14. Procedural Step: Clean the earpieces and the diaphragm of the stethoscope with an alcohol sponge.
Reason: The equipment will be ready for use the next time.

15. Procedural Step: Remove your gloves if it was necessary to put them on.
Reason: Standard Precaution.

16. Procedural Step: Wash your hands before providing care to another patient.
Reason: Standard Precaution.

Chart it like this, indicating which arm was used and whether the patient was sitting or lying down: **BP=160/90 RA, sitting** meaning the blood pressure was 160 mm Hg systolic and 90 mm Hg diastolic, and the reading was taken on the right arm with the patient in a sitting position.

Note: When listening for the diastolic pressure, you will notice a change in the quality of the sounds before they completely disappear. Some physicians consider this change to be the first diastolic blood pressure. If you are asked to record this sound, chart it as follows: B/P 180/100/90. This would mean that the first sound you heard was 180 (systolic blood pressure), a change or muffled sound was noted at 100 (first diastolic sound), and the last sound you heard was at 90 (final diastolic pressure).

Continuous Monitoring of Blood Pressure Automatically

Automatic continuous blood pressure monitoring is common practice in the Emergency Department. There are less errors using the automated method than with the traditional method because it is done by a machine. This method also is convenient and is easily used by all medical staff. One type of monitor has the capability of monitoring not only the blood pressure, but also of continuous monitoring of an electrocardiograph tracing, heart rate, and the pulse oximetry, or oxygen level of the blood. Always observe the equipment carefully and alert the nursing staff to changes in the system or any alarms you hear.

As a prudent healthcare worker, you must be able to recognize situations in which blood pressure readings from a machine are not consistent with the patient's signs and/or symptoms. Always manually verify an abnormal blood pressure reading. Remember, assess the patient, not the machine!

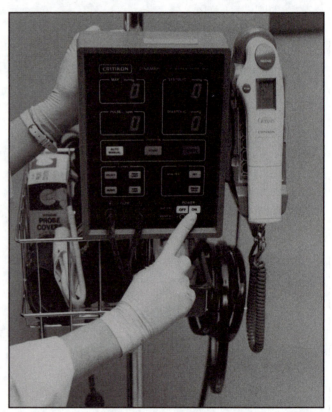

Figure 10-4: Automatic monitoring of the blood pressure is possible with an automatic sphygmomanometer.

Continuous Monitoring of Blood Pressure Automatically

Materials needed:

✓ an automated blood pressure monitoring device
✓ an automatic blood pressure cuff
✓ an electrical outlet
✓ gloves (if blood or other body fluids are present)

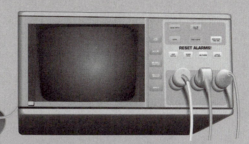

1. Procedural Step: Wash your hands.
   Reason: Standard Precaution.

2. Procedural Step: Put on gloves if there is any blood or other body fluid present.
   Reason: Standard Precaution.

3. Procedural Step: Identify the patient.
   Reason: This confirms that you are assessing the correct patient.

4. Procedural Step: Explain the procedure to the patient using terms he or she will understand.
   Reason: This keeps the patient calm and provides the information necessary for the patient to give informed consent.

5. Procedural Step: Connect the tubing to the monitor and the cuff.
   Reason: Air tubing must be connected to the monitor to obtain a blood pressure reading.

6. Procedural Step: Make sure the cuff is deflated.
   Reason: This will ensure an accurate reading.

7. Procedural Step: Apply the automatic blood pressure cuff to the patient. Make sure it is the correct size and that it fits the patient properly.
   Reason: Proper fit and placement of the cuff is essential for correct measurement.

8. Procedural Step: Press the power ON button located on the front of the monitor.
   Reason: The machine must be turned on in order for it to work. The digital display will light up when it is receiving power.

9. Procedural Step: Select the AUTO or MANUAL mode.
   Reason: For a one-time reading, use the manual setting. For frequent readings at specified intervals (from 1 to 60 minutes) select the automatic setting.

Continuous Monitoring
of Blood Pressure Automatically (Cont.)

10. Procedural Step: To change the time interval between readings, press the appropriate button (according to the manufacturer's instructions) and enter the desired amount of time between readings.
    Reason: The physician may decide that less frequent readings are appropriate. Machines vary from model to model, so you will need to study the manufacturer's manual to learn which button to use for setting the time interval.

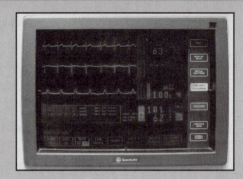

11. Procedural Step: Set the alarms for the high and low limits of blood pressure according to the manufacturer's instructions.
    Reason: The alarms will alert the medical staff to a sudden, critical change in the blood pressure.

12. Procedural Step: To read the blood pressure look at the display.
    Reason: The display will indicate the blood pressure and the time it was obtained.

13. Procedural Step: Remove your gloves if it was necessary to put them on.
    Reason: Standard Precaution.

14. Procedural Step: Wash your hands.
    Reason: Standard Precaution.

15. Procedural Step: Record the results of each reading on the patient's chart according to the physician's orders.
    Reason: For documentation.

Chart it like this, indicating which arm was used and whether the patient was sitting or lying down:

8:00 a.m. BP=160/90 RA, lying down
8:30 a.m. BP=160/90 RA, lying down
9:00 a.m. BP=160/90 RA, lying down

Weight and Height

In addition to assessing vital signs, you may be required to obtain the weight and height of a patient. Both of these measurements give the primary healthcare provider important information. If a patient is on a special medical diet, then weight becomes important. Some medications a patient may be taking can influence either a weight gain or a loss. For example, patients with certain heart conditions may be given a medication to help them eliminate excess fluid. Others may be undergoing treatment for life-threatening eating disorders. So it will be important to monitor a patient in these situations. Moreover, infants and children sometimes have diseases that do not allow them to grow. You can see why nurses and physicians rely on accurate measurements!

Children 2 years and older can also be weighed on the adult scale. Infants and children younger than 2 years old must be weighed using a baby scale that has ounces. If the child is uncooperative, have one of the parents hold the child and step on the scale. Record this weight. Have the parent put the child down and step back up on the scale. Record this weight. Subtract the second weight from the first weight and this will give you the approximate weight of the child. Infants should be undressed, including the diaper, and placed on their back on the scale. Be sure to record the weight on the patient's chart.

An infant's length is recorded using a cloth measuring tape. The length is measured from the top of the infant's head to the heel. Accurately record the length.

For adult patients, it may be facility policy to convert the weight from pounds (lbs) to kilograms (kg). Kilograms are part of the metric system that is universally used in the medical field. To do this, divide the weight by 2.2. For example:

$$150 \text{ lbs} \div 2.2 = 68.18 \text{ kg}$$

The scale used in hospitals often contains a sliding device that is attached to the scale used for determining height. Use the guidelines on the following pages for measuring an adult patient's weight and height.

Measuring the Weight of an Adult

Materials needed:

✓ a scale with a
measuring device

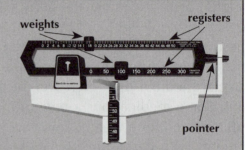

weights · registers · pointer

---

1. Procedural Step: Identify the patient.
   Reason: To confirm that you are assessing the correct patient.

2. Procedural Step: Ask the patient if he or she knows his or her correct weight.
   Reason: This will assist you in setting the weight on the scale in the general area; it also avoids embarrassment if you judge the patient to weigh more than he or she actually does.

3. Procedural Step: Ask the patient to remove any heavy outer wear such as coats and sweaters. If the patient wishes, shoes may be removed too.
   Reason: Clothing and footwear can add 3-6 lbs.

4. Procedural Step: Make sure both the weights on the scale are pushed completely to the left. They should be at the zero position.
   Reason: To prevent an inaccurate reading.

5. Procedural Step: If the patient is barefoot, place a paper on the scale for him or her to stand on.
   Reason: Aseptic technique.

6. Procedural Step: Inform the patient the scale may move and assist him or her onto the scale by gently taking an arm for extra support.
   Reason: To prevent the patient from falling.

7. Procedural Step: Always be ready to physically assist the patient. Constantly watch for any unsteadiness.
   Reason: To prevent a fall if the patient loses his or her balance.

8. Procedural Step: Instruct the patient to stand still, with arms at sides. The patient should not hold on to any part of the scale or on to you.
   Reason: If the patient touches you, the scale, or anything else, some of his or her weight will be displaced, causing an inaccurate reading.

9. Procedural Step: The bottom weight on the scale marks increments of 50 lbs. Slide this weight to the mark (50, 100, 150, or 200) that is closest to, but not over, the patient's stated weight. Make sure the weight rests securely in the incremental groove on the register.
   Reason: Unless this bottom weight is properly set, your measurement may be off by several pounds.

Measuring the Weight of an Adult

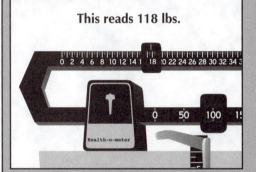

This reads 118 lbs.

Health-o-meter

10. <u>Procedural Step:</u> Gradually move the upper weight, which indicates individual pounds, across the upper register until the pointer on the right end of the set of registers rests in the center of the metal frame. The registers should not touch the sides of the frame.
<u>Reason:</u> *When the set of registers balances in the center of the metal frame, the scale is set to the patient's correct weight.*

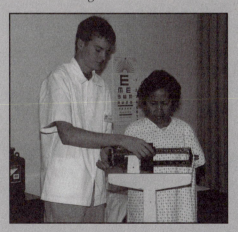

11. <u>Procedural Step:</u> Assist the patient from the scale.
<u>Reason:</u> *To prevent the patient from falling.*

12. <u>Procedural Step:</u> Return the weights to the *zero* setting.
<u>Reason:</u> *To prepare the scale for the next patient.*

13. <u>Procedural Step:</u> Record the patient's weight in kilograms or pounds to the nearest fraction of a pound and indicate whether the patient was weighed in a hospital gown or while wearing street clothes.
<u>Reason:</u> *To provide documentation. Street clothes are usually heavier than a hospital gown and may affect the physician's interpretation of the patient's weight.*

14. <u>Procedural Step:</u> Remove and discard the paper you placed on the scale.
<u>Reason:</u> *Aseptic technique.*

15. <u>Procedural Step:</u> Assist the patient back to bed.
<u>Reason:</u> *Patient safety.*

16. <u>Procedural Step:</u> Wash your hands before providing care to another patient.
<u>Reason:</u> *Standard Precaution.*

Chart it like this:

9:00 a.m. 45 kg, wearing hospital gown

Measuring the Height of an Adult

Materials needed:
✓ a scale with a measuring device

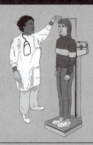

1. Procedural Step: Identify the patient.
   Reason: To confirm that you are assessing the correct patient.

2. Procedural Step: Have the patient step on the scale and face away from it.
   Reason: To obtain the most accurate measurement.

3. Procedural Step: With the hinged arm in the lowered position, raise the height bar above the patient's head.
   Reason: To prevent the arm from injuring the patient.

4. Procedural Step: Instruct the patient to look straight ahead.
   Reason: This will keep the top of the head level.

5. Procedural Step: Extend the hinged arm and gently slide the measuring bar down until it rests lightly on the patient's head.
   Reason: If done too quickly, the patient may be injured.

6. Procedural Step: Read the last digit or fraction of a digit that is visible on the moveable portion of the bar, just above the stationary portion.
   Reason: This is the patient's height.

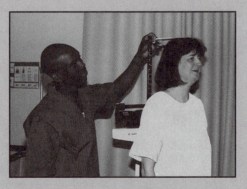

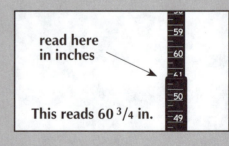

read here in inches

This reads 60 $^3/_4$ in.

7. Procedural Step: Record the patient's height in inches.
   Reason: To provide documentation.

Chart it like this:

9:00 a.m. 60 $^3/_4$ in.

Chapter Summary

The clinical healthcare worker is responsible for providing competent and quality patient care. One of the most basic and important skills is proper measurement and interpretation of vital signs. Although the nurse or physician is responsible for interpreting those values, the allied healthcare worker must learn to recognize changes.

The four basic vital signs include the patient's core temperature, pulse, respiratory rate, and noninvasive blood pressure (T, P, R, and BP). There are specific procedures for obtaining accurate measurements of each of these vital signs. Make sure you know what these procedures are, and practice them until you are confident that you can perform them quickly and accurately. Understanding the traumatic and medical conditions that can affect each vital sign also will help ensure the quality of the care you provide to your patients. Other fundamental skills include the measurement of the patient's height and weight. This information may provide important information about the patient's condition.

Name _____

Date _____

Student Enrichment Activities

Complete the following statements.

1. _____ _____ provide the healthcare worker with information concerning the health status of the body.

2. _____, _____, and _____ are methods of heat loss.

3. The maintenance of equilibrium within the body through internal and external functions is called _____.

4. The oral or rectal methods are preferred for measurements of the _____ _____.

5. The _____ temperature registers approximately 1° higher than the oral temperature.

6. The rhythmic throbbing caused by the regular contraction and expansion of an artery is the _____.

7. The blood flow supplied to the vital organs is the _____ circulation.

8. Gas exchange involves exchanging _____ _____ for _____.

9. The temporary cessation of breathing is _____.

10. A sphygmomanometer is used in taking a _____ blood pressure reading.

11. When charting the weight of an adult patient, pounds should be converted to

   _____.

12. Write this Fahrenheit thermometer reading in the blank below.

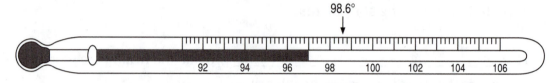

   _____

13. Write this Fahrenheit thermometer reading in the blank below.

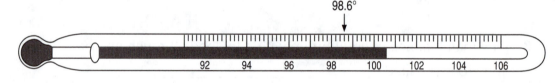

   _____

14. Draw a line to indicate where the mercury will end for a temperature of 103.2°F.

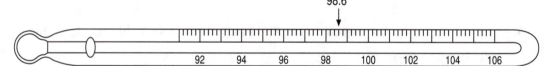

15. Write this Celsius thermometer reading in the blank below.

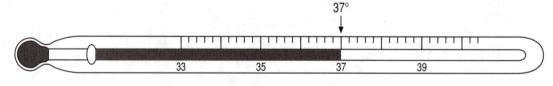

   _____

16. Write this Celsius thermometer reading in the blank below.

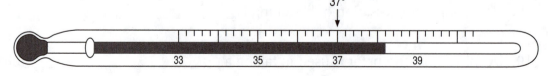

   _____

Name _____

Date _____

17. Draw a line to indicate where the mercury will end for a temperature of 39.4°C.

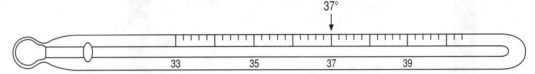

Write the sphygmomanometer readings in the spaces below.

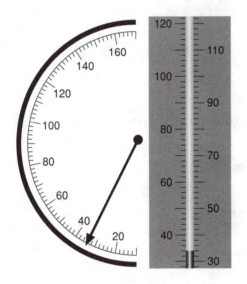

18. _____

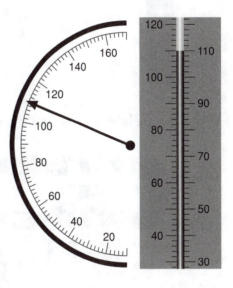

19. _____

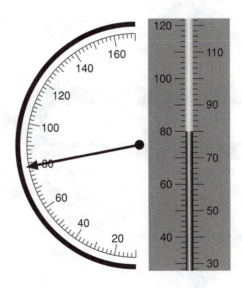

20. _____

Write the height measurements in the spaces below.

21. _____ in   **22.** _____ in

Write the weight measurements in pounds and kilograms in the spaces below.

23.
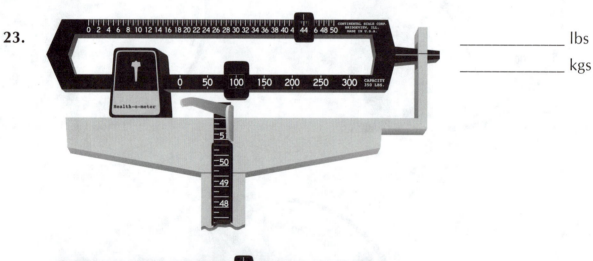
_____ lbs

_____ kgs

24.
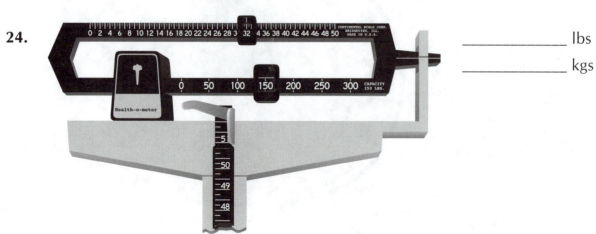
_____ lbs

_____ kgs

Name _____

Date _____

Unscramble the following terms.

25. PEAX   _____

26. ROADTIC   _____

27. AGS ECXNGHAE   _____ _____

28. TRIADANIO   _____

29. SUMALSKUS   _____

30. ERSIOPATIRN   _____

31. SCHOOPTESTE   _____

32. PYATHECAN   _____

33. RYDEATH   _____

34. NEVI   _____

35. YCNEHE KSOTSE   _____ _____

Chapter Eleven
Fundamental Patient Care Equipment

Objectives

After completing this chapter you should be able to
do the following:

1. Define and correctly spell each of the key terms.

2. List at least three basic ambulation devices.

3. Describe the universal method for identifying oxygen.

4. Explain the components of a urinary catheter.

5. Explain the procedure for using a patient lift.

6. List at least six items found on the crash cart.

7. Name three reasons why a patient may be in a private room.

8. List five items that can be found in a patient unit.

Key Terms

- activities of daily living
- ambulation
- bedside commode
- call light
- cardiopulmonary arrest
- cardiopulmonary resuscitation
- Code Blue
- crash cart
- eggcrate mattress

- gurney
- indwelling catheter
- intercom system
- IV infusion pump
- patient lift
- patient unit
- traction
- wheelchair

The Importance of Proper Equipment Identification and Operation

When you care for patients in the hospital you will see many different kinds of patient care equipment. In addition to equipment that aids in the treatment of patients, there are many items that are used to make the patient comfortable as well. As an allied healthcare worker you must be familiar with the basic hospital equipment you may be asked to use. Valuable time may be wasted if you are forced to search for an item with which you are not familiar. Furthermore, a patient's confidence in you may decrease if you must stop what you are doing to locate someone who knows how to operate the equipment. However, even though admitting uncertainty to a patient is difficult, it is even more undesirable to try to fake your way through a procedure. This can be dangerous! For your patients' safety as well as your own, NEVER use a piece of equipment without instruction! Instead, gain self-confidence and earn the trust of patients by learning the proper way to use equipment now and during your orientation.

Beds and Gurneys

A **gurney** is a stretcher, usually with an aluminum frame and wheels, that is used to transport patients. You will use them frequently if you work in a hospital, but rarely if you work in a doctor's office. Before using a gurney, be sure you understand how it locks and unlocks, how to raise and lower the siderails, how to adjust the head and feet, how to maneuver the IV poles, and how to steer it. Operating instructions for beds and gurneys vary from manufacturer to manufacturer. The patient's safety is your responsibility—KNOW YOUR EQUIPMENT!

Different kinds of patient beds are used throughout the hospital. Patients who have sustained full-body burns or spinal cord injuries usually will be placed on a special bed called a **Stryker frame**, or on a **circular double frame bed**. These beds can be rotated along the patient's long axis, allowing you to turn the patient over without his or her assistance. By rotating the patient, you can relieve the pressure on a particular area of the body. Be especially attentive to the needs of the patients on these beds. Their arms and legs are secured in place, making it impossible for the patient to do simple tasks such as scratching his or her nose.

gurney:
a stretcher with wheels used for transporting patients

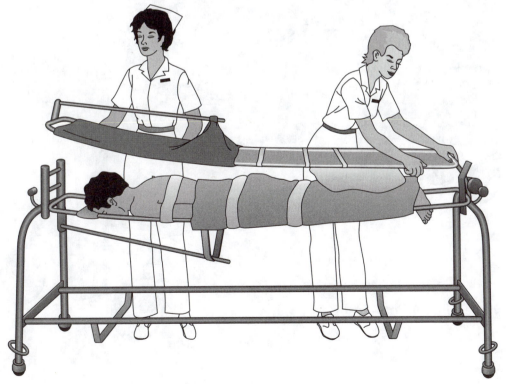

Figure 11-1: A Stryker Frame Bed

Other specially designed devices that help prevent skin breakdown are the Roto-Rest bed, alternating pressure mattress, and the eggcrate mattress. When a patient remains in the same position for too long, circulation to a particular area may become restricted by the pressure exerted from the bones against the mattress. Human tissues cannot live without oxygen, which circulates to all parts of the body through the blood. Elderly patients, obese patients, malnourished patients, and those with debilitating diseases (such as diabetes and cancer) usually need one of these special beds or mattresses. The Roto-Rest bed can eliminate pressure points and prevent bedsores by allowing the patient to be rotated periodically, thereby shifting the patient's weight from one part of the body to another. The **alternating pressure mattress** is filled with air that changes pressure in various locations. This constantly changes the pressure over the patient's back, buttocks, head, arms, and legs, allowing the blood to circulate properly. The **eggcrate mattress** is a foam mattress that looks like the bottom of an egg carton. It covers the entire mattress of the bed. This mattress helps keep constant pressure off of specific areas of the patient's body.

eggcrate mattress: a special mattress made from foam that is shaped like the bottom of an egg carton, and which is used to prevent skin breakdown

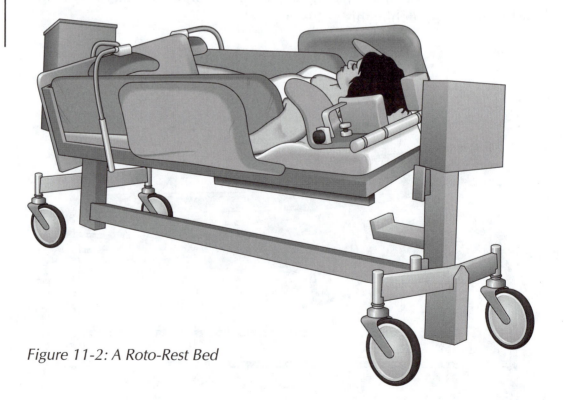

Figure 11-2: A Roto-Rest Bed

Traction Devices

Patients in different departments of the hospital may be in **traction**. A traction device is an apparatus consisting of pulleys and weights that keep broken bones in alignment. It is connected to the patient's bed. Frequently, a triangular piece of equipment called a **trapeze** hangs from an overhead bar above the patient's head. By reaching up and grasping it, the patient can shift position by moving the upper body around when he or she becomes uncomfortable. Only a doctor can order traction for the patient.

traction:
the process of pulling a part of the body into proper alignment

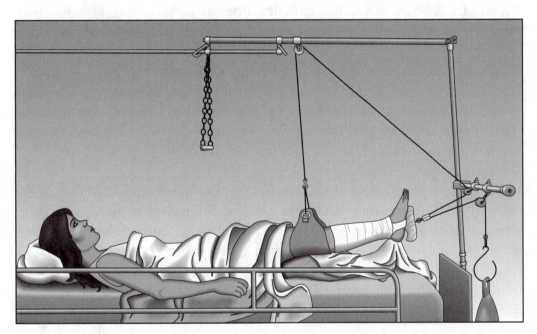

Figure 11-3: Traction can help keep broken bones in alignment as they heal.

Ambulation Equipment

Ambulation refers to a patient's ability to move about when he or she is not confined to a bed or **wheelchair**. If a patient is unable to walk without assistance, but is not restricted to bed, then he or she will need to be assisted by an ambulation device. One of the most common items for patient ambulation is the wheelchair. There are two sizes of wheelchairs: pediatric and adult. All wheelchairs are equipped with wheel brakes. Apply the brakes whenever a patient is being seated or leaving the wheelchair. If the brakes are not secure, the wheelchair may move away from the patient as he or she attempts to sit or rise. If the chair moves, the patient may fall and be injured.

ambulation:
the process of walking

wheelchair:
a special chair that is equipped with wheels for transporting patients

Most wheelchairs have several moving parts. For example, most foot rests can be moved out of the patient's way when he or she enters or exits the chair. Furthermore, most chairs have folding legs that may be extended in front of the patient, allowing him or her to elevate one or both legs. Vertical poles also are on most wheelchairs, so that intravenous (IV) fluid bottles can be hung on them while transporting the patient. Chapter Seven discussed safety guidelines for transferring patients into and out of wheelchairs.

Crutches frequently are used by patients with an orthopedic injury such as a broken bone or a severe sprain, or by patients who have had an amputation. Patients must be trained to use crutches properly before using them independently. Improper use of crutches can lead to additional patient injuries.

Canes can assist patients who need help with walking. They are usually constructed of wood and may have one, two, three, or four prongs. The more prongs the cane has, the more support the patient receives. Canes with one prong can usually be purchased in a drug store, but hospitals usually have four-pronged canes because they reduce the risk of the patient falling.

Walkers usually are made of aluminum and offer more support to the patient than a cane because they have two handles. Some walkers have two small wheels, which allow the patient to scoot the walker in front of them. The walkers without wheels must be lifted and moved in front of the patient with each step, requiring more effort and strength from the patient. Some walkers also have a built-in seat, which gives the patient a place to rest.

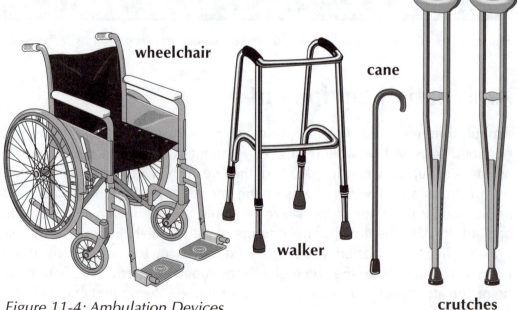

Figure 11-4: Ambulation Devices

Respiratory Devices

Many patients throughout the hospital must receive oxygen. Oxygen, or O_2, is given to the patient via a green tube attached to an outlet in the wall or to a portable oxygen tank, which is either green, chrome, or stainless steel. All oxygen outlets in the wall and portable oxygen tanks are also green. Green is the universal color for identifying oxygen. Patients may receive oxygen from a variety of methods. Two of the most common are the **oxygen mask** and the **nasal cannula.** The oxygen mask covers the mouth and the nose of the patient, whereas the nasal cannula is placed just inside each nostril. Either method may be used depending on the severity of the patient's condition. Be sure *NO SMOKING* signs are visible to all patients and visitors wherever oxygen is in use! Never adjust a patient's oxygen level—this is the nurse's responsibility!

Other special respiratory devices used in a hospital include nebulizers, respirators or ventilators, intermittent positive pressure breathing (IPPB) machines, and incentive spirometers. A **nebulizer** is an apparatus that delivers a fine mist of medication to the patient's nose, mouth, or both. This method allows the medication to be transported deeply into the lungs. **Respirators**, or **ventilators** are machines that mechanically breathe for a patient when he or she is unable to do so. These machines may be used to assist the patient with his or her own breathing, or to force every breath.

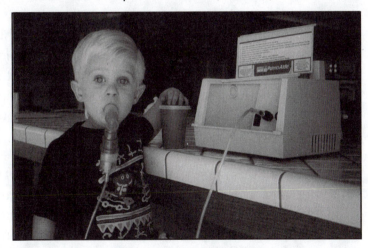

Figure 11-5: Children who have asthma often use a portable nebulizer.

Intermittent positive pressure breathing machines are used to assist those who are unable to inhale deeply. These devices use pressure to force mucus (phlegm) out of the air sacs in the lungs, which allows the patient to cough up the sputum. The oxygen that is pumped into the lungs replaces the fluid that is being forced out. These machines usually are used along with nebulizers.

Incentive spirometers are hand-held devices that encourage the patient to take a deep breath. Postsurgical patients use them to strengthen the lungs and promote proper ventilation. This greatly reduces the risk of contracting pneumonia. The incentive spirometer has three clear columns, each containing a ping pong ball, and a small flexible hose with a mouth piece. The patient inhales until one of the ping pong balls rises to the top of its column. The deeper the breath, the greater the number of ping pong balls that rise. When the patient elevates all three balls, his or her lungs are fully expanded.

Intravenous Therapy

Most of the patients in the hospital receive intravenous, or IV, fluids. The **IV fluid** is a combination of water and other substances, such as dextrose (sugar), and other electrolytes (eg, sodium, potassium, chloride, or lactate). This fluid replenishes essential elements or compounds that are lost from the body. All IV solutions are sterile. They come prepared from the manufacturer in bottles or plastic bags. The solution must be suspended above the patient so that the fluid can be administered accurately to the patient. This is usually done by hanging the IV solution on an IV pole. IV poles usually are attached to the patient's bed, but if the patient is ambulatory a portable IV pole will be used. This is a wheeled, metal pole with either two or four prongs to hold the solution.

IV infusion pump: a machine that, when attached to IV tubing via an IV pole, allows accurate administration of a solution

Most IV solutions are administered through an **IV infusion pump**. These are machines that, when attached to an intravenous pole, allow accurate administration of the solution. The pump is equipped with alarms and settings that control the flow of the IV fluid and notify caregivers when the bag is nearly empty. Whenever you hear an infusion pump beeping, notify the charge nurse. Do not adjust the settings and never turn off the pump!

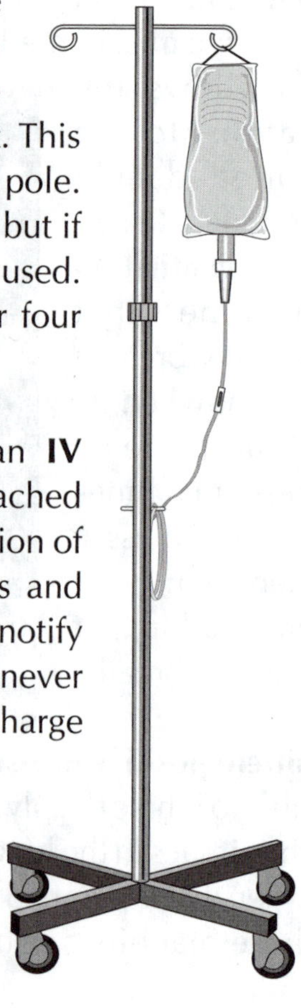

Figure 11-6: A Portable IV Pole

Excretory Equipment

There are many different kinds of equipment used to assist patients with urination, defecation, and the elimination of mucus and sputum. The urinary, digestive, and respiratory systems all participate in excretion by creating urine, stool, and sputum.

Some hospital patients are restricted to using a **bedside commode**, a portable toilet that is kept near the patient's bedside. This allows him or her more privacy than a bedpan, which requires assistance in placement, removal, and emptying. The bedside commode has four wheels, each with its own lock that must be secured before the patient attempts to use the commode. After the commode has been used, it must be thoroughly cleaned with the cleaning solution recommended by the healthcare facility. Other patients have a tube inserted through the external urinary opening, to drain the urinary bladder. This **indwelling catheter** is connected to a **drainage bag**, which may be attached to the patient's leg, bed, or chair to collect the urine. This combination of a catheter and drainage bag is called a urinary catheter. Be sure to unhook the drainage bag from the bed, chair, or other piece of equipment when the patient leaves the bed and don't hold the bag higher than the patient's bladder! To do so could cause the urine to drain back into the patient's bladder.

Suctioning assists the respiratory system by preventing patients from inhaling solids or liquids and keeps them from choking on secretions. It also can be used to aide the digestive system by removing the contents of the stomach. Most of the patient units are equipped with wall suction, but if the unit does not have this feature, a portable suction unit can be placed at the patient's bedside. A patient can be suctioned only by personnel trained in that procedure. If done incorrectly, serious harm may befall the patient.

Suctioning equipment includes tubing, a special suction catheter, and a receiving canister with markings that show the amount of secretions that have been removed. If a patient needs to be suctioned, notify the charge nurse. NEVER SUCTION A PATIENT UNLESS YOU HAVE BEEN PROPERLY TRAINED IN THE PROCEDURE.

bedside commode: a portable toilet usually kept by the patient's bedside

indwelling catheter: a catheter inserted into a particular area of the body such as the urinary bladder

The Patient Lift

Some patients, particularly those in a long-term care facility or in a geriatric unit in an acute care hospital, must be confined to bed due to their state of health. However, these patients, and patients who are paralyzed sometimes need to be moved from the bed to a chair to prevent complications from immobility. A **patient lift** is a device that makes this transfer easier on the patient and on the healthcare worker. The lift usually has a metal frame and contains a canvas or fabric seat resembling a hammock. This seat, which is secured to the lift with four hooks attached to the corners of the seat, will be put under the patient while he or she is still in bed. After the brake on the lift is secured and the hooks are attached, the handle on the frame will be either turned or jacked until the patient is clear of the bed and can be positioned above the receiving chair. The receiving chair must be locked before lowering the patient into it. Do not attempt to use the lift to move a patient until you have been trained in its use!

patient lift:
a piece of equipment used to transfer a bedridden patient out of bed into a chair or bath

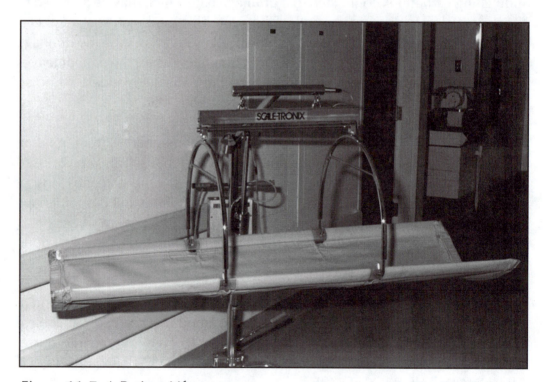

Figure 11-7: A Patient Lift

The Crash Cart

Every nursing unit and some of the allied health departments, such as Radiology and Physical Therapy, will be equipped with a **crash cart**. This is a cart stocked by the nursing and pharmacy staff with emergency medications, advanced breathing supplies, intravenous solutions and appropriate tubing, needles, a heart monitor and **defibrillator**, an oxygen tank, and a suction machine. This cart, which is usually red or blue, is used when a patient stops breathing (respiratory arrest), his or her heart stops beating (cardiac arrest), or both (**cardiopulmonary arrest**). All hospitals use the term **Code Blue** when a cardiopulmonary arrest occurs. This is an emergency situation to which hospital personnel must be prepared to react at all times. Part of this preparation includes training in **cardiopulmonary resuscitation (CPR)**. In fact, all hospital employees MUST be certified or recognized in CPR. Make sure you are proficient in this procedure and that you know the hospital's Code Blue number to notify the operator.

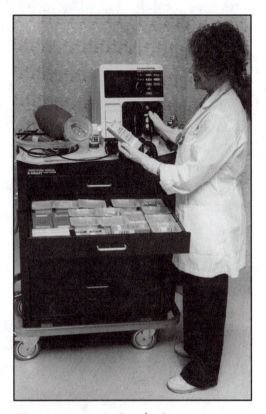

Figure 11-8: A Crash Cart

crash cart:
a portable supply cabinet that contains all of the emergency equipment necessary to treat a full arrest, or Code Blue

cardiopulmonary arrest:
the sudden absence of a pulse and respirations

Code Blue:
the emergency call signal in the hospital for a full arrest situation, which alerts all emergency resuscitation team members to respond to a specific location

Special Patient Care Items

There are other items designed for the patient with which every healthcare worker must become familiar. These include elastic stockings, bed cradles, aqua-K pads, warming blankets, and foot boards.

Elastic stockings are also called TED hose. They are usually white, and provide heavy support to the lower extremity to which they are applied. Physicians prescribe these for patients who may be confined to bed for an extended length of time or for patients who are suspected of having a blood clot in one or both legs. TED hose may extend from the toes to the knee or from the toes to the upper thigh.

cardiopulmonary resuscitation (CPR):
the basic life-saving procedure of artificial ventilation and chest compressions that is done in the event of a cardiac arrest

A bed cradle and a foot board often are used at the same time. The **bed cradle** is placed over a part of the patient's body, such as the legs, in order to keep linen from coming in contact with the patient's skin. Patients with burns, open skin lesions, or painful skin often use a bed cradle. The **foot board**, when placed at the end of the mattress, keeps the patient's feet in proper alignment. This helps prevent a condition called **footdrop**. This condition, which may require surgery to correct, limits the patient's ability to walk because the foot often drags along the floor.

Sometimes physicians prescribe heat therapy for their patients. One method of applying dry heat is through the use of a special pad, called an **aqua-K pad**, that contains heated water that is circulated electrically through the pad. The water temperature is preset and secured so that the patient's skin will not get burned. A **warming blanket** is for patients who have an extremely low body temperature. It resembles a large aqua-K pad because it also circulates electrically heated water throughout the blanket. However, the blanket is the size of the hospital bed mattress. Only nurses and doctors may regulate the temperature setting on a warming blanket.

The Patient Care Unit

Each nursing unit has a charge nurse who is responsible for assigning each patient to a patient care unit, or room. It is this nurse's job to keep the patient-to-nurse ratio at a safe level.

Most private hospitals offer private or semiprivate rooms for patients. *Semiprivate* means there is more than one bed, or patient care unit, in the room. Patients in semiprivate rooms must not have communicable diseases, which are capable of being transmitted from one individual to another from direct or indirect contact. Private hospitals usually have two patient care units in the same room. State funded hospitals, such as the teaching institutions, may have wards that contain at least four patient care units in one room.

A patient's privacy is important at all times, but in a semiprivate atmosphere, it is imperative that a special effort be made to guarantee physical privacy and to limit the nature of conversation to subject matter that does not invade the patient's privacy. Usually a private room is more expensive than a semiprivate room. Almost all patients are admitted to semiprivate rooms, but a patient may be assigned to a private room for any of the following reasons.

1. The patient may have a communicable disease and must be isolated so that other patients or staff members don't contract the illness.

2. The patient may request a private room.

3. The admitting physician may order a private room.

4. The patient may need to be protected from the public (ie, the patient is a celebrity or is in police custody).

Perhaps one of the greatest problems for the hospitalized patient is the interruption in his or her **activities of daily living**. These activities include sleep habits, eating habits, bowel and bladder habits, sexual activity, and other aspects of life. One of the ways in which hospitals have tried to help patients cope with hospitalization is to equip the patient units with basic supplies for the patients' use.

The **patient unit** includes the bed, an overbed light, an overbed table with storage area and personal mirror, a closet, a bathroom, a bedside table, a television, a radio, and a telephone. Almost all hospitals provide a Bible at each bedside and offer chaplain services as well. Most of the beds in the units are electric, and are equipped with positioning controls on the siderail for patient convenience. The call light control also may be on the siderail, or it may be on the wall or on the bedside table.

The **call light** is directly connected to the **intercom system**, and notifies personnel of the need for assistance. When a patient uses the call light, it will automatically trigger the main intercom control panel at the nurses' station and activate a light above the patient's door in the hallway. If the light is flashing it means the button in the

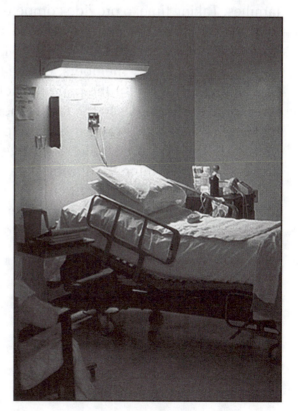

Figure 11-9: A Patient Unit

activities of daily living (ADL): normal, everyday actions, such as self care, communication, and mobility skills that are required for independent living

patient unit: a patient's room, including the bed, overbed table, bedside table, call light, telephone, television, radio, bathroom, and closet

call light: a communication device, located by the patient's bed, that is used by patients to notify the nurses' station of the need for assistance

intercom system: a communication system between the patient's bedside and the nurses' station

patient's bathroom has been pressed and the patient is in there. This is to alert the healthcare workers that an emergency may be in progress. This system provides a means of direct communication between the patient and the staff. Be familiar with the operation of the intercom and call light system; IT COULD BE THE PATIENT'S ONLY MEANS OF COMMUNICATION!

The television set may be mounted on the wall, or it may be a small personal television mounted on an adjustable pole on the wall. This allows more privacy for the patient and less disturbance to the other patients in the same room. The bedside table, overbed table, and the closet provide storage areas for the patient's personal items. Be sure to label the patient's loose items with his or her name and unit location to help prevent loss. All personal items should be documented on the appropriate form used by the healthcare facility. This will help provide a way of tracking any items that may become misplaced during the hospital stay.

Although equipment items are important elements of the patient care unit, so are the healthcare workers. As you carry out your various responsibilities, try to make meaningful use of the time you spend with the patients and their families. Taking time to provide competent and compassionate patient care will greatly affect the patient's course of recovery as well as his or her impression of that healthcare facility. Make time to talk and listen to your patient and the family members. Before leaving the bedside, ask if there is anything you can get for the patient, such as an extra pillow or blanket, or offer some refreshments to the family members. These gestures of kindness mean more than words can express. If a procedure requires you to move the bedside table or overbed table, or change the angle of the television, be sure and replace everything within the patient's reach and vision. Elderly and surgical patients often have difficulty in moving and reaching. Always leave the patient unit in better condition than when you entered the room and always leave the patient in a safe environment!

Chapter Summary

It is important to be familiar with the basic patient equipment that exists in a hospital environment. Although you may not use some of the items, you may be asked to locate them for another area of the hospital. Patients depend on you for competent and quality care! Learning how to operate each piece of equipment makes you more efficient in providing quality patient care and encourages the patient to place his or her trust in you, the healthcare worker. DO NOT OPERATE ANY EQUIPMENT OR PERFORM ANY PROCEDURE IF YOU ARE NOT TRAINED TO DO SO.

The development of a compassionate bedside manner is as important as knowing how to operate the equipment. As you work, remember that the patient is a person! He or she is special to someone, so take good care of your patient. After all, you or someone special to you may be a patient one day!

Name _____

Date _____

Student Enrichment Activities

Complete the following statements.

1. The word _____ refers to the process of walking.

2. Three examples of commonly used ambulation devices are _____,
   _____ , and _____.

3. An eggcrate mattress helps prevent skin _____.

4. The universal color indicating oxygen is _____.

5. Most intravenous solutions are administered through an _____
   _____ pump.

6. A tube that is inserted to drain the urinary bladder is an _____
   _____.

7. A _____ _____ is a specially-equipped cart used for
   cardiopulmonary arrests.

8. An _____ _____ is often used to apply heat therapy
   to a patient.

9. Patients with an extremely low body temperature are often placed on a
   _____ _____.

10. A patient communication device contained within the patient care unit is the
    intercom and _____ _____ system.

Unscramble the following terms.

11. LAMBTAUNIO   _____

12. RCSAH TCRA   _____ _____

13. LINGLINDEW THEATERC _____ _____

14. TSKRYER EARFM   _____ _____

15. CLEAHWERHI   _____

16. DBE CELDAR   _____ _____

17. PLAYDARIONCRUOM STARRE _____ _____

18. RUNGEY   _____

19. SLIEBURZEN   _____

20. ICONRATT   _____

21. ECDO ULEB   _____ _____

22. DEISBDE MOEMDOC   _____ _____

23. TEPANIT FLIT   _____ _____

24. LASAN CANLANU   _____ _____

Chapter Twelve
Introduction to Medical Terminology

Objectives

After completing this chapter you should be able to
do the following:

1. Define and correctly spell each of the key terms.

2. Correctly spell, define, and use all of the medical
   abbreviations.

3. Identify prefixes, suffixes, and combining forms from
   selected medical terms.

4. Identify medical abbreviations from a selected list.

Key Terms

- combining form
- combining vowel
- prefix
- root word
- suffix

The Importance of Accurate Terminology

The purpose of this book is to prepare you for employment in the hospital environment. An important part of any career is the terminology used in that particular line of work. Medicine, nursing, and allied health are no exceptions; in fact, proper terminology is ESPECIALLY important in healthcare, because human lives depend upon accurate **communication**. The provision of high quality patient care requires the mastery of medical terminology. Without it, documentation and verbal communication become flawed. This chapter will help you learn the more commonly used medical terms, but it cannot serve as a medical dictionary.

Determining the Meaning

There are a number of medical, nursing, and allied health dictionaries on the market today, all of which can be helpful to health occupations students. Because there are so many medical terms, it is virtually impossible to memorize all of them; but by dividing the words into their basic building blocks (**prefixes**, roots, and **suffixes**), the meaning will be easier to determine.

A great number of medical words are created by combining smaller words or word elements. If a word element is placed at the front of the main word, or **root word**, it is called a prefix. Prefixes change the meaning of the root word and help to further define it. If a word element is placed at the end of the root word, it is known as a suffix. Like a prefix, a suffix modifies the root word.

The letters *a, e, i, o,* and *u* are called vowels. The letter *y* is also sometimes called a vowel. All the other letters in the alphabet are called consonants. For spelling and pronunciation purposes, a vowel (usually *o*) is added between certain word elements. This vowel is called the **combining vowel**, and the root plus the vowel is called the **combining form**. The rule for using the combining vowel is as follows:

Use a combining vowel between a root and a suffix that begins with a consonant. Do not use a combining vowel before a suffix that begins with a vowel.

prefix:
a word element placed in front of a root to modify its meaning

suffix:
a word element placed at the end of a root to modify its meaning

root word:
the main part of a word

combining vowel:
a vowel that is placed between two word elements to join the two word parts

combining form:
a root word plus a combining vowel

Here are some examples of how this concept works.

Combining Word Elements

PREFIX	+	COMBINING FORM (Root/Combining Vowel)	+	SUFFIX	=	MEDICAL TERM
PERI (around)	+	CARD (heart)	+	ITIS (inflammation of)	=	PERICARDITIS (inflammation of the area around the heart)
		MY/O (muscle)	+	LOGY (study of)	=	MYOLOGY (study of muscles)
		HEMAT (blood)	+	URIA (urine)	=	HEMATURIA (blood in urine)
HYPO (under)	+	DERM (skin)	+	IC (pertaining to)	=	HYPODERMIC (pertaining to the area under the skin)
		GASTR (stomach)	+	ECTOMY (surgical removal)	=	GASTRECTOMY (surgical removal of the stomach)
		ARTHR/O (joint)	+	PLASTY (surgical repair)	=	ARTHROPLASTY (surgical repair of a joint)

Note: *Myology* and *arthroplasty* are the only words in the above example that require a combining vowel. This is because their suffixes begin with a consonant.

Figure 12-1: How Word Elements Combine to Form Medical Terms

Sometimes more than one combining form will be used to create a word:

COMBINING FORM		COMBINING FORM		SUFFIX		MEDICAL TERM
GASTR/O (stomach)	+	ENTER/O (intestine)	+	LOGY (study of)	=	GASTROENTEROLOGY (study of stomach and intestines)

Complete mastery of these medical terms can only be achieved through constant practice and drills. When documenting patient information, use as many of the CORRECT terms that you are familiar with as possible. The more often you use them, the easier it will become to document information accurately and appropriately. It is extremely important that you are 100% accurate in the context in which you use the term, AND in the spelling of the term. As you will learn, what may appear to be only a *slight error*, can communicate a completely inaccurate picture of the patient's condition to another member of the healthcare team. You must not only think—YOU MUST KNOW!

The Word Elements

The following glossary terms are some of the word elements that are used to create words commonly used in the healthcare environment. Terms that usually appear as prefixes are shown below with a hyphen following them (ie, *ab-*); while common suffixes are shown following a hyphen (ie, *-algia*). You will find that, at times, some of them are used as roots words too. Roots followed by a slash and a vowel (usually *o*) indicate combining forms.

a-, an-: absent; deficient; without; not; lack of.
ab-: away from; absent.
abdomin/o: abdominal area.
ad-: near; toward.
aden-, adeno-: gland.
-algia: painful.
ambi-: both; two-sided.
angi/o: vessel.
ante-: before; preceding.
anter/o: in front of; ahead of; before.
anti-: against.
arteri/o: artery.
arthr/o: joint.
-ase: enzyme.
audi/o: sound.
auto-: self.

bi-: two.
bi/o: life.
brachi/o: arm.
brachy-: short.
brady-: slow.
bronch/o, bronchi/o: bronchial tubes (air tubes in the lungs).
bucc/o: cheek.

carcin/o: cancer.
cardi/o: heart.
-cele: swelling; tumor; hernia.
cephal/o: head.
cerebr/o: cerebrum (part of the brain).
chol/e, chol/o: bile; gall.
chondr/o: cartilage.
-cid, -cide: kill or destroy.
circum-: surrounding; around.
contra-: opposite; opposed; against.
cost/o: rib.
crani/o: skull.
cyan/o: blue.
cyst/o: fluid-filled sac; urinary bladder; bag.
-cyte, cyt/o: cell.

dactyl/o: digits (the fingers or toes).
dent-, dent/o: teeth.
-derma, derm/o, dermat/o: skin.
dextr/o: right side.
di-, dipl/o: two; twice; double.
dia-: through; complete.
dorsi-, dors/o: back of body.
duoden/o: duodenum (first part of the small intestine).
-dynia: pain.
dys-: painful; difficult; bad; disordered.

-ectasis: dilation; expansion; stretching.
ecto-: external; outside.
-ectomy: surgical removal; excision.
-emesis: vomiting.
-emia: blood.
encephal/o: brain.
end/o: inside; within.
enter/o: intestine; small intestine.
epi-: upon; over; upper.
erythr/o: red.
-esthesia: sensation; feeling.
ex-, exo-: out; outside; away from.
extra-: in addition to; outside of.

-ferous: producing.
fibr/o: threadlike structures; connective tissue.
fore-: in front of; before.
-form: resembling; having the form of; shape.
-fuge: pushing or driving away.

gaster-, gastr-, gastr/o: stomach.
gen/o, -genetic, -genic: an originating or producing agent; produced from; pertaining to heredity.
genit/o: genitalia; male and female reproductive organs.
gloss/o: tongue.
gluc/o, glyc/o: sugar; glucose.
-gram: record.
-graph: instrument used for recording.
-graphy: process of recording.
gyne-, gynec/o: woman or female.

hem-, hem/o, hemat/o: blood.
hemi-: half.
hepat/o: liver.
heter/o: unlike; different; other.
hist/o: tissue.
hom/o, home/o: alike; the same.
hydr/o: water.
hyper-: excessive; above; increased.
hypo-: below; deficient; under.
hyster/o: uterus; womb.

-iasis: abnormal condition.
-ic: pertaining to.
idi/o: one's own; distinct; not known.
ile/o: ileum (last part of small intestine).
ili/o: ilium (part of hip bone).
inter-: between.
intra-: within.
-itis: inflammation.

jejun/o: jejunum (second part of small intestine).
juxta-: near.

-kenesis, **kinesi/o:** movement.
kerat/o: cornea of eye; horny; hard.

labi/o: lips.
lacrim/o: tears; lacrimal duct.
lact/o: milk.
later/o: side.

leuk/o: white.
lingu/o: tongue.
lip/o: fat.
lith/o: stone or calculus.
-logist: specialist; one who studies.
-logy: science of; study of.
-lysis: loosen; dissolve; destruction.

macro-: large; long.
mal-: abnormal; bad; disordered.
-malacia: softening.
masto-: breast.
-megaly, **mega-**, **megal/o:** enlarged.
men-, **men/o:** menstruation; monthly.
mening/o: meninges (membranes that cover the brain and the spinal cord).
micro-, **micr/o:** small.
mono-, **mon/o:** one; single.
multi-: many.
my/o: muscle.

necr/o: death.
neo-: new.
neph-, **nephr/o:** kidney.
neur/o: nerves or nervous system.

ocul/o: eye.
odont/o: teeth.
olig/o: few; less than normal; a deficiency.
-oma: tumor.
onc/o: tumor.
oophor/o: ovary.
ophthalm/o: eye.
orth/o: straight.
-osis: abnormal condition.
oste/o: bone.
ot/o: ear.

para-: beside; beyond; apart from; near; abnormal.
-para: to bring forth; to bear.
-pathy, **path/o:** disease.
ped/o: child; foot.
-penia: lack of; deficiency.
per-: through.
peri-: surrounding; around.
-phage, **phag/o:** ingest; eat; swallow.
-phasia, **phas/o:** speech.
phleb/o: vein.
phob/o: dread; abnormal fear.
-plasty: surgical repair.
pleur/o: pleura.
-pnea: breathing.
pneum/o: lung; air.
pod/o: foot.
poly-: many.

post-: following; after.
pre-: in front of; before.
pro-: in front of; before; for.
proct/o: rectum.
pseud/o: false.
psych/o: mind.
pulm/o, **pulmon/o:** lung.
py/o: pus.
pyel/o: pelvis of kidney.

quadri-: consisting of four.

ren/o: kidney.
retr/o: located behind; backwards.
-rhage, **-rhagia:** bursting forth; excessive flow of blood.
-rhaphy: suture or sew up a defect.
-rhea: flow or discharge.
rhin/o: nose.

salping/o: oviduct, uterine tube, or fallopian tube; auditory tube.
scler/o: hardening; sclera (white of eye).
scoli/o: twisted; curved.
-scope: instrument used to examine or look into a part.
-scopy: visual examination.
semi-: half.
sept/o: poison.
-sis: condition or process.
somat/o: the body.
sten-, steno-: contracted; narrow.
-stomy: surgical creation of an opening.
sub-: under; below.
super-, supra-: over; above.
sym-, syn-: with; together.
syring/o: fistula; tube.

tachy-: fast; rapid; swift.
tars/o: tarsal (ankle bone).
tax/o: order; arrangement; coordination.
tend/o, ten/o: tendon.
tens/o: stretch; strain.
therm/o: heat.
thromb/o: clot.
-tomy: cutting into; incision.
tox/o: poison.
trache/o: trachea (windpipe).
trans-: across; through.
tri-: three.
-trophy: nutrition; development; growth.
-tropia: to turn.

ultra-: excess; beyond.
uni-: one.
-uria, **uro-:** presence in urine.

vas/o: duct; vessel; vas deferens.
ven/o: vein.
ventr/o: front or belly side of body.
viscer/o: viscera (internal organs).

xanth/o: yellow.
xer/o: dryness.

The glossary of terms provided in this chapter does not include all of the roots (combining forms), prefixes, and suffixes that exist. These are only some of the most common ones. As procedures and techniques continue to progress and change in this field, so does the medical language. Be sure and stay current!

As you progress in your work, pay attention to particular medical terms used during verbal communication and written documentation. Practice writing and speaking medical terminology. If there is a term that is unfamiliar to you, LOOK IT UP! NEVER GUESS THE MEANING OF A MEDICAL TERM!

Abbreviations for Use in Documentation

Throughout the medical field, abbreviations are used either alone or in combination to give specific directions and provide certain information. You MUST learn the acceptable abbreviations in order to communicate properly with other healthcare workers. The following list of acceptable abbreviations is an introduction. There are specific, approved abbreviations in all of the medical specialties, but be sure to use only abbreviations that are acceptable to the healthcare facility. NEVER USE AN UNAPPROVED ABBREVIATION! No one will know what you are trying to communicate if you do.

NOTE: It is recognized that sources differ regarding the use of periods with abbreviations. In this series, we have elected to follow the guidelines set forth by the *American Medical Association Manual of Style, 8th Edition,* which states that periods in abbreviations are to be omitted.

A

ā: before.
ABC: airway, breathing, & circulation.
abd: abdomen.
ABGs: arterial blood gases.
ABP: arterial blood pressure.
ac: before meals.
Ac: acetest.
Ac and Cl: acetest and clinitest.
ADA: American Diabetic Association; American Dietetic Association; American Dental Association.
ADL: activities of daily living .
ad lib: as desired.
adm: admission.
AF: atrial fibrillation.
AIDS: acquired immune deficiency syndrome.
AM: before noon; morning hours.
AMA: against medical advice; American Medical Association.
AMI: acute myocardial infarction.
amt: amount.
ant: anterior.
Ap: apical.
AP: anteroposterior.

APGAR: a test for newborns based on appearance, pulse, grimace, airway, and reflex.
appy: appendicitis.
AQ or **aq:** water; aqueous base.
ARDS: adult respiratory distress syndrome.
ARF: acute renal failure; acute respiratory failure.
ARN: authorized radio nurse.
ASHD: arteriosclerotic heart disease.
AT: atrial tachycardia.

B

Bac T: bacteriology.
BBB: bundle branch block.
B and C: biopsy and conization.
BCP: birth control pills.
BE: barium enema; below elbow.
Be: beryllium.
BID or **bid:** twice daily.
bil: bilateral.
bl: blood.
BLE: both lower extremities.
BM: bowel movement.
BMR: basal metabolic rate.
BP: blood pressure.

BR: bathroom or bedrest.
BRP: bathroom privileges.
BS: blood sugar.
BSC: bedside commode.
BUE: both upper extremities.
BUN: blood urea nitrogen.
Bx: biopsy.

C

C: Centigrade or Celsius.
c̄: with.
CA: cancer.
Ca: calcium.
CABG: coronary artery bypass with graft.
Cal: large Calorie.
cal: small calorie.
cap: capsule.
CAT scan: computerized axial tomography scan.
cath: catheter.
CBC: complete blood count.
CBR: complete bedrest.
cc: cubic centimeter.
CC: chief complaint.
CCU: Coronary Care Unit.
CDA: certified dental assistant.
CE: cardiac enzymes.
CEN: certified emergency nurse.
CHF: congestive heart failure.
CHO: carbohydrate.
cl: clinitest.
Cl: chloride; chlorine.
Cl and Ac: clinitest and acetest.
CL or Cl liq: clear liquids.
cm: centimeter.
CNA: certified nursing assistant; Canadian Nurses Association.
CNS: central nervous system.
co or c/o: complaining of.

CO₂: carbon dioxide.
CODE III: lights and sirens.
comp: complete.
cont: continue.
COPD: chronic obstructive pulmonary disease.
CP: cerebral palsy or chest pain.
CPK: creatinine phosphokinase.
CPR: cardiopulmonary resuscitation.
CRF: chronic renal failure.
CS: Central Supply.
C & S: culture and sensitivity.
CSF: cerebrospinal fluid.
CT: computerized tomography.
CTA: clear to auscultation.
CT scan: computerized tomography scan.
CVA: cerebrovascular accident.
CVR: controlled ventricular rate.
Cx: cervix.
CXR: chest x-ray.

D

d: day.
/d: per day.
DAT: diet as tolerated.
DC: doctor of chiropractic; discharge.
dc: discontinue.
D & C: dilatation and curettage.
DCA: directional coronary atherectomy.
DDS: doctor of dental surgery.
dept: department.
diff: differential white blood cell count.
dil: dilute.
DM: diabetes mellitus.
DNR: do not resuscitate.
DO: doctor of osteopathy.
DOA: dead on arrival.
DPM: doctor of podiatry medicine.
Dr: doctor.

dr: drainage; dram.
DTs: delirium tremens.
DW: dextrose in water.
Dx: diagnosis.
Dz: disease.

E

ea: each.
ECG: electrocardiogram.
ECU: Emergency Care Unit.
ED: Emergency Department.
EEG: electroencephalogram.
EENT: eye, ear, nose and throat.
EKG: electrocardiogram.
EMS: Emergency Medical Services.
EMT: emergency medical technician.
ER: Emergency Room.
ERT: emergency room technician.
ESR: erythrocyte sedimentation rate.
ETOH: ethanol.
exc: excision.
exp: exploratory.
ext: extract, extraction, external.

F

F: Fahrenheit.
FB: foreign body.
FBS: fasting blood sugar.
FBW: fasting blood work.
FC: foley catheter.
Fe: iron.
FF or **F Fl:** force fluids.
FH or **FHB:** fetal heart beat.
FHTs: fetal heart tones.
FL or **Full Liq:** full liquids.
Fl or **fl:** fluids.
FUO: fever of undetermined origin.
Fx or **Fr:** fracture.

G

GB: gallbladder.
GC or **Gc:** gonococcus, gonorrhea.
GI: gastrointestinal.
Gm or **gm:** gram.
gr: grain.
Gtt or **gtt:** drops.
GU: genitourinary.
GYN or **gyn:** gynecology.

H

h: hour.
HBV: hepatitis B virus.
Hep B: hepatitis B.
Hct: hematocrit.
Hg: mercury.
HIV: human immunodeficiency virus.
H_2O: water.
HOH: hard of hearing.
HS: hour of sleep.
HSV: herpes simplex virus.
ht: height.
HTN: hypertension.
HUC: health unit coordinator.
HX: history.
hypo: hypodermic.
hyst: hysterectomy.

I

IABP: intra-aortic balloon pump.
IBP: invasive blood pressure.
ICU: Intensive Care Unit.
I & D: incision and drainage.
IDDM: insulin dependent diabetes mellitus.
IJ: internal jugular.
IM: intramuscular.
inf: infusion or inferior.

ing: inguinal.
inj: injection.
int: internal, interior.
I & O: intake and output.
IUD: intrauterine device.
IV: intravenous.
IVP: intravenous pyelogram.

J

JR: junctional rhythm.
JVD: jugular vein distention.

K

K: potassium.
KCl: potassium chloride.
kg: kilogram.
KO'd: knocked out.
KUB: kidney, ureter, and bladder.

L

L or l: liter.
LA: left atrium; left arm.
lab: laboratory.
lap: laparotomy.
lat: lateral.
lb: pound.
LBP: low back pain.
LCTA: lungs clear to auscultation.
L&D: labor and delivery.
LFT: left frontotransverse fetal position.
LFTs: liver function tests.
liq: liquid.
LLE: left lower extremity.
LLL: left lower lobe.
LLQ: left lower quadrant.
LOC: level of consciousness; loss of consciousness.

LOM: left otitis media.
LP: lumbar puncture.
LPN: licensed practical nurse.
LR: lactated ringers.
LS: lumbosacral.
Lt: left.
LUE: left upper extremity.
LUQ: left upper quadrant.
LV: left ventricle.
LVN: licensed vocational nurse.
LWBS: left without being seen.

M

m: minim or meter.
MA: medical assistant.
MAE: moves all extremities.
MAST: military antishock trousers.
mat: maternity.
MD: medical doctor.
med: medical.
mEq: milliequivalent.
Mg: magnesium.
mg: milligram.
MI: myocardial infarction.
MICN: mobile intensive care nurse.
ml: milliliter.
mm: millimeter.
MOM: milk of magnesia.
MRI: magnetic resonance imaging.
MT or Med Tech: medical technologist.
MVA: motor vehicle accident.

N

N: nitrogen.
n: nausea.
Na: sodium.
NA: nursing assistant.
NaCl: sodium chloride.
nc: nasal cannula.

Neur: neurology.
NIBP: non-invasive blood pressure.
NO: Nursing Office.
no: number.
noc: night.
np: nasal prongs.
NPN: nonprotein nitrogen.
NPO: nothing by mouth.
NS: normal saline.
nsy: nursery.
NWB: no weight bearing.

O

O₂: oxygen.
OB or **Obs:** Obstetrics.
OD: right eye; overdose.
OP: outpatient.
OR: operating room.
ord: orderly.
ORIF: open reduction and internal fixation.
ortho: orthopedics.
OS: left eye.
os: mouth.
OT: occupational therapy.
OTC: over the counter.
OU: each eye.
oz: ounce.

P

p̄: after; post.
P: phosphorous; pulse.
PAC: premature atrial contraction.
PACU: Post Anesthesia Care Unit.
PAST: pneumatic antishock trousers.
PAT: paroxysmal atrial tachycardia.
path: pathology.
PBI: protein bound iodine.
pc: after meals.

PCXR: portable chest x-ray.
PDR: Physician's Desk Reference.
peds: pediatrics.
per: by or through.
PERL: pupils equal and react to light.
PERLA: pupils equal and react to light and accommodation.
PET: positron emission tomography.
pharm: pharmacy.
PI: present illness.
PID: pelvic inflammatory disease.
PJC: premature junctional contraction.
PKU: phenylketonuria.
pm: afternoon or evening.
PMD: primary medical doctor.
PMH: past medical history; personal medical history.
po: by mouth.
PO: phone order.
post: posterior; after.
post-op: after the surgery.
PR: paced rhythm.
pre-op: before the surgery.
PRN: whenever necessary or as needed.
psy: psychology, psychiatry.
PT: physical therapy or prothrombin time.
PTCA: percutaneous transluminal coronary angioplasty.
pt: patient.
PTT: partial thromboplastin time.
PVC: premature ventricular contraction.

Q

Q or **q̄:** every.
QD or **qd:** every day; daily.
qh: every hour.
q2h: every 2 hours.

q3h: every 3 hours.
q4h: every 4 hours.
q6h: every 6 hours.
q8h: every 8 hours.
q12h: every 12 hours.
QHS or **qhs:** every night at sleep.
QID or **qid:** four times per day.
QOD or **qod:** every other day.
QS or **qs:** quantity sufficient.
Qt or **qt:** quart.

R

R: rectal; respirations.
RA: right atrium, right arm.
RBC: red blood cell/count.
RLE: right lower extremity.
RLQ: right lower quadrant.
RML: right middle lobe.
RN: registered nurse.
ROM: right otitis media or range of motion.
RR: Recovery Room; respiratory rate.
Rt: right.
RTB: respiratory tract burn.
RUE: right upper extremity.
RUQ: right upper quadrant.
RV: right ventricle.
Rx: prescription; take.

S

S: sacral.
s̄: without.
SAC: short arm cast.
SBO: small bowel obstruction.
SC or **sc:** subcutaneous.
SGOT: serum glutamic-oxaloacetic transaminase (test).
SGPT: serum glutamic pyruvic transaminase (test).

SIDS: sudden infant death syndrome.
Sig: give the following directions.
SL: sublingual.
SOB: short of breath.
Sod: sodium.
sol: solution.
sos: if necessary.
spec: specimen.
Sp Gr or **sp gr:** specific gravity.
SN: student nurse.
s̄s̄: one-half.
SSE or **SS enema:** soap solution, or soap suds, enema.
stat: at once; immediately.
STD: sexually transmitted disease.
sup: superior.
surg: surgical; surgery.
syp: syrup.

T

T or **temp:** temperature.
T & A: tonsillectomy and adenoidectomy.
tab: tablet.
TAH: total abdominal hysterectomy.
Tbs or **tbsp:** tablespoon.
TC: traffic collision.
TEMP: temperature.
TIA: transient ischemic attack.
TIBC: total iron binding capacity.
TIB-FIB: tibia-fibula.
TID or **tid:** three times daily.
TLC: tender loving care.
TO: telephone order.
TPR: temperature, pulse, and respiration.
tr or **tinct:** tincture.
tsp: teaspoon.
TURP: transurethral resection of the prostate.
tx: traction; treatment; transmit.

U

UA: urinalysis.
UCVR: uncontrolled ventricular rate.
ung: ointment.
Ur or **ur:** urine.
URI: upper respiratory infection.
US or **Uz:** ultrasound.
UTI: urinary tract infection.

V

vag: vaginal.
VD: venereal disease.
VDRL: blood test for syphilis;
     Venereal Disease Research
     Laboratories.
VO or **vo:** verbal order.
vol: volume.
VS: vital signs.

W

WBC: white blood cell/count.
WC: ward clerk.
w/c: wheelchair.
wt: weight.

X

x: times (3x means 3 times).
XR: x-ray.

Y, Z

None at present.

Symbols

The following symbols are used frequently in medical documentation. They, too, are abbreviations that you will need to know.

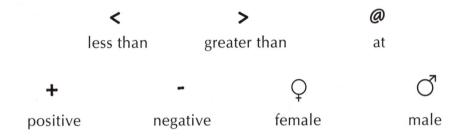

<	**>**	**@**
less than	greater than	at

+	**-**	♀	♂
positive	negative	female	male

These lists are challenging; however, mastery of the terms and definitions can be attained through persistent and accurate study. You also will find that to interpret some of the meanings, you will have to look at the context in which the abbreviations are used. Practice writing and speaking in medical jargon as much as possible, and above all—DO NOT BECOME DISCOURAGED! Learn the terms accurately and use them correctly.

Chapter Summary

As with any profession, medicine has its own terminology and approved abbreviations. Root words can be changed by adding prefixes and/or suffixes. The slightest letter change can result in a completely different meaning.

It is extremely important to be accurate and precise when documenting and interpreting the medical terminology. Be sure to use only those abbreviations that are universally approved and are accepted by your hospital. Perseverance and practice will ensure competent and correct patient care!

Name _____

Date _____

Student Enrichment Activities

Define the following prefixes, roots (combining forms), and suffixes.

1. arteri/o: _____ .

2. -algia: _____ .

3. anti-: _____ .

4. arthr/o: _____ .

5. audi/o: _____ .

6. cephal/o: _____ .

7. chol/o: _____ .

8. derm/o: _____ .

9. cyan/o: _____ .

10. circum-: _____ .

11. cyst/o: _____ .

12. dys-: _____ .

13. epi-: _____ .

14. -ectomy: _____ .

15. glyc/o: _____ .

16. -gram: _____ .

17. enter/o: _____ .

18. gynec/o: _____ .

19. hydr/o: _____ .

20. hepat/o: _____ .

21. intra-: _____ .

22. -itis: _____ .

23. lip/o: _____ .

24. -logy: _____ .

25. mal-: _____ .

26. nephr/o: _____ .

27. oste/o: _____ .   29. -tomy:_____ .

28. -stomy: _____ .   30. peri-:_____ .

Define the following.

31. cholecystectomy: _____ .

32. dysuria: _____ .

33. glycosuria: _____ .

34. hepatitis: _____ .

35. hydrocephalus: _____ .

36. hysterectomy: _____ .

37. appendicitis: _____ .

38. lipase:_____ .

39. ABGs:_____ .

40. AMI: _____ .

41. BCP: _____ .

42. BP: _____ .

43. BUE:_____ .

Name _____

Date _____

44. epicardial: _____ .

45. pericarditis: _____ .

46. gynecology: _____ .

47. arteriogram: _____ .

48. nephritis: _____ .

49. CNS: _____ .

50. DAT: _____ .

51. pleuritis: _____ .

52. EKG: _____ .

53. FBS: _____ .

54. GI: _____ .

55. gastritis: _____ .

56. AIDS: _____ .

57. dermatitis: _____ .

58. myalgia: _____ .

59. IM: _____ .

60. OTC: _____ .

61. OR: _____ .

62. pathology: _____ .

63. RN: _____ .

64. TPR: _____ .

65. XR: _____ .

66. pleur/o: _____ .

67. -pnea: _____ .

68. path/o: _____ .

69. phleb/o: _____ .

70. pseud/o: _____ .

71. retr/o: _____ .

72. -scopy: _____ .

73. sub-: _____ .

74. supra-: _____ .

Name _____

Date _____

75. thromb/o: _____ .

76. -uria: _____ .

77. vas/o: _____ .

78. viscer/o: _____ .

Unscramble the following terms.

79. DEAMCIL TROMINGLOEY   _____   _____

80. FREXIP   _____

81. FUFSIX   _____

82. MONTIOMUNCIAC   _____

83. NOACTEMDUNTOI   _____

84. CIDARRESITIP   _____

85. TOMASEGRYTC   _____

Chapter Thirteen
An Introduction to the Human Body

Objectives

After completing this chapter, you should be able to do the following:

1. Define and correctly spell each of the key terms.

2. Name and explain the function of at least four cellular components.

3. Explain the function of enzymes.

4. Describe two kinds of reproductive processes.

5. Name and describe the four different types of tissue groups.

6. Name the three kinds of muscle tissue.

7. Explain the requirements of a body system.

8. Identify the three directional planes.

9. Name the three sections of the anterior cavity.

10. Name the two sections of the posterior cavity.

11. Identify the body organs that are contained within each of the body cavities.

Key Terms

- anatomy
- cell
- connective tissue
- edema
- epithelial tissue
- meiosis
- mitosis

- muscle tissue
- nerve tissue
- organ
- physiology
- semipermeable
- system

Understanding Human Body Function

anatomy:
the study of
the structure
of the body

Since the goal of the healthcare team is to provide complete care to patients, it is important to understand the **anatomy** (how the body is put together) and **physiology** (how the body works) of the human body. This section will serve as an introduction to the highly detailed and intricate anatomy and physiology of the human body.

physiology:
the study of
the function
of the body

Cells: The Basis of Life

cell:
the basic unit
of life

The most basic unit of life is the **cell**. Cells are made up of a jelly-like material known as **cytoplasm** (**protoplasm**), meaning original substance. Cytoplasm is composed of carbon, hydrogen, calcium, nitrogen, oxygen, and phosphorus. The composition of organisms vary in complexity; from single-celled organisms such as an egg, to multicelled **organisms** such as human beings. Cells are the basis for all living objects, including plants and animals. In order to appreciate the magnificent, intricate functions of the living cell, you must understand its various parts.

semipermeable:
the ability to
permit certain
substances
to enter and
exit through a
membrane

The outer covering of the cell is known as the **cell membrane**. The membrane is **semipermeable**. This means that it is selective in permitting certain substances to enter and/or to exit. This is another method the body uses to maintain **homeostasis**, or balance. The main substance of the cell is cytoplasm, which, in addition to the already named elements, contains water, nutrients, and pigment. Tiny structures called **organelles** also are found in the cytoplasm.

Mitochondria are a type of organelle that release energy and are responsible for the chemical reactions that occur within the cell. **Enzymes** are contained within the mitochondria and influence the amount of energy released during these chemical reactions. Enzymes are very complex proteins that increase the speed of the reaction without changing themselves. At the center of the cell is the **nucleus**. The nucleus controls vital functions of the cell such as metabolism, growth, and reproduction. The **chromosomes** are found within the nucleus of the cell and contain the **genes**. Chromosomes and genes determine the physical and mental characteristics of the human being.

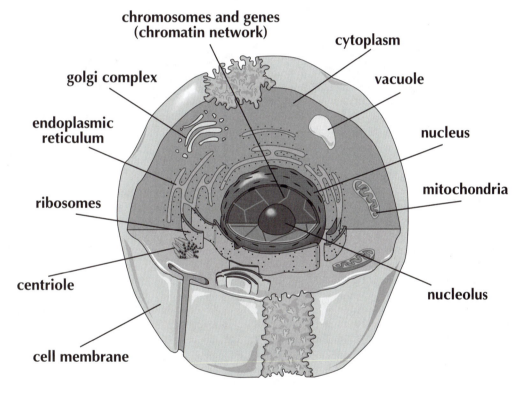

Figure 13-1: The Parts of a Human Cell

Cellular reproduction occurs through actual cell division. Within the human reproductive organs this division is called **meiosis**. This type of cell division is specific for the ovaries and the testes only, and creates cells that contain half the number of chromosomes that nonreproductive cells contain. This type of division is necessary for proper fertilization and reproduction. Cell division that occurs elsewhere in the body, such as skin cells producing more skin cells, is called **mitosis**. (See Figure 13-2.) Cells of the same type divide and form **tissues**.

meiosis:
cell reproduction specific for the ovaries and testes

mitosis:
cell reproduction in which a cell divides, forming two daughter cells that are identical to the original cell

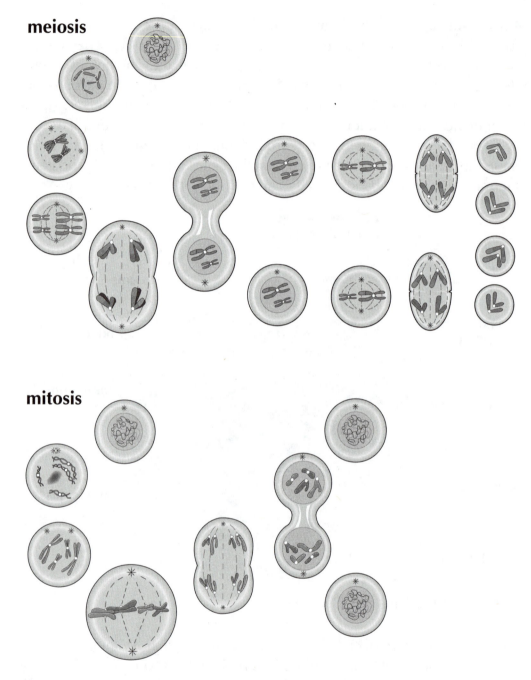

Figure 13-2: There are two types of cell division that take place in the human body.

Tissues

Tissues are a group of similar cells and their cell products. Surrounding the cells is tissue fluid (**interstitial fluid**), which performs particular functions. This tissue fluid is composed of water, salt, and various other substances. The main component of the interstitial fluid is water. In fact, water accounts for about 60% of the body's weight. Tissue fluid plays a vital role in the overall health of an individual. If there is not enough tissue fluid, the patient is **dehydrated**. Signs and symptoms may include dry mucous membranes, thirst, weakness, and tenting (when the skin is pinched, it remains in that position—like a tent.) On the other hand, if a patient has too much tissue fluid, **edema** (swelling) occurs and the patient is said to have **fluid overload**. There are four main types of tissue groups: 1) epithelial, 2) connective, 3) nerve, and 4) muscle.

edema: swelling due to fluid in the tissues; fluid retention

The main tissue of the skin is called **epithelial tissue**. This specific type of tissue lines the cavities of the body and the principal tubes and passageways that lead to the outside, such as the trachea, esophagus, vagina, rectum, and so on. Epithelial tissue plays an important role in maintaining homeostasis by protecting the internal organs and helping to regulate body temperature. Epithelial tissue also forms the glands which produce hormones responsible for regulating various bodily functions.

epithelial tissue: tissue that lines the cavities of the body and the principal tubes and passageways that lead to the exterior of the body

Connective tissue supports and connects other tissues and parts. There are two types of connective tissue: *soft* and *hard*. **Adipose**, or fatty tissue, is soft connective tissue. Fatty tissue stores fat as a food reserve, insulator, and energy source. Adipose tissue also forms **fibrous connective tissue** (ie, tendons and ligaments) that serves to support the joints of the body and helps hold particular structures together. Bone and cartilage are made up of hard connective tissue. The skeletal system of the body is composed of bone. Bone is also known as **osseous tissue**, which is made up of blood vessels, calcium, and nerves. **Cartilage** is a dense connective tissue with characteristics that resemble an elastic band. It is found between the spinal discs, at the end of long bones where it acts as a shock absorber, and in the nose, the ears, and the **larynx** (voice box).

connective tissue: tissue that supports and attaches other tissues and parts to each other

The third type of tissue is **nerve tissue**. Nerve tissue is the substance that comprises the **nervous system** (ie, the brain, spinal cord, and the nerves). Nerve tissue is made up of special cells called **neurons**, which carry commands and information between the brain and the rest of the body. The nervous system is very complex!

nerve tissue: tissue, made up of neurons, that comprises the nervous system

muscle tissue:
tissue that is
responsible for
body movement

The fourth type of tissue is **muscle tissue**. Contraction of muscle fibers allows the muscles to produce movement and power. There are three main types of muscle tissue: **skeletal**, which attaches to the bones and permits movement; **cardiac**, which causes the heart to contract; and smooth, or **visceral**, muscle that is found principally in the organs.

organ:
a structure
within the
body made
up of tissues
that allow it
to perform
a particular
function

Just as cells combine to form a particular type of tissue, two or more tissues that combine to perform a specific function form an **organ**. The lungs, heart, stomach, and liver are examples of organs, or **viscera**. When organs and other body structures combine to perform a common function, they form a body **system**, such as in the circulatory, respiratory, gastrointestinal, and reproductive systems. The following chapters will provide you with basic anatomical and physiological information about each of the body systems.

system:
a group of
organs that
work together
to perform a
common
function

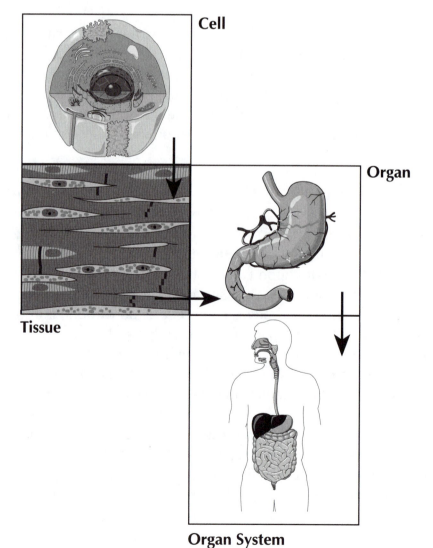

Cell

Organ

Tissue

Organ System

Figure 13-3: From Cell to System

Body Planes And Directional Terms

One of the most important aspects of accurate documentation and patient assessment involves the use of the appropriate anatomical terms. Using imaginary lines, the body can be separated into sections.

The **transverse plane** refers to an imaginary, horizontal line that divides the body into a top half and a bottom half. (See Figure 13-4.) The transverse plane also has two other directional terms associated with it. The first term, **cranial**, refers to body parts that are located near the head. The second term, **caudal**, refers to the body parts that are located near the lower back or sacral area.

Another directional plane that is used in the medical field is the **midsagittal plane**. This refers to the imaginary line that divides the human body exactly into right and left halves. This plane also has two other terms associated with the location of body areas: **medial** and **lateral**. Medial pertains to those parts located near the middle, or center, of the body. Lateral refers to those parts located near the side.

The third and last directional plane used when referring to the location of body parts is the **frontal**, or **coronal**, **plane**. This plane uses an imaginary line to separate the body into a front and back section. The body parts located on the front are referred to as **ventral**, or **anterior**. Parts located on the back are referred to as **dorsal**, or **posterior**.

Body parts that are located above another are said to be **superior** to those located below. Body organs or parts that are located below others are **inferior** to those located above. For example, the thigh is inferior to the chest, but superior to the foot.

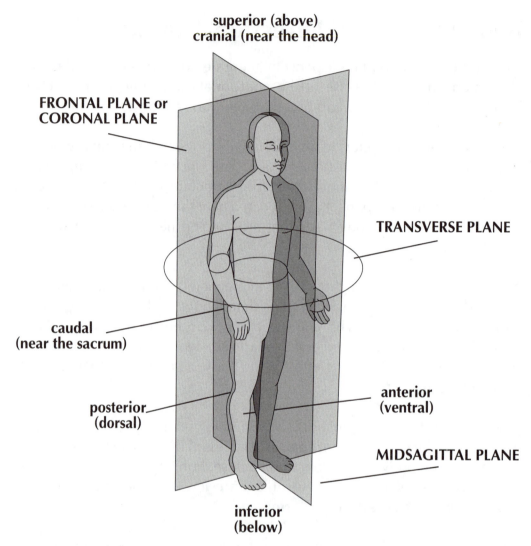

superior (above)
cranial (near the head)

**FRONTAL PLANE or
CORONAL PLANE**

TRANSVERSE PLANE

caudal
(near the sacrum)

posterior
(dorsal)

anterior
(ventral)

MIDSAGITTAL PLANE

inferior
(below)

Figure 13-4: Directional Planes and Terms

Other locational terms used extensively in the healthcare field are distal, proximal, external and internal. **Distal** indicates that something lies distant to the point of attachment or original reference point (ie, the radial pulse is distal to the upper arm). **Proximal** means the opposite of distal; the body part (or something else, such as a wound, incision, etc.) is close to the reference point. For example, in reference to the shoulder, the elbow is proximal and the wrist is distal. **External** generally refers to a location outside of, or near to the surface of the body. For example, the ribs are said to be external to the heart because they surround the heart. **Internal** refers to a location that is inside the body. For example, the stomach is an internal organ. Internal wounds or incisions are said to be *deep* and external wounds are described as *superficial*. Make sure you understand these terms and use them correctly.

The Body Cavities

There are many cavities (hollow spaces) within the body. Each contains specific organs. For example, the **posterior**, or **dorsal**, **cavity** is located along the back of the body and is divided into two sections. The **cranial cavity** contains the brain, and the **spinal cavity** contains the spinal cord. The spinal cord and the brain, along with cranial and spinal nerves and their branches, make up the nervous system.

The **anterior**, or **ventral**, **cavity** is located along the front part of the body and is separated into three distinct sections: the **thoracic cavity**, which is located within the chest and contains the heart, lungs, and large blood vessels; the **abdominal cavity**, which is subdivided into the upper and lower regions; and the **pelvic cavity** which contains the urinary bladder, the last part of the large intestine, and the reproductive organs. The abdominal cavity contains several organs. Their location is simplified by further separating the upper and lower regions into four quadrants. The four quadrants are created by the imaginary lines formed from both the midsagittal and the transverse directional planes.

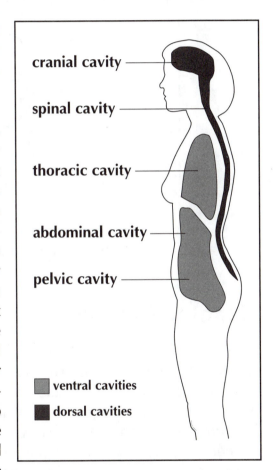

Figure 13-5: The Body Cavities

The **left upper quadrant**, often abbreviated **LUQ**, contains the pancreas, stomach, and spleen. The **right upper quadrant (RUQ)** contains such organs as the liver and gallbladder. The **right lower quadrant (RLQ)** contains the appendix and, in the female, some of the reproductive organs. The **left lower quadrant (LLQ)** contains part of the intestines and, in the female, other organs of the reproductive system. Both the large and small intestines are found throughout the entire abdominal cavity.

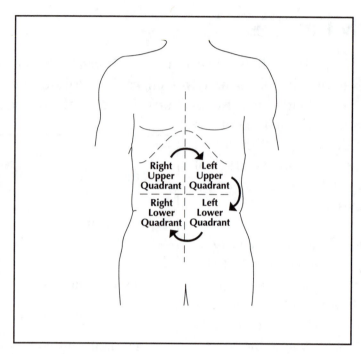

Figure 13-6: The Abdominal Quadrants

Chapter Summary

Studies in anatomy must include learning about the directional planes as well as the body cavities. The basis of all living organisms is the cell. Common cells form together and become tissues; common tissues combine and form organs; and similar organs form systems. The following chapters will provide basic anatomy and physiologic information concerning each of the body's systems. This information will help you understand the patient's illness as well as changes in his or her condition.

Name _____

Date _____

Student Enrichment Activities

Complete the following statements.

1. The jelly-like material contained within a cell is called _____.

2. The _____ is the basis of all living things.

3. The two types of cell division are _____ and _____.

4. The amount of energy released during the chemical reactions that occur in cells is determined by _____.

5. The four types of tissues are _____, _____, _____, and _____.

6. _____ muscle attaches to bones and permits movement.

7. Imaginary lines that separate the body into sections are called _____ _____.

8. The _____, or _____, cavity is the body cavity located along the front part of the body.

Unscramble the following terms.

9. MEADE   _____

10. POISADE   _____

11. EOSSUOS   _____

12. THLIAPEIEL   _____

13. SVRETRENSA LAPEN   _____ _____

14. GLIATTDISAM LAPNE   _____ _____

15. SODRLA CYTIVA   _____ _____

16. CITRHOAC AVTICY   _____ _____

Chapter Fourteen
Support, Movement, and Protection: The Skeletal, Muscular, and Integumentary Systems

Objectives

After completing this chapter, you should be able to
do the following:

1. Define and correctly spell each of the key terms.

2. Identify the components of the integumentary system.

3. Name and explain four main functions of the skin.

4. Identify the sections of the skeletal system and describe the function and components of each.

5. Identify and describe three types of joints found within the body.

6. Describe five types of muscle movement.

7. Describe some of the most common diseases that can affect the described systems.

8. Name and describe some of the most common diagnostic tests for diseases of each of the described systems.

Key Terms

- alimentary canal
- appendicular skeleton
- axial skeleton
- constrict
- dilate

- gland
- joint
- peristalsis
- synovial fluid

The Systems That Shape Our Bodies

This chapter is devoted to providing you with information regarding basic anatomy and physiology for each of the body's systems concerned with support, movement, and protection. Each system builds upon the other systems. The **skeletal** system provides a framework of support and shape for the body, and protects the internal organs from damage. The **muscular** system provides shape and support for the **integumentary** system, and provides additional protection for the internal organs. The integumentary system helps protect the body from infection and illness by preventing the entry of pathogens. Each of these systems will be examined in more detail throughout this chapter.

The Skeletal System And Joints

The skeletal system provides a framework of support for the soft tissues of the body. Each of the 206 bones that form the human skeleton plays a passive, but essential, role in movement. The skeletal system performs five specific functions.

1. Provides support for the muscles, fat, and soft tissues.

2. Protects the internal organs.

3. Provides leverage for lifting and movement through the attachment of muscles.

4. Produces blood cells.

5. Stores the majority of the body's calcium supply.

Bones, which are composed primarily of calcium and phosphorous, are classified into four groups.

1. **Long:** bones in which the length is greater than the width, such as the femur, humerus, tibia, and radius.

2. **Short:** blocky bones that are closely joined and those in which there is no relationship between their length and width, such as the wrist (carpal) and ankle (tarsal) bones.

3. **Flat:** bones that are composed of two relatively parallel plates of compact bone that are separated by a layer of spongy bone, such as the scapula (shoulder) and skull.

4. **Irregular:** bones of complex shape and structure, such as the facial bones and vertebrae.

The long bones have four basic parts. The long shaft is known as the **diaphysis**, and at each of its ends is an **epiphysis**. The **medullary canal** is the cavity in the diaphysis that is filled with yellow marrow (fat cells). The **endosteum** is the lining of the medullary canal that keeps the yellow marrow intact.

The outside layer of every bone is called the **periosteum**. The specialized cells in this layer promote bone growth (**ossification**), nutrition, and repair.

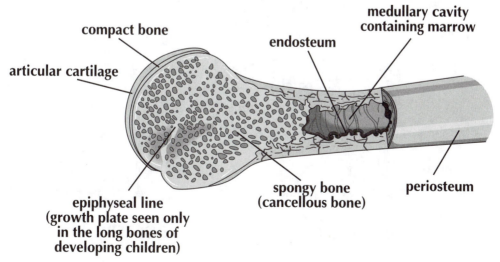

Figure 14-1: The Parts of a Bone

Some bones contain **red bone marrow**, which is the primary site for the formation of all blood cells: **erythrocytes** (red blood cells), **leukocytes** (white blood cells), and **thrombocytes** (platelets). The bones that contain red bone marrow are the ribs, **sternum** (breastbone), **vertebrae** (spinal bones), **scapula** (shoulder), and the proximal ends of the **femur** (thigh bone) and **humerus** (upper arm bone).

axial skeleton: a division of the skeletal system that includes the main trunk of the body, the skull, the spinal column, the ribs, and the sternum

The skeletal system is divided into two distinct sections: the **axial skeleton** and the **appendicular skeleton**. The axial skeleton is the main trunk of the body and includes the skull, spinal column, ribs, and sternum. The appendicular skeleton is formed from the extremities (arms and legs), shoulder girdle, and the pelvic girdle. (See Figure 14-2.)

appendicular skeleton: the part of the skeletal system formed by the extremities, shoulder girdle, and pelvic girdle

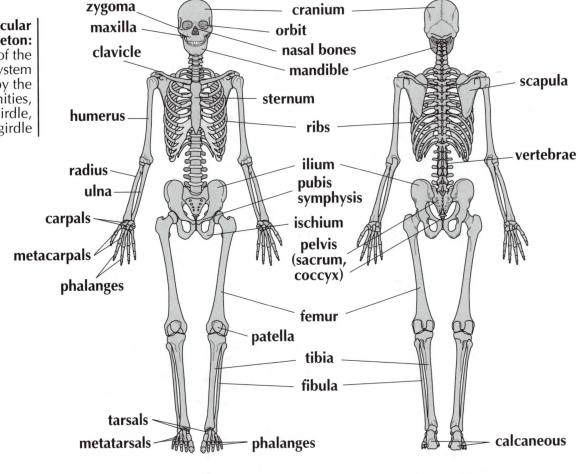

zygoma
maxilla
clavicle
humerus
radius
ulna
carpals
metacarpals
phalanges

cranium
orbit
nasal bones
mandible
sternum
ribs
ilium
pubis
symphysis
ischium
pelvis (sacrum, coccyx)
femur
patella
tibia
fibula
phalanges

scapula
vertebrae
calcaneous

tarsals
metatarsals

ANTERIOR   **POSTERIOR**

Figure 14-2: The Major Bones of the Skeletal System

Disorders of the Skeletal System

A variety of disorders can affect the skeletal system. Some are listed below.

- **fracture:** a break in the continuity of a bone; usually results from a direct or indirect force, or a twisting of forces.

- **osteomyelitis:** severe inflammation of bone and bone marrow, resulting from a bacterial infection. This can occur if an infection that has been introduced through the skin goes untreated.

- **osteoporosis:** a condition that describes bones that have calcium and phosphorous deficiencies. Bones affected by osteoporosis are very porous and fracture easily. This condition naturally occurs in women as they age due to estrogen and other hormonal and mineral deficiencies.

Diagnostic Tests for the Skeletal System

There are a variety of diagnostic tests that allow the physician to check the health of the skeletal system. Some of the more common tests are listed below.

- **bone density studies:** a method of determining how porous bone is, using radiographic techniques.

- **bone marrow biopsy:** the extraction of a small amount of bone marrow for microscopic examination.

- **bone scan:** a nuclear medicine procedure, in which a special kind of medication is either ingested orally or injected directly into the vein. A machine is then scanned over the particular area of the body to detect the amount of radiant energy released from the medication. This information allows the physician to detect fractures, osteoporosis, cancer, and, growths.

- **computerized tomography (CT) scan:** a technique for examining transverse planes of internal structures of the body in which x-rays are used to construct a precise image and show the relationship of structures.

- **magnetic resonance imaging (MRI):** a diagnostic procedure in which parts of the body are exposed to an electromagnetic field to produce an image.

- **x-rays:** radiographs; film images, created by the projection of high energy electromagnetic waves through an area of a patient's body onto a photographic plate, which show the bony structures and specific organ outlines in that area of the body.

Joints: Articulation and Movement

joint:
a place where
two or more
bones meet

Joints allow movement according to their range of motion. There are three types of joints.

1. **fibrous:** (immovable) includes the bones of the cranium, or skull.

2. **cartilaginous:** (slightly moveable) includes the vertebrae in the spine.

3. **synovial:** (freely moveable) includes the elbow, knee, fingers, etc.

Mobile joints are grouped according to the way in which they work. For example, **pivot** joints allow rotation on a single axis and **hinge** joints allow the adjoining parts to bend and straighten. See Figure 14-3 for examples of the different groups of joints.

synovial fluid:
the clear fluid
surrounding a
joint; like
all other body
fluids, this fluid
is capable of
transmitting the
AIDS virus

Special bands of white connective tissue attach bone to bone to form a joint. These connective tissues are called **ligaments**. **Tendons** are fibrous connective tissues that attach muscle to bones. The joint is enclosed in a protective capsule that contains **synovial fluid**. This fluid is colorless and contains mineral salts, fat, and other substances. It acts as a shock absorber and cushions both ends of the bone so they do not irritate each other. There are other structures that protect the bones too. A **bursa** is a sac full of synovial fluid that reduces friction between tendons, bones, ligaments, and other structures. A **meniscus** is a fluid-filled disc that also reduces friction during movement.

Diseases and Injuries of the Joints

Because joints are in constant use, they are susceptible to injuries, inflammation, and stress. The following are the most common disorders affecting the joints.

*   **arthritis:** inflammation of the joint.

*   **bursitis:** inflammation of a bursa.

*   **dislocation:** the separation of a joint and the malposition of an extremity.

*   **gout:** the accumulation of uric acid crystals in a joint.

*   **sprain:** injury to the soft tissues of a joint, characterized by the inability to move, deformity, and pain.

Motion Groups for Joints

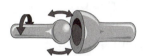

ball & socket

A round end of one bone fits into a cup-like end of another bone, allowing a wide range of movement. The shoulder and the hip are examples of ball and socket joints.

pivot

A projection fits through a ring made up of bone and ligament, allowing only pivoting movement. The first and second cervical vertebrae (the atlas and the axis) are pivot joints.

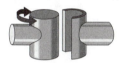

hinge

A joint in which the two surfaces are molded together closely, allowing a wide range of flexion and extension along a single plane. The elbow is a hinge joint.

saddle

A joint in which two surfaces, one convex and the other concave, fit together. A saddle joint can be found in the thumb.

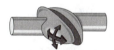

condyloid (ellipsoid)

A rounded or oval end of a bone fits into an oval cavity, allowing all types of movement except pivoting. One of the wrist joints is a condyloid joint.

gliding

Two facing bone surfaces meet, allowing only gliding movements. Motion is limited by surrounding tissues and ligaments. The wrist and the ankles contain examples of gliding joints.

Figure 14-3: Motion Groups for Joints

Diagnostic Tests for Joints

Patients who experience disorders of the skeletal system often seek care from physical therapists and other rehabilitation specialists. The following are the most common tests for diagnosing diseases and injuries of the joints.

- **arthrogram:** the injection of dye into a specific joint followed by a series of x-rays.

- **arthroscopy:** the visual examination of all aspects of a joint using a special instrument that contains a light and camera.

- **aspiration:** the removal of excessive fluid from the synovial space through a needle.

- **x-rays:** film images, created by the projection of high energy electromagnetic waves through an area of the patient's body onto a photographic plate, which show the bony structures and specific organ outlines in that area of the body.

The Muscular System

The human body is composed of over 600 muscles. Each of these muscles helps us move in different ways. They are made up of bundles of tiny contractile muscle fibers, which are held together by connective tissue. These highly conductive muscle fibers initiate movement when they are stimulated by nerve endings. This stimulation causes the muscle fibers to become short and thick (contract) causing movement of the organs and parts of the body.

There are many types of movement, and different muscles are capable of causing different types of movement. **Rotation** is the turning, or circular motion, of a body part on its axis. The movement of a body part toward the middle of the body is called **adduction**; and the opposite motion, the movement of a body part away from the middle of the body, is called **abduction**. **Extension** is the movement which results in an increased angle between two bones, or straightening of a body part; and the movement which results in a decreased angle between two bones, or bending a body part, is known as **flexion**. The muscular system performs hundreds of movements daily; many times without a person consciously thinking about them!

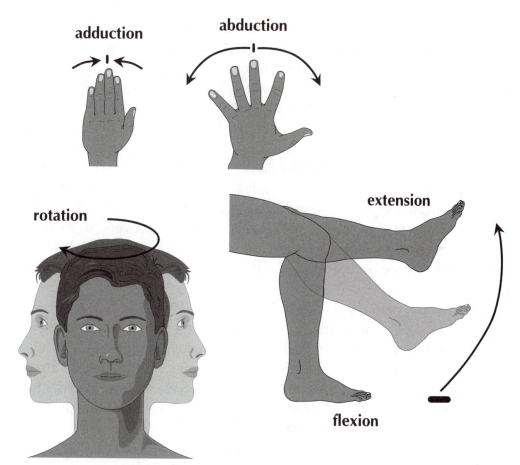

Figure 14-4: Types of Movement

As you learned in Chapter Thirteen, the body is composed of three types of muscle tissue. The first is called **cardiac** muscle. This special type of muscle fiber makes up the walls of the heart. Cardiac muscle is involuntary; that is, the brain controls it automatically. The heart continues to beat and pump blood to the lungs and throughout the body without you having to think about it.

The second type of muscle fiber found in the body is known as smooth, or **visceral**, muscle and is found throughout the body in the internal organs. Visceral muscle is found in the respiratory and digestive tracts, the blood vessels, and in the eyes. Smooth muscles are made up of long and circular fibers. This special arrangement allows for wavelike movement, called **peristalsis**, to occur throughout the digestive tract, or **alimentary canal**. Like the cardiac muscle, this type of muscle is involuntary.

peristalsis: rhythmic, wavelike motion that occurs throughout the digestive tract, and which causes the contents of the alimentary canal to be forced onward

alimentary canal: a general term for the digestive tract

The third kind of muscle is known as skeletal, also called **striated** or voluntary. These muscles are attached to the bones, and produce movement upon command from the brain. There are two points of attachment: the **point of origin** and the **point of insertion**. The point of origin is the end where movement does not occur. The point of insertion is the end where movement occurs. Skeletal muscles are attached to bones by **tendons**. A tendon is a very strong, fibrous connective tissue that acts as an anchor. An example of a tendon securing a muscle to a bone is the **Achilles tendon**. This tendon is located at the bottom of the calf, on the **gastrocnemius muscle**, and secures that muscle to the heel bone, or **calcaneus**. Some muscles are attached to other body parts or other muscles by **fascia**. Fascia is a fibrous membrane that covers, supports, and separates muscle. For example, lumbodorsal fascia surrounds and protects the deep muscles of the back. Fascia also connects the skin to underlying tissues.

Muscles remain partially contracted at all times. This is true even when the muscles are at rest. This partial state of contraction is known as **muscle tone**. Proper muscle tone means that the muscles are ready for action. When muscles are not used over a period of time, they lose their tone. This is known as **atrophy**, and occurs with paralysis and other conditions. When atrophy exists for an extended period of time, a joint may become damaged and remain in a flexed position. This is known as a **contracture**. If this occurs, the patient is unable to extend those muscles or move those joints.

Muscles throughout the body are different sizes and shapes. This is part of what gives the body its contour or form. For example, the muscles of the trunk are long, broad, flat, and expanded; however, the muscles of the extremities are long and round. The major muscles of the body are shown in Figure 14-6.

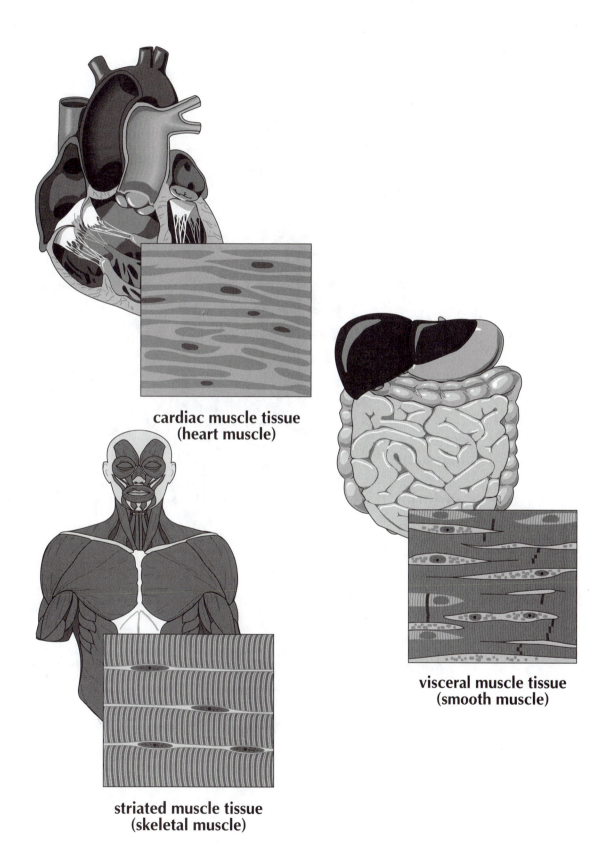

**cardiac muscle tissue
(heart muscle)**

**visceral muscle tissue
(smooth muscle)**

**striated muscle tissue
(skeletal muscle)**

Figure 14-5: The Muscle Types

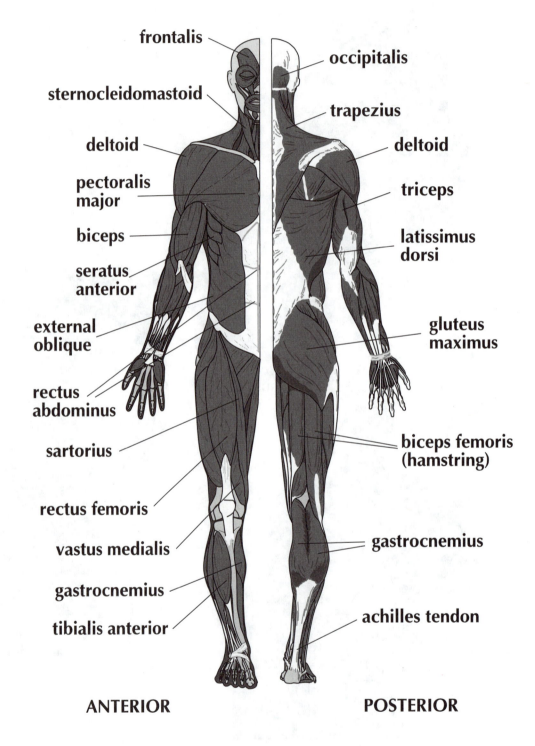

frontalis

occipitalis

sternocleidomastoid

trapezius

deltoid

deltoid

pectoralis major

triceps

biceps

latissimus dorsi

seratus anterior

external oblique

gluteus maximus

rectus abdominus

sartorius

biceps femoris (hamstring)

rectus femoris

vastus medialis

gastrocnemius

gastrocnemius

tibialis anterior

achilles tendon

ANTERIOR

POSTERIOR

Figure 14-6: The Major Muscles of the Body

Muscular Diseases

There are many disorders that may affect the muscle tissue of the body. The body's muscles may be adversely affected by disease processes that result in generalized muscle weakness, **atrophy**, disfigurement, and in some diseases, death. Death can result due to atrophy and paralysis of muscles involved with breathing and circulation. Remember—the heart is a muscle. If it becomes diseased, a life-threatening situation is possible. The following are examples of muscular disorders.

- **muscular dystrophy:** a **congenital**, progressive disease that results in wasting and atrophy of muscles.

- **myositis:** inflammation of muscle that may be caused by irritation or a pathogen.

- **myalgia:** muscle pain that may be caused by any number of reasons.

Diagnostic Tests for the Muscular System

Because so much depends on the proper functioning of our muscles, several tests have been developed to evaluate the condition of the muscular system. A **biopsy** involves the removal of a sample of living tissue for microscopic examination to assist with diagnosis of medical problems. **Strength testing** is the process of determining the strength of specific muscles through the use of weights. Strength testing is often used to monitor disease progression as well as muscular rehabilitation following an injury.

The Integumentary System

The integumentary system is comprised of the external portion of the body: the skin, hair, nails, **glands**, and receptors. This is the largest system of the human body. The skin is very pliable and forms a protective covering on the external surface of the body.

There are three main layers of skin: the epidermis, the dermis, and the subcutaneous. The **epidermis** is the outer layer of skin. It is actually made up of six smaller layers. The epidermis does not contain any blood vessels. This is the layer of skin that constantly sheds old skin cells and reproduces new ones. The coloring, or **pigmentation** of the skin, is determined from the amount of **melanin** contained within the epidermis. The more melanin a person has, the darker his or her skin color will be. The **dermis** also is known as the true skin, or **corium**. This is the layer of skin that contains the elastic framework, where the skin's strength comes from, as well as the blood vessels, nerves, hair follicles, sweat glands, and involuntary muscles. The **subcutaneous tissue** is the innermost layer of skin. It is composed of elastic, fibrous, and adipose connective tissue. This layer of skin actually connects the other layers of skin to the underlying muscles.

A gland is a structure within the body that secretes a substance used elsewhere in the body. Two types of glands are found within the integumentary system: **sudoriferous** (sweat) and **sebaceous** (oil). The pores of the epidermis are the actual openings of the sudoriferous glands. These glands are coiled tubes that extend through the dermis to the epidermis. They produce perspiration, which cools the body. The sebaceous glands most frequently open into the end of a **hair follicle**. The production of oil helps keep the hair soft. If, for some reason, a sebaceous gland on the scalp or the face becomes closed, the oil is not allowed to be released; thereby causing a fluid-filled sac, or **cyst**, to form. Cysts may or may not be surgically removed, depending on the size, the location, and whether it is painful.

Two other parts of the integumentary system are the hair and the nails. Each strand of hair is composed of a root, which grows in a hollow tube called a hair follicle, and the hair shaft. The main purpose of hair is to help protect the skin. **Nails** are dead epithelial cells. These cells are packed together closely to form a very thick surface, which protects the ends of the phalanges from injury. If a nail becomes injured or is removed, it can grow again if the nail bed has not been damaged.

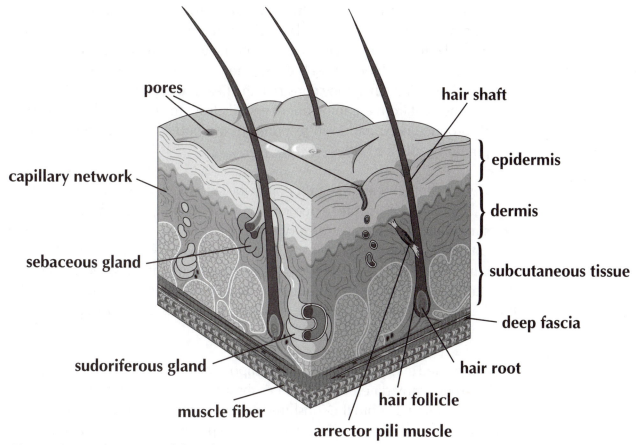

Figure 14-7: The Parts of the Skin

The skin has the following functions:

- protection
- temperature regulation
- sensory perception
- absorption and excretion

Each of these functions are closely related. In Chapter Nine you learned that many different pathogens occur naturally on the surface of the skin. When it is intact, the skin provides a protective barrier. Once that barrier has been broken by a laceration, puncture wound, or abrasion, pathogens can enter into the deeper layers of the skin and may begin to multiply. This can result in a localized infection or an infection that spreads throughout the circulatory system.

dilate:
to become
larger

constrict:
to become
smaller

The skin also helps maintain **homeostasis** through two mechanisms: the **sudoriferous** glands and the blood vessels contained within the skin. The blood vessels will either **dilate** or **constrict** according to the temperature demands of the body. When the blood vessels dilate, more heat is allowed to escape to the surface of the skin. When they constrict, the heat is directed internally; thereby keeping the heat from escaping unnecessarily from the body. The sudoriferous glands produce perspiration in response to the body's elevated temperature. Perspiration cools the body.

Sensory perception is another function of the skin. The skin contains numerous nerves that make it possible to perceive pain, heat, cold, and different levels of pressure. Many times these sensory receptors prevent extensive injury to the skin layers. A simple example of this occurs whenever a person touches something hot. The sensory nerves in the fingers send the message of pain and heat to the brain, which sends a motor message to remove the hand from the hot item. This helps reduce the risk of developing burns through all the skin layers.

Absorption and excretion are two other important functions. The skin is capable of absorbing many different substances through its surface including medications and Vitamin D from the sunshine. Because of the sudoriferous glands, the body can excrete waste products in the form of perspiration. Perspiration serves two purposes; it helps maintain appropriate body temperature, and it aids in the excretion of waste by-products.

Skin colors vary greatly. Caucasian and Oriental skins contain melanin in the first two layers of skin; however, African and African-American skin contains melanin in all three layers. Prolonged exposure to the ultraviolet rays of the sun results in tanning, or an increase in the amount of melanin. Tanning is the skin's method of protecting itself from those ultraviolet rays.

Skin Diseases and Disorders

As with any of the other body systems, the integumentary system can develop certain problems. A common skin disturbance is a rash, which generally refers to a skin eruption. The degree of **erythema** (skin redness) usually depends on the severity of the rash and/or the causes. Certain communicable diseases and allergic reactions can cause a rash. A rash may appear as **macules**, which are flat skin eruptions, or **papules**, which are firm red areas on the skin. Another common skin eruption is a **wart**, which is an eruption of the epidermis that resembles a cauliflower in shape. Warts are caused by a particular type of virus.

Other skin disorders include dermatitis and various kinds of skin cancer. **Dermatitis** is an inflammation of the skin that often affects the epidermis. There are varying degrees of dermatitis as well as different causes, including severe allergic reactions and bacterial infections. For example, the skin's appearance may range from erythema to **pustules**. Pustules are skin elevations that are filled with a liquid that contains white blood cells and bacteria. Skin cancer most frequently occurs in those body areas that receive excessive exposure to the sun. **Malignant melanoma** is a very serious form of skin cancer. *Malignant* indicates that it is cancer and *melanoma* refers to a pigmented mole or tumor. This is a very fast-spreading cancer and frequently is fatal if early and adequate treatment is not received.

The following are additional disorders that can affect the skin.

- **acne:** an inflammatory disease of the sebaceous glands; usually on the face.

- **burns:** tissue damage from excessive exposure to heat, chemical, electricity or radiation. Depending on the number of skin layers affected, burns may be classified as superficial, partial thickness, or full thickness burns.

- **decubitus ulcers:** (commonly known as pressure, or bed sores) tissue damage resulting from reduced circulation of blood to a given area.

Disorders that affect other parts of the integumentary system include alopecia, commonly known as baldness, and onychia, a bacterial disease of the nails.

Diagnostic Tests for the Skin

The treatment of skin disorders depends upon the cause of the disorder. For instance, skin cancer may be treated through surgery, whereas acne is usually treated with an oral or topical medication. Therefore, diagnosing the disorder is the first step in the treatment of any type of skin disease. Two of the tests that are done to determine specific skin disorders are listed below.

- **culture and sensitivity:** a laboratory test for bacterial growth that involves instilling microorganisms in special media, monitoring them for the growth of pathogens, and then determining how susceptible the patient's bacterial infection is to certain antibiotics or antibacterial drugs.
- **skin scrapings:** epithelial cells that are scraped onto a glass slide and examined for diagnosis.

Skin disorders, because they are so visible, can be quite traumatic for the people who experience them. Self-consciousness is common among sufferers of skin diseases, leading to behavior that is directly related to their altered self-esteem. Be especially compassionate and understanding with these patients; an extra kind word or touch can make a world of difference! Diagnostic tests can be frightening to the patient; after all, hospital procedures are unfamiliar to most patients. Take time to answer patients' questions with simple, but accurate explanations.

Chapter Summary

The skeletal system provides the framework for the body. There are four basic shapes of bones. Bones attach to each other by ligaments, forming a joint. Joints allow for various body parts to move. The muscular system provides strength and helps control movement. Muscles are attached to bones by tendons. The integumentary system acts as a protective barrier from pathogens and holds everything in its place. Through the skin, the body is able to maintain homeostasis.

All of the systems have specific diseases that can affect them. Learning to recognize these diseases and the way they affect the body systems will help you better understand the patient's condition.

Name _____

Date _____

Student Enrichment Activities

Complete the following statements.

1. The two main types of glands contained within the integumentary system are
    _____ and _____.

2. Four functions of the skin are _____, _____,
    _____, and _____.

3. The integumentary system includes _____, _____,
    _____, _____ and _____.

4. _____ _____ is a serious form of skin cancer.

5. The human skeleton contains _____ bones.

6. Bones are made up primarily from two minerals: _____ and
    _____.

7. Name the five functions of the human skeleton.
    A. _____ .
    B. _____ .
    C. _____ .
    D. _____ .
    E. _____ .

8. The skeleton is divided into the _____ and the _____
    sections.

9. Name the four types of bone and provide one example of each:

    A. _____ .

    B. _____ .

    C. _____ .

    D. _____ .

10. Name three kinds of joints and provide one example of each.

    A. _____ .

    B. _____ .

    C. _____ .

11. The body is made up of over _____ muscles.

12. The three kinds of muscle tissue are _____, _____,

    and _____.

13. Name five types of movement of which muscles are capable.

    A. _____   D. _____

    B. _____   E. _____

    C. _____

Unscramble the following terms.

14. SHOASSMEIOT   _____

15. PRATHOY   _____

16. XELIFON   _____

17. SLAMCUE   _____

Name _____

Date _____

18. SUMEHUR

_____

19. SLAPRIESTIS

_____

20. SLUUPTES

_____

21. CAUBSEOSE

_____

22. MEITISLOSTYEO

_____

23. ITALED

_____

24. CNSRTOICT

_____

25. MSYTIISO

_____

Chapter Fifteen
Transporting and Transmitting: The Circulatory, Lymphatic, and Nervous Systems

Objectives

After completing this chapter you should be able to
do the following:

1.　Define and correctly spell each of the key terms.

2.　Name and define the three types of blood vessels and at least four kinds of blood cells.

3.　Describe the path of a drop of blood through the body.

4.　Identify and explain the diseases that can affect the circulatory, lymphatic, and nervous systems.

5.　Describe the common diagnostic tests for the circulatory, lymphatic, and nervous systems.

6.　Name the primary functions of the circulatory, lymphatic, and nervous systems.

7.　Identify the three nervous systems and their components.

8.　List and describe the five main parts of the brain.

Key Terms

- alveoli
- artery
- atrium
- autonomic nervous system
- capillaries
- central nervous system
- cerebrospinal fluid
- gas exchange
- meninges
- motor neurons
- nerve
- parasympathetic nervous system
- peripheral nervous system
- sensory neurons
- sinoatrial node
- somatic nervous system
- sympathetic nervous system
- vein
- ventricle

The Body's Transportation Systems

The circulatory, lymphatic, and nervous systems are responsible for transporting or transmitting in the body. Both the circulatory and lymphatic systems transport substances throughout the body. The nervous system, through its complex and intricate composition, acts as the computer for the body. Each system is important to the health and well-being of every person. If all or part of a system fails, medical intervention will be needed.

The Circulatory System

The circulatory system also is known as the **cardiovascular** system. **Cardi/o** is a combining form that refers to the heart, and **vascular** refers to blood vessels. The cardiovascular system is a closed transportation system; it does not have an outlet to the outside of the body. The purpose of this system is to transport blood from the heart to the lungs, back to the heart, and to all other body parts. Many miles of blood vessels help accomplish this amazing process.

Blood Vessels

There are several types of blood vessels in the body, and each of them performs a specific function. The three main kinds of vessels are arteries, capillaries, and veins. **Arteries** are the blood vessels that carry highly **oxygenated** blood away from the heart to all the other body parts. Oxygenated blood contains oxygen from the lungs. The largest artery in the body is the **aorta**. It branches directly off the heart. Throughout its length, it divides into arteries that nourish specific organs and tissues of the body. This is known as the **systemic** circulation. The **pulmonary**, or lung, circulation receives low-oxygenated blood from the right side of the heart and includes all parts of the lungs. As the blood circulates through the lungs, it receives oxygen from the **alveoli**. The oxygen then can be transported to other body parts. Arteries contain three muscular layers: the **tunica intima**, or inner lining; the **tunica media**, or middle layer; and the **tunica adventitia**, or outer layer. The strength of these layers allows the arteries to receive the blood that is being pumped under high pressure from the heart. Arteries further subdivide into smaller branches called **arterioles**. These, in turn, join with even smaller vessels known as capillaries.

Capillaries are the smallest blood vessels in the body. A capillary has only one thin wall that allows oxygen and nutrients to pass through into each cell. It is at this level where the **gas exchange** occurs. Cells receive oxygen from the bloodstream and tissues, and release carbon dioxide as a waste product. One end of the capillary is joined to the arteriole, and the other end is joined to one of many small veins, known as venules.

Venules accept the blood from the capillaries and transport it directly into the veins. **Veins** are composed of three layers; however, the total thickness of the wall is thinner than an artery. Since veins are transporting blood back to the heart, they contain one-way valves that keep blood from flowing backwards. Because of the low concentration of oxygen in the veins, the blood is a deep, dark red. In contrast to this, the blood contained in the arteries has a high oxygen concentration and is bright red. **Lacerations**, or cuts, often result in active bleeding. If only veins have been lacerated, the blood will resemble a stream; however, if an artery is lacerated, the blood will be spurting. Moreover, pulses are only felt in arteries, not veins. These differences in the force of blood through the different vessels are due to the pumping action of the heart.

artery: a blood vessel that carries highly oxygenated blood away from the heart to the tissues

alveoli: microscopic air sacs within the lungs responsible for the exchange of oxygen and carbon dioxide

capillaries: tiny blood vessels in the circulatory system that link arteries and veins

gas exchange: the process of exchanging oxygen for carbon dioxide in the blood during breathing; this process takes place in the alveoli in the lungs

vein: a blood vessel that carries low-oxygenated blood to the heart

Blood and Blood Cells

Blood is composed of several different types of blood cells, fluid, and many different chemical substances. It is approximately 78% water and about 22% various solids. The fluid portion of the blood is known as **plasma**. Plasma contains many different substances including special proteins like **fibrinogen** and **prothrombin**. These proteins cause the blood to clot, which stops active bleeding. Other specific substances contained in the plasma include carbohydrates, proteins, calcium, sodium, gases (such as oxygen and carbon dioxide), hormones, **enzymes**, and waste products. The blood performs many important functions to sustain life. It transports nourishment, hormones, vitamins, oxygen, and heat to the tissues, and removes waste products and carbon dioxide.

Erythrocytes, or red blood cells (RBCs), are the largest part of the solids contained in the blood. Erythrocytes live only for about 120 days. Therefore, they are continually being reproduced by the **red bone marrow** located in the femur (the thigh bone), the hip, the sternum (breast bone), humerus (upper arm bone), some of the cranial bones, and in the vertebrae (spinal column). The main function of erythrocytes is to carry oxygen and carbon dioxide. They are red because of a very complex protein contained within each red blood cell. This protein is known as **hemoglobin**. Once oxygen connects to it, each cell becomes red. The more oxygen there is, the brighter red the erythrocytes become. Consequently, the opposite also is true; when less oxygen is present, the erythrocytes become a darker red.

A **platelet** or **thrombocyte** is an extremely specialized type of blood cell. This cell is produced to coagulate, or clot, the blood. A delicate balance of platelets and erythrocytes must be maintained within the blood—life depends on it!

Leukocytes, or white blood cells (WBCs), are another type of blood cell. There are two different kinds of leukocytes: **granulocytes**, which contain granules in their cytoplasm, such as neutrophils, basophils, and eosinophils; and **agranulocytes** (leukocytes that do not have granules in their cytoplasm), such as lymphocytes and monocytes. Leukocytes are produced in various locations throughout the body. For example, the granulocytes are produced in the bone marrow; the lymphocytes are formed mostly in the lymph nodes; and the monocytes are produced from the cells that line the walls of the capillaries and are found in specific body organs such as the spleen. The main function of leukocytes is to fight various infections. They act as scavengers and destroy

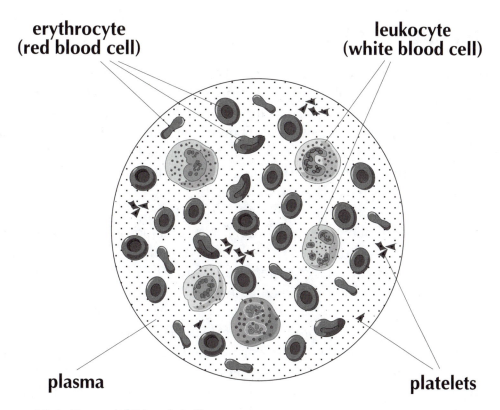

Figure 15-1: Types of Blood Cells

bacteria, viruses, fungi, and other pathogens. Sometimes the leukocytes are outnumbered by the pathogens. When this happens, the leukocytes die and clump together. This collection of dead leukocytes and other cells that result from infection is known as **pus**. If the dead white blood cells are unable to escape from the body, they form an **abscess**. Leukocytes are the basis of the immune system and are necessary for good health.

An average adult has 5 to 6 quarts of blood in the body. This blood is circulated throughout the vascular system every 20 seconds. This is accomplished by the amazing pumping capacity of the heart.

The Pump of Life

Located in the middle of the anterior chest and slightly on the left side, the heart is a four-chambered, hollow, muscular organ that automatically pumps 60 to 100 times a minute in an average adult. If a person's pulse is 72 beats per minute, then that person's heart beats 104,000 times a day, and 38 million times during one year. The natural pacemaker of the heart is located in the **right atrium** and is called the **sinoatrial node**. The electrical activity conducted by the heart determines the pulse rate of each individual.

The heart, which is about the size of your fist, is contained in the **thoracic cavity** of the body, and is tilted slightly to the left of the sternum. It is located between the lungs and surrounded by the **pericardial sac**. The pericardial sac is a thin layer of tissue that surrounds the entire heart.

The heart is composed of three layers of tissue: the smooth innermost layer, called the **endocardium**; the muscular middle layer, called the **myocardium**; and the outermost layer, called the **epicardium**, which is serous (watery) in appearance. The heart contains four chambers, and is divided into right and left halves. The right and left halves of the heart are separated by a **myocardial septum**. This prevents blood from flowing between the right and left sides. The upper chambers of the heart are separated from the lower chambers by several one-way valves. A one-way valve also separates the heart from the lungs and prevents blood leaving the heart from backflowing into the lungs. The upper chambers of the heart are receiving chambers. The left receiving chamber is known as the left **atrium**, and the right receiving chamber is called the right atrium. Together they are called the atria. The lower chambers are the pumping chambers, and are known as the **ventricles**. It is important to note that the heart has its own blood supply, consisting of arteries and veins, known as the **coronary circulation**.

---

sinoatrial node:
the natural pacemaker of the heart, located in the upper part of the right atrium

atrium:
either the upper right or left chamber of the heart, also known as a receiving chamber

ventricle:
one of the two pumping chambers of the heart, located inferior to the atria

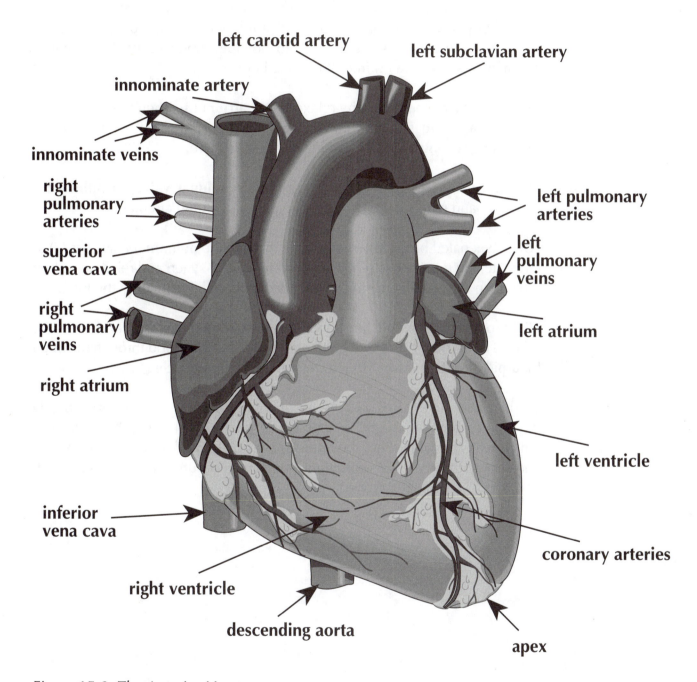

Figure 15-2: The Anterior Heart

The Circulatory Path

Figure 15-3 illustrates the path a drop of blood takes through the heart to all parts of the body. Oxygen-poor (low oxygenated) blood from the peripheral veins enters from the head, neck, and arms into the **superior vena cava** (1), and enters the **inferior vena cava** (2) from the lower body.

Both vena cava empty into the relaxed **right atrium** (3). Then the right atrium contracts and forces blood through the open **tricuspid valve** (4) and into the relaxed **right ventricle** (5), closing the tricuspid valve.

The right ventricle contracts and opens the **semilunar valve**, or **pulmonary valve** (6), and marks the beginning of pulmonary (lung) circulation.

Low-oxygenated blood enters the lungs through the **pulmonary arteries** (7) to circulate and receive oxygen. The blood receives oxygen and releases carbon dioxide in the **alveoli** (air sacs surrounded by capillaries) within the lungs.

Highly oxygenated blood then flows into the **pulmonary veins** (8) and enters the relaxed **left atrium** (9), which contracts and forces the blood through the open **bicuspid** or **mitral valve** (10) into the relaxed **left ventricle** (11).

The bicuspid valve closes, and the left ventricle contracts. This forces the highly oxygenated blood through the open **aortic valve** (12) and into the **aorta** (13), which feeds the blood into the arteries, arterioles, capillaries, venules, veins, and back to the heart. This complete blood cycle occurs with every heart beat.

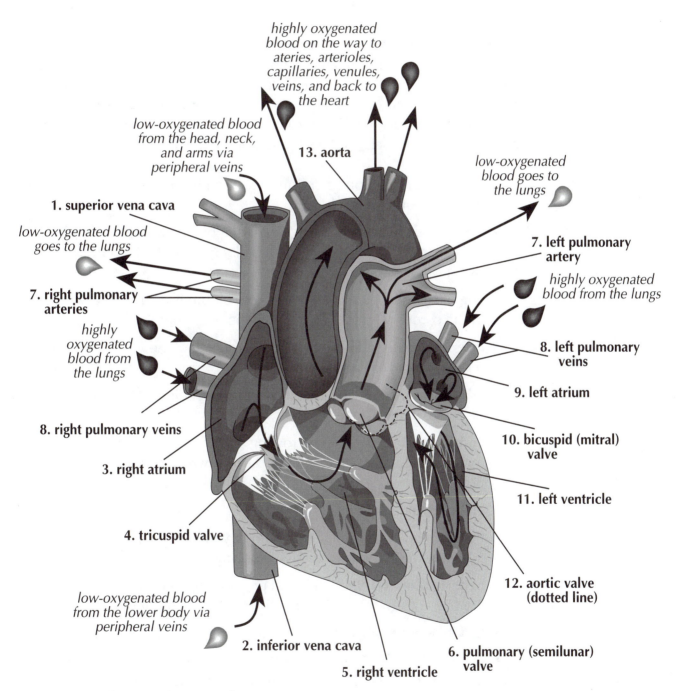

highly oxygenated blood on the way to ateries, arterioles, capillaries, venules, veins, and back to the heart

low-oxygenated blood from the head, neck, and arms via peripheral veins

13. aorta

low-oxygenated blood goes to the lungs

1. superior vena cava

low-oxygenated blood goes to the lungs

7. left pulmonary artery

7. right pulmonary arteries

highly oxygenated blood from the lungs

highly oxygenated blood from the lungs

8. left pulmonary veins

8. right pulmonary veins

9. left atrium

3. right atrium

10. bicuspid (mitral) valve

11. left ventricle

4. tricuspid valve

12. aortic valve (dotted line)

low-oxygenated blood from the lower body via peripheral veins

2. inferior vena cava

6. pulmonary (semilunar) valve

5. right ventricle

Figure 15-3: The Circulatory Path

Conditions of the Circulatory System

Genetics and preventive healthcare affect the overall condition of the circulatory system. Diseases and conditions such as arteriosclerosis, atherosclerosis, coronary artery disease, and hypertension (HTN) may be prevented or reduced beginning in infancy with good dietary habits, regular exercise, managing stress, and not smoking. If these conditions are not prevented, serious illnesses and even death may result by progressing to an aneurysm, angina, or myocardial infarction. These and other conditions that may affect the blood, blood vessels, and heart are listed and defined below.

- **anemia:** a reduction in erythrocytes (red blood cells) or the amount of hemoglobin in the blood.

- **aneurysm:** a weak section of a wall of a blood vessel, that results in the expansion of the vessel like a balloon. If this balloon ruptures, death can result.

- **angina:** cardiac pain caused by a low blood oxygen level (hypoxemia) in the coronary arteries that supply the heart muscle.

- **arteriosclerosis:** a thickening and hardening of the arterial walls that results in poor elasticity.

- **atherosclerosis:** an accumulation of fat or cholesterol that forms a blockage in the arteries.

- **coronary artery disease:** narrowing of the coronary artery lumen (opening), usually due to atherosclerosis, which restricts the blood flow to the myocardium.

- **embolus:** a circulating clot.

- **hemophilia:** a congenital condition in which the blood does not clot normally, resulting in excessive bleeding.

- **hypertension (HTN):** high blood pressure that has been diagnosed on the basis of several random readings of 140/90 or above.

- **hypotension:** an abnormally low blood pressure that impairs functioning.

- **myocardial infarction (MI):** a condition caused by the blockage of one or more coronary arteries, which prevents oxygenated blood from nourishing the myocardium; a heart attack.

- **phlebitis:** inflammation of a vein.

- **thrombus:** a blood clot.

Diagnostic Tests for the Circulatory System

Some of the common diagnostic tests used to evaluate conditions of the circulatory system are listed and defined below.

- **angiography:** a test using x-rays or fluoroscopy that permits a physician to see and evaluate the heart's pumping performance as well as the flow of blood through the coronary arteries following the injection of contrast medium.

- **arterial blood gas test:** a blood test used to determine acidity or alkalinity as well as the oxygen and carbon dioxide levels in the arterial blood.

- **cardiac catheterization:** insertion of a catheter through a chamber of the heart or great vessels for the purpose of diagnostic testing.

- **cardiac enzymes test:** blood tests that confirm that a myocardial infarction has occurred.

- **chest x-ray:** a diagnostic test that produces a view of the position, size, and shape of the heart and the great vessels (the pulmonary arteries, pulmonary veins, and the aorta), as well as the condition of the lungs, through the use of radiation.

- **computerized tomography (CT) scan:** a technique for examining transverse planes of internal structures of the body in which x-rays are used to construct a precise image and show the relationship of structures.

- **echocardiography:** a process that uses ultrasound (sound waves) to reveal the structure of the heart and its valves and evaluate their function.

- **electrocardiography:** the process of recording or tracing the electrical activity of the heart.

- **magnetic resonance imaging (MRI):** a diagnostic procedure in which parts of the body are exposed to an electromagnetic field to produce an image.

- **stress test:** a diagnostic test that is done to evaluate a patient's cardiovascular fitness. The patient's heart and lungs are carefully monitored while the patient performs a controlled physical activity such as walking on a treadmill.

- **venography:** the process of taking an x-ray of a vein to confirm the presence of deep vein thrombosis through the injection of iodine into the vein and observation of the progression of the dye.

The Lymphatic System

The circulatory system and the lymphatic system work together to remove excess fluid and waste products from the tissues. **Lymph** is a colorless fluid that is formed in tissue spaces throughout the body and carried in the lymphatic vessels. The main cells that compose lymph are leukocytes; lymph does not contain erythrocytes.

Lymph is produced at different locations throughout the body. It is picked up by small tubes called **lymphatic capillaries**. These, in turn, join and form larger vessels called **lymphatic vessels**. The lymphatic vessels pass through **lymph nodes**, which also are contained in several different locations throughout the body. Lymph nodes are commonly called glands and range in size from that of a pinhead to the size of an almond. Their main function is to filter impurities, such as pathogens and cancer cells, from the lymph.

Lymphocytes (a type of leukocyte) and **antibodies** (substances produced by the body to use in fighting infection) are produced in the lymph nodes. The purified lymph leaves the lymph node through a single lymph vessel to join other lymph vessels, which continue to combine and eventually form large lymphatic vessels. These larger vessels drain into one of the two lymphatic ducts. The right side of the head and neck, the right side of the chest, and the right upper extremity drain into the **right lymphatic duct**. This particular duct empties the purified lymph into the vein directly underneath the right clavicle (collar bone), called the subclavian vein. The rest of the body releases its purified lymph into the larger duct, called the **thoracic duct**. This empties into the left subclavian vein. At this point the purified lymph enters the bloodstream.

There are several sources of lymphatic tissue throughout the body. It can be found in the **tonsils**, the **spleen**, and the **thymus**. The tonsils are located in three areas of the throat: the **palatine tonsils** are on each side of the palate (the roof of the mouth); the **pharyngeal tonsils**, also called the **adenoids**, are located on the back of the throat; and the **lingual tonsils** are on the back of the tongue. The spleen, located in the left upper abdominal quadrant posterior to the stomach, produces lymphocytes and monocytes in adults, but it can produce erythrocytes if the bone marrow becomes damaged. During pregnancy and until three weeks after birth, the spleen forms all kinds of blood cells. The thymus, located in the center of the chest, produces lymphocytes and antibodies during early life. After **puberty**, however, it **atrophies** (shrinks) and is replaced by fat, connective tissue, or both.

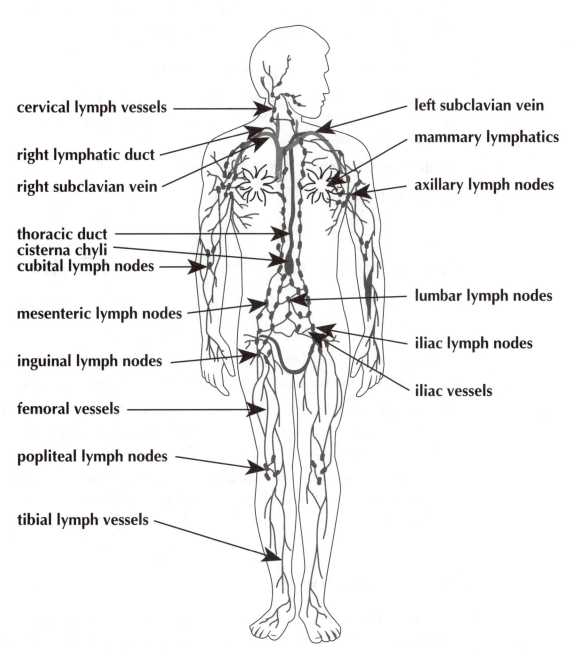

cervical lymph vessels

right lymphatic duct

right subclavian vein

thoracic duct
cisterna chyli
cubital lymph nodes

mesenteric lymph nodes

inguinal lymph nodes

femoral vessels

popliteal lymph nodes

tibial lymph vessels

left subclavian vein

mammary lymphatics

axillary lymph nodes

lumbar lymph nodes

iliac lymph nodes

iliac vessels

Figure 15-4: The Lymphatic System

Conditions of the Lymphatic System

The lymphatic system, like the other body systems, can be affected by certain health conditions and diseases. Some of these are listed below.

- **adenitis:** inflammation of the lymph nodes.
- **Hodgkin's disease:** a type of cancer that begins in the lymphoid tissue and, if untreated, will be fatal to the patient by invading or obstructing the vital organs.
- **splenomegaly:** enlargement of the spleen.
- **tonsillitis:** inflammation of the tonsils.

Diagnostic Tests for the Lymphatic System

The following diagnostic tests may be used to identify a disease of the lymphatic system.

- **biopsy:** the removal of a small piece of living tissue for examination under a microscope. This test is usually done if cancer is suspected.
- **complete blood cell count:** a blood test that determines the number of erythrocytes, leukocytes, and platelets that are present in the patient's blood as well as the hemoglobin and hematocrit.
- **culture:** a laboratory test for bacterial growth that involves instilling microorganisms in special media and monitoring it for the growth of pathogens.

The Nervous System

One of the most complex and fascinating systems of the human body is the **nervous system**. The main components of this system are the brain, cranial nerves, spinal cord, spinal nerves, and peripheral nerves. This is a highly organized and intricate system, the main function of which is to coordinate and regulate the body's many responses to internal and/or external environmental changes. The nervous system also determines the body's response to stimuli. A stimulant is anything that produces a temporary increase in the functional activity or efficiency of an organism.

The basic structural unit of the nervous system is the nerve cell, or **neuron**. Neurons differ from common cells in their design and specific function. A neuron has a cell body that contains a nucleus, several **dendrites** (cytoplasmic branches off the cell body that transmit impulses to the body of the cell), and an **axon** (a branch off of the cell body that conducts impulses away from the body of the cell). The main function of the neuron is to cause the body to react to its environment.

Two types of neurons exist in different areas of the body. **Sensory neurons**, or **afferent neurons**, are found in the skin and in the sensory organs. These neurons transmit messages, or impulses, from the sensory organs and the skin to the brain and spinal cord. The second kind of neuron is the **motor**, or **efferent**, **neuron**. Motor neurons originate in the brain or spinal cord and carry impulses to the muscles and glands of the body. They enable the body to react to its environment. For example, sensory neurons detect heat, and motor neurons cause the body to remove the affected part away from the heat source. **Mixed nerves** are a combination of sensory and motor neurons.

sensory neurons: afferent neurons; nerve cells that transmit impulses from the sensory organs and the skin to the brain and spinal cord

motor neurons: efferent neurons; nerve cells that carry impulses from the brain or spinal cord to the muscles or gland tissue

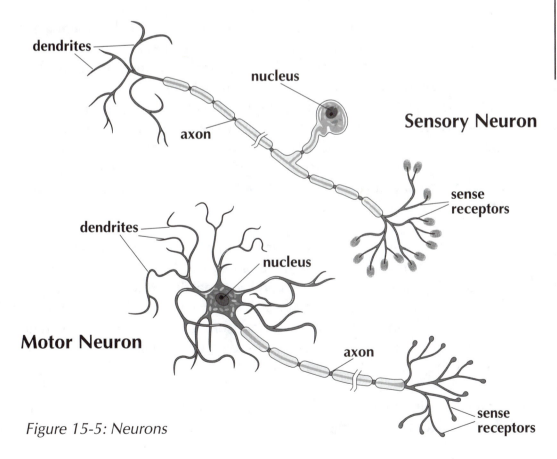

Figure 15-5: Neurons

nerve:
a combination of nerve fibers located outside the brain or spinal cord, and that connect those structures with various parts of the body

central nervous system (CNS):
the body system composed of the brain and the spinal cord

peripheral nervous system:
the nervous system outside the central nervous system that is responsible for gathering information and carrying the response signals

meninges:
the three protective membranes covering the brain and the spinal cord

ventricle:
one of the four cavities of the brain

cerebrospinal fluid (CSF):
the clear, watery fluid that flows through the brain and spinal column, protecting the brain and spinal cord

Nerves originate in a specific nerve center, either the brain or the spinal cord, and infiltrate other organs as well as the muscles and skin. They convey impulses from one part of the body to another.

The Central Nervous System

The nervous system is more easily understood when it is broken down into the special functions it performs. There are actually two main divisions within the nervous system: the **central nervous system** (**CNS**) and the **peripheral nervous system** (**PNS**).

The central nervous system consists of the **brain** and the **spinal cord**. The brain is located within the skull and performs numerous functions. It is the main center for controlling and coordinating the body's activities. The average weight of the brain is about 3 pounds. The brain requires **dextrose** (a form of sugar) and oxygen to perform at its highest potential.

The brain is surrounded by a protective barrier of membranes called **meninges**. There are three layers of meninges: the outer layer, called the **dura mater**, is thick and strong; the middle layer, called the **arachnoid membrane**, is very delicate and resembles a spider's web; and the inner layer, called the **pia mater**, is directly connected to the brain and the spinal cord. The pia mater contains many blood vessels that provide nourishment to both structures. Between each of these layers is a space. The space between the dura mater and the skull is the **epidural** space; the **subdural** space is beneath the dura mater and above the arachnoid membrane; and the **subarachnoid** space is beneath the arachnoid membrane and above the pia mater.

Contained within the brain are four hollow spaces, called **ventricles**, that connect to each other and the subarachnoid space. The ventricles are constantly producing a special fluid called **cerebrospinal fluid** (**CSF**). This is a clear, colorless, watery fluid that acts as a shock absorber to protect the brain and the spinal cord. Cerebrospinal fluid provides nourishment to and removes different waste products from the brain and spinal cord. Eventually, CSF becomes absorbed by the veins of the dura mater.

The brain contains many specialized areas. However, because this is an introductory text, only the larger sections will be addressed.

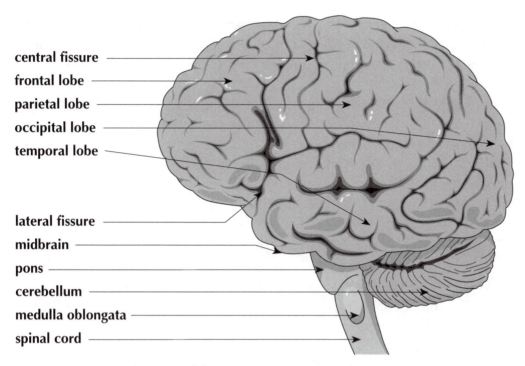

central fissure
frontal lobe
parietal lobe
occipital lobe
temporal lobe

lateral fissure
midbrain
pons
cerebellum
medulla oblongata
spinal cord

Figure 15-6: Lateral View of the Brain

The **cerebrum** controls willful actions, interprets **sensory** messages gained from sound, sight, smell, touch, etc., and governs thought and speech. The cerebrum is the largest part of the brain, and it takes up most of the cranial cavity. It is separated into two halves and is made up of two layers: **gray matter**, the outer layer, which is approximately one-eighth of an inch thick; and **white matter**.

The **cerebellum** is responsible for muscle coordination and tone, and for maintaining balance and posture. It is located inferior to the cerebrum and posterior in the cranial cavity.

The **midbrain** is located inferior to the cerebrum and anterior to the brain stem. It is responsible for conducting impulses throughout the brain, and for conducting certain visual and auditory reflexes.

The **pons** is located within the brain stem inferior to the cerebrum. It acts mainly as a bridge between two or more sections of the brain, and is responsible for conducting certain impulses throughout the brain and for some reflexive actions, such as chewing and producing saliva.

The **medulla oblongata** is located at the base of the brain stem and protrudes slightly over the spinal cord. It controls involuntary actions like respirations, heartbeat, blood pressure, swallowing, and coughing.

The spinal cord is attached to the medulla oblongata and continues down to the second lumbar vertebrae of the back. It is protected by the vertebrae, cerebrospinal fluid, and the meninges. The spinal cord's two major functions are to conduct impulses through afferent and efferent nerves, and to connect the body parts to the brain.

The Peripheral Nervous System

This section of the nervous system is composed of the nerves located outside the brain and spinal cord. The peripheral nervous system is subdivided into the **somatic nervous system** and the **autonomic nervous system**.

There are 12 pairs of **cranial nerves** within the brain. Each pair is responsible for one or more functions, such as sight, taste, hearing, smell, and smiling. The spinal cord contains 31 pairs of special nerves called **spinal nerves**. The axons and dendrites of the cranial and spinal nerves extend into the outer parts of the body. This makes up the part of the peripheral nervous system known as the **somatic** (pertaining to the body) nervous system. The right side of the brain controls the left side of the body and vice versa. When the spinal cord sustains injury, the degree of damage depends on where the spinal cord was injured.

The autonomic nervous system is responsible for the **involuntary** functions of the body. This particular system also is broken down into two divisions that maintain homeostasis within the body. The **sympathetic nervous system** prepares the body for a *fight or flight* response to an emergency situation. When this occurs, the respiratory rate and heart rate increase, blood pressure is raised, and the digestive tract slows down. The **parasympathetic nervous system** has the opposite effect on the body. It acts as a brake by slowing the heart rate and respiratory rate, lowering blood pressure, and increasing the activity of the digestive system. These two systems help balance each other.

somatic nervous system: the part of the peripheral nervous system that controls skeletal muscles responsible for voluntary movement

autonomic nervous system: a division of the peripheral nervous system that regulates the balance between the involuntary functions of the body and causes the body to react in emergency situations

sympathetic nervous system: the part of the autonomic nervous system that controls many involuntary activities of the glands, organs, and other parts of the body

parasympathetic nervous system: the part of the autonomic nervous system that acts in specific ways to complement the activities of the sympathetic nervous system

Parasympathetic Nervous System		**Sympathetic Nervous System**
constricts pupils	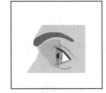	*dilates pupils*
stimulates salivation		*inhibits salivation*
slows heart rate		*accelerates heart rate*
constricts bronchi		*dilates bronchi*
stimulates gastric juice production		*inhibits gastric juice production*
no action		*stimulates release of epinephrine and norepinephrine*
accelerates digestive process and relaxes the rectum		*inhibits digestive process and contracts the rectum*
contracts bladder muscles	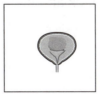	*relaxes bladder muscles*

Figure 15-7: Divisions of the Autonomic Nervous System

Nervous System Conditions

As with all other systems in the body, there are certain types of conditions that can impair the **nervous system**. Some of these conditions are listed below.

- **cerebrovascular accident (CVA):** the blockage, hemorrhage, or compression of a blood vessel in the brain, often resulting in weakness or paralysis of one or more body part, slurred speech, absence of speech, etc. (Also known as a stroke.)

- **cerebral palsy:** a congenital condition that results in a lack of muscle function and coordination due to brain damage.

- **concussion:** an injury or loss of function resulting from a blow to the head or a fall.

- **contusion of the brain:** bruising of the brain as the result of a blunt force, such as from being hit with a baseball bat or hitting one's head on concrete.

- **epilepsy:** a term that describes a group of nervous system disorders that involve disturbed rhythms of the electrical impulses that fire throughout the cerebrum, resulting in seizure activity or abnormal behavior.

- **hemiplegia:** paralysis of half of the body, such as that which may occur from a cerebrovascular accident (CVA).

- **meningitis:** inflammation of the membranes covering the spinal cord and brain, marked by severe headache, vomiting, fever, and a stiff neck, and usually caused by infection.

- **neuralgia:** severe pain along the length of a nerve.

- **paraplegia:** paralysis of the lower part of the body, including both legs.

- **poliomyelitis:** an acute viral disease that inflames parts of the spinal cord and may result in muscular atrophy, deformity, and paralysis. It is characterized by a sore throat, headache, vomiting, possible stiffness of the neck and back, and atrophy of the muscles.

- **quadriplegia:** paralysis of the body from the neck down.

Diagnostic Tests for the Nervous System

There are different tests used by healthcare professionals for the nervous system. Some of them are described below.

- **computerized tomography (CT) scan:** a technique for examining transverse planes of internal structures of the body in which x-rays are used to construct a precise image and show the relationship of structures.

- **lumbar puncture:** a procedure in which a specimen of cerebrospinal fluid is removed and analyzed for diseases such as meningitis. (Also known as a spinal tap.)

- **magnetic resonance imaging (MRI):** a diagnostic procedure in which parts of the body are exposed to an electromagnetic field to produce an image.

- **myelogram:** an x-ray of the spinal cord and associated nerves after an injection of contrast medium.

- **nerve conduction studies:** studies that aid in the discovery of peripheral nerve injuries and diseases by electrically stimulating nerves and measuring the response.

Chapter Summary

The circulatory and lymphatic systems are the two main transportation systems of the body. The human heart automatically pumps 5 to 6 liters of blood through the entire body with each heartbeat. Through this pumping action, oxygen and nutrients are transported to the different areas of the body, and carbon dioxide and other waste products are removed from the system. The human body cannot survive without this system of transportation.

The lymphatic system is concerned with cleansing and filtering the blood from toxins and other impurities. It is composed of leukocytes. This system is a vital part of our immune system for fighting infection and illness.

The nervous system is composed of the brain, the spinal cord, and the nerves. Through this system, messages are received, interpreted, and transmitted via electrical impulses throughout the body. When these impulses reach the muscles, an appropriate action occurs in response to the stimulus.

As a healthcare worker, a basic understanding of these systems is essential to your ability to provide quality care to your patients. If a patient exhibits signs or symptoms that are unfamiliar to you, report your findings to the primary healthcare provider.

Name _____

Date _____

Student Enrichment Activities

Complete the following statements.

1. Highly oxygenated blood is transported to the body through _____.

2. The smallest blood vessels in the body are _____.

3. Blood is made up of approximately _____% water.

4. Blood cells that help the blood to clot are called _____.

5. The normal pacemaker of the heart is located in the _____ _____.

6. Name the three layers of cardiac tissue: _____,
   _____, and _____.

7. _____ occurs due to a low oxygen level in the blood in the
   coronary arteries.

8. Impurities are filtered from lymph by the _____ _____.

9. The primary structural units of the nervous system are the _____.

10. _____ neurons are located in the skin and in the sensory organs.

11. _____ neurons originate in the brain and spinal cord and carry
    impulses to the muscles and glands.

12. The brain is surrounded by three layers of membranes called _____.

13. The three layers of meninges are the _____, the
    _____, and the _____.

14. The _____ nervous system prepares the body for
    fight or flight.

15. The _____ nervous system has a calming effect on the body.

Unscramble the following terms.

16. GREATCLEORADCRIOPHY   _____

17. DOCYMARILA TRAFIONCIN _____ _____

18. STAMOIC   _____

19. BRIOPTHORMN   _____

20. DRAMIUCRIPE   _____

21. SAIDIENT   _____

22. VIOLEAL   _____

23. SLUVEEN   _____

24. PRESIOUR NEAV AVAC   _____ _____ _____

Name _____

Date _____

25. STINGMIENI   _____

26. ANAING   _____

27. SPUDIBIC LAVVE   _____ _____

28. SCLAUVAR   _____

29. PRETENSNYOHI   _____

30. MULLEBCREE   _____

Chapter Sixteen
Excretion: The Respiratory, Digestive, and Urinary Systems

Objectives

After completing this chapter you should be able to do the following:

1. Define and correctly spell each of the key terms.

2. Identify and describe all the parts of the respiratory system.

3. Describe the breathing process.

4. Describe at least four diagnostic tests for the respiratory system.

5. Name two enzymes produced in the stomach.

6. Trace the course of a bite of food through the entire digestive system.

7. Name and explain at least three functions of the liver.

8. Name the three enzymes produced by the pancreas.

9. Briefly explain the disease process of diabetes.

10. Describe the three main functions of the kidneys.

11. Describe the path of a drop of urine as it passes through the urinary system.

Key Terms

- alveoli
- chyme
- cilia
- diaphragm
- insulin
- kidneys
- larynx
- metabolism
- nephron

- pancreas
- peristalsis
- trachea
- ulcer
- ureter
- urinary bladder
- ventilation
- vermiform appendix
- vocal folds

Excretion: The Body's Disposal Systems

The body is an extraordinary machine. It must use fuel effectively to make energy. The body also must **excrete** the waste products from the conversion of fuel to energy, and what it cannot use, it must eliminate, or excrete. Excretion is necessary for the proper performance of the body as a whole. The respiratory, digestive, and urinary systems will be discussed together since they have the common function of excretion. While these systems are discussed in this chapter as they relate to excretion, it is important to note that they perform other functions as well.

The Respiratory System

The human body can store enough food for weeks and enough water for 5 to 7 days, but only enough oxygen for 4 to 6 minutes. All cells need oxygen (O_2). Carbon dioxide (CO_2) is a gaseous waste produced by cellular activity that must be removed from the body. This process takes place in the urinary and respiratory systems.

The respiratory system consists of the nose, pharynx, larynx, trachea, bronchial tubes, alveoli, and the lungs. This intricate system can be described as a pathway between the atmosphere and the blood. When we inhale through our nose, air from the atmosphere enters the body through two openings called **nares**. The nares are separated by cartilage called the **nasal septum**. The nasal passages are lined with a mucous membrane and tiny, hairlike structures called **cilia**. The nose warms, moistens, and filters particles and pathogens from the air before they enter the bronchial tubes and lungs. In addition to the moisture provided by the mucous membrane of the nose, the **lacrimal ducts** drain fluid into the nose. This explains why a person's nose *runs* when he or she cries.

The **pharynx**, or throat, is directly attached to the nose. The pharynx can be divided into three sections. The upper section, called the **nasopharynx**, is directly posterior to the nasal cavities and contains the pharyngeal **tonsils**. The opening from the **eustachian tube**, the canal leading from the outer ear to the throat, is also found in this area. The middle section, called the **oropharynx**, is located in the posterior mouth and inferior to the nasopharynx. It receives air from the nose as well as food and air from the mouth. The third section, called the **laryngopharynx**, is located inferior to the oropharynx and contains the opening to the **esophagus** (the tube that leads directly into the stomach) and the trachea (the tube that leads into the bronchi and lungs). The trachea is located anterior to the esophagus.

The **larynx,** or voice box, is located between the pharynx and the trachea. It is composed primarily of muscles and nine layers of cartilage. The largest layer of cartilage, known as the **thyroid cartilage**, is commonly called the Adam's Apple. The larynx also houses the **vocal folds**, which vibrate to produce a certain pitch of sound. The larger the larynx, the deeper the voice. Located between the two vocal folds is an opening called the **glottis**. It is protected by a flap of cartilage called the **epiglottis**. When a person swallows, the epiglottis closes to prevent the introduction of a foreign substance into the trachea and lungs.

Extending from the larynx down the center of the chest is the **trachea**, or windpipe. The trachea is made of C-shaped cartilage and is 4 to 5 inches long in an adult, approximately $1\frac{1}{2}$ inches long in an infant, and $2\frac{1}{2}$ inches long in a toddler. The dorsal aspect (the back) of the trachea is soft and flexible, which allows the esophagus to expand when food is present. The main function of the trachea is to allow air to pass from the atmosphere to the lungs.

cilia:
tiny, hairlike structures projecting from the epithelial cells, that propel mucus, pus, and dust particles

larynx:
the upper end of the trachea; the voicebox

vocal folds:
the edges of the lips of the larynx that vibrate to pro- duce a certain pitch of sound

trachea:
the windpipe; a tube of cartilage that extends from the larynx to the bronchial tubes, and which leads air into the lungs

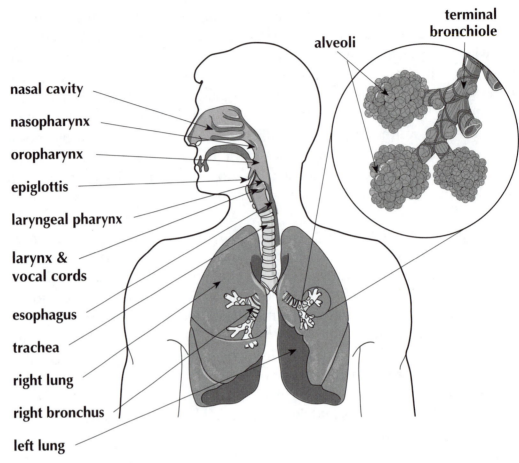

Figure 16-1: The Respiratory Tract

The trachea divides into two tubes called **bronchi** at approximately the center of the chest. Each bronchus enters into a lung. The bronchi continue to decrease in size and form **bronchioles** that enter tiny air sacs called **alveoli**. Oxygen and carbon dioxide can easily pass through the capillary walls surrounding the alveoli, so it is within these structures that the **gas exchange** occurs. The shape of alveoli resembles a bunch of grapes. Because of the vast number of alveoli and because they are filled with air, lung tissue is light in weight.

The **lungs** make up the largest part of the respiratory system. The right lung is made up of three lobes: the superior, the middle, and the inferior lobes. Because of the position of the heart within the thoracic cavity, the left lung is smaller and has only two lobes: the superior and the inferior. Each lung is surrounded by a layer of thin tissue called the **pleura**. The thoracic cavity is separated from the abdominal cavity by a large muscle called the **diaphragm**, which is the main breathing muscle.

alveoli:
microscopic air sacs within the lungs responsible for the exchange of oxygen and carbon dioxide

diaphragm:
the dome-shaped muscle separating the thoracic cavity from the abdominal cavity

The Breathing Process

Breathing (respiration) consists of two phases: **inspiration** and **expiration**. These two phases form one **respiratory cycle**. Another term used interchangeably with respiration is **ventilation**.

The process of breathing air into the lungs is called inspiration, or inhalation. During this phase of respiration, the intercostal (rib) muscles and the diaphragm contract and cause the chest cavity to increase in size. The lungs expand in order to accommodate the air that has been inhaled. Once the gas exchange (external respiration) has occurred in the alveoli, oxygen is used by the cells and carbon dioxide, a waste product, is produced. This gas exchange is also called **cellular respiration**. At this point, the second phase of ventilation (internal respiration) must occur.

Expiration takes place when the respiratory center in the medulla oblongata of the brain receives a message concerning the increasing level of carbon dioxide in the blood. At this time, the intercostal muscles and the diaphragm relax and the carbon dioxide is forced out of the lungs and through the air passages. When the carbon dioxide is unable to be adequately released from the body, the respiratory rate will increase above the normal level, as in a patient having an asthma attack. This is one way in which the body attempts to adapt to, or compensate for, an abnormal condition. Although the ventilation process is mostly involuntary, a person can control the voluntary muscles and deliberately increase or decrease the respiratory rate.

ventilation: the exchange of air between the lungs and the atmosphere; breathing

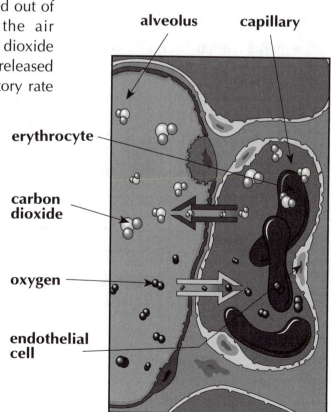

Figure 16-2: Cellular Respiration

Conditions of the Lung and Associated Structures

The following are conditions which affect the respiratory system.

- **anoxia:** a lack of oxygen.

- **apnea:** the temporary cessation of spontaneous breathing.

- **asthma:** a lung disorder that causes breathing difficulty, wheezing, and coughing, and that can lead to airway obstruction.

- **atelectasis:** a condition in which the lung tissue is airless; a collapsed lung.

- **bronchitis:** inflammation of the bronchial lining.

- **dyspnea:** difficult or painful breathing.

- **emphysema:** a chronic lung disease that destroys the alveoli.

- **epistaxis:** a nosebleed.

- **hemothorax:** blood within the pleural cavity.

- **hyperventilation:** prolonged, deep, and rapid breathing, resulting in decreased levels of CO_2 in the blood.

- **influenza:** a highly communicable disease of the upper respiratory tract; the flu.

- **laryngitis:** inflammation of the larynx.

- **lung cancer:** malignant tumors involving the lung tissue.

- **pleurisy:** inflammation of the pleura.

- **pneumonia:** inflammation of the lungs.

- **rhinitis:** inflammation of the lining of the nasal cavity.

- **upper respiratory infection:** a general term used to describe an infectious disease process involving the nasal passages, pharynx, and bronchi.

Diagnostic Tests for the Respiratory System

The following is a list of some of the diagnostic tests for the respiratory system.

- **arterial blood gas (ABG) test:** a blood test used to determine acidity or alkalinity as well as the oxygen and carbon dioxide levels in the blood.

- **bronchoscopy:** the visual examination of the bronchial tubes and trachea through the introduction of a flexible tube equipped with a light called a bronchoscope.

- **chest x-ray (CXR):** a diagnostic test that permits visualization of the position, size, and contour of the structures within the thoracic area through the use of radiation.

- **computerized tomography (CT) scan:** a technique for examining transverse planes of internal structures of the body in which x-rays are used to construct a precise image and show the relationship of structures.

- **fluoroscopy:** a method of viewing the internal structures while they are in motion through the use of x-rays.

- **lung scan:** a test that reveals whether lung tissue is receiving enough blood, in which medication is introduced into the body and a machine measures the amount of radiant energy that is released.

- **magnetic resonance imaging (MRI):** a diagnostic procedure in which parts of the body are exposed to an electromagnetic field to produce an image.

- **pulmonary angiography:** a diagnostic test that allows the physician to view the pulmonary system through the use of radiopaque dye.

- **pulmonary function tests:** tests that are used to determine the capacity of the lungs to take in oxygen and release carbon dioxide.

- **ventilation lung scan:** the diagnostic examination of the lungs following the inhalation of a radioactive gas.

The Digestive System

All food substances taken into the body must be broken down into chemical parts that can be absorbed and used by cells. The digestive system performs this function and others. This system includes the **alimentary canal**, which begins at the mouth and ends at the anus, and other accessory organs, which secrete certain chemicals to assist with digestion and absorption.

The mouth receives food and contains many important parts of the alimentary canal: the tongue contains taste buds that taste the food; the teeth masticate (chew) the food into smaller pieces; and **saliva** moistens and begins to partially digest the food before it is swallowed. Saliva also contains an **enzyme** called **ptyalin**, which is a very complex protein capable of causing chemical reactions to occur in another substance. Ptyalin breaks down starches into simpler sugars, thereby allowing the body to fully use this source of energy. The roof of the mouth, or **hard palate**, separates the mouth from the nasal cavities. Once the food is ready for further digestion, it is pushed back into the pharynx, or throat, by the tongue. The pharynx accepts both air and food. Sensory receptors tell the pharynx which tube to open or close.

peristalsis: rhythmic, wavelike motion that occurs throughout the digestive tract, and which causes the contents of the alimentary canal to be forced onward

The **esophagus** is a large muscular tube that extends from the pharynx to the stomach. The esophagus is posterior to the **trachea**. Food is moved throughout the length of the esophagus to the **stomach** by a rhythmic, wave-like motion called **peristalsis**. The entire alimentary canal, which is about 30 feet long, functions with this type of action. After traveling down the esophagus, the food enters the first of many accessory organs, the stomach. This organ is capable of being filled with approximately one-half gallon of food and liquid. It resembles a gourd in shape and functions both as a pouch and a churn. The stomach is closed at both ends by valves. The first valve is the **cardiac sphincter**, located between the stomach and the esophagus. This valve normally only permits food to enter the stomach; however, there are times when it will open and allow food to be expelled from the stomach. This is what happens when a person vomits. The second valve is called the **pyloric sphincter**. It remains closed until the contents of the stomach are ready to be emptied into the small intestine.

The stomach contains digestive juices that are composed mainly of **hydrochloric acid** and enzymes. The hydrochloric acid (HCl) kills pathogens, softens connective tissue contained in meat, assists in the absorption of iron, and activates one or more of the enzymes. There are two main enzymes produced by the stomach: **pepsin**, which helps break down proteins, and **lipase**, which is responsible for helping to break down **fats.** Once food has been mixed with the gastric secretions produced by glands on the stomach wall, it forms a semisolid mass called **chyme.** Food generally remains in the stomach for 30 minutes to 4 hours.

chyme:
a semisolid mass found in the stomach, which is formed by the mixture of the gastric secretions and food

Digestive Juices and Their Enzymes

Juice	Gland	Place of Action	Enzymes	Effect on Foods
Saliva	Salivary Glands (3 pairs)	Oral Cavity	Ptyalin	Begins digestion of starch.
Gastric Juice	Stomach Wall	Stomach	Pepsin Lipase Rennin	Begins digestion of protein. Aids in digestion of fats. Aids in curdling milk protein.
Pancreatic Juice	Pancreas	Small Intestine	Amylopsin Trypsin Lipase	Acts on starches. Acts on proteins. Acts on fats.
Intestinal Juice	Tubular Glands (in the small intestine)	Small Intestine	Lactase Maltase Sucrase	Break down complex sugars into simpler sugars.
Bile	Liver	Small Intestine	None	Breaks down fats so that lipase can digest them.

Figure 16-3: Digestive Juices and Enzymes

There are certain conditions that specifically affect the stomach. The following is a short list of some of the more common disorders.

- **gastritis:** inflammation of the stomach lining.

- **heartburn:** a burning sensation in the area of the esophagus and stomach.

- **nausea:** a sensation leading to the urge to vomit.

- **ulcer:** a lesion on skin or mucous membrane (in this case the membrane of the stomach or duodenum) accompanied by sloughing of inflamed, dead tissue. A stomach ulcer is caused by the effect of gastric acid and pepsin.

- **vomiting:** reverse peristalsis that results in the expulsion of the stomach contents through the mouth.

ulcer:
a lesion on skin or mucous membrane accompanied by sloughing of inflamed, dead skin

As food is expelled from the stomach, the **pyloric sphincter** will open and the contents will enter the **small intestine** via peristalsis. The small intestine is the longest part of the alimentary canal. Uncoiled, it is about 20 feet long and 1 inch in diameter. The lining of the small intestine contains many finger-like projections called **villi**. These projections contain capillaries and **lacteals**. Lacteals absorb most of the digested fats and transport them into the lymphatic system, which releases them into the bloodstream. The capillaries contained within the villi absorb digested nutrients and transport them to the liver for storage or release into the body's general circulation.

The first 10 inches or so of the small intestine is known as the **duodenum**. It contains ducts that allow digestive juices from the pancreas and the liver to flow into the small intestine. **Pancreatic juice** arrives from the pancreas and **bile** comes from the liver. Both of these secretions assist with digestion. The middle section of the small intestine is the **jejunum**, which is approximately 8 feet long. The last section is called the **ileum**. It is separated from the large intestine by a muscle called the **ileocecal sphincter**. This sphincter remains closed until only wastes, water, and indigestible products remain. At that time, the remaining products are passed into the large intestine.

vermiform appendix:
the worm-like tube of tissue directly connected to the cecum

The large intestine, or colon, is about 2 inches in diameter and approximately 5 feet long when uncoiled. The materials to be eliminated from the body will enter the proximal portion of the large intestine known as the **cecum**. The cecum is located in the right lower quadrant of the abdomen and is attached to the ileum of the small intestine. Below the cecum is the **vermiform appendix**, commonly referred to as the *appendix*. It contains large amounts of lymphoid tissue. The remaining sections of the colon travel across the abdomen as their names indicate: the **ascending colon** extends up from the cecum along the right side to the inferior portion of the liver; the **transverse colon** continues across the abdomen, superior to the small intestine and inferior to the stomach and liver; and the **descending colon** continues down the left side of the abdomen. The functions of the large intestine (the colon) include absorption of water and any remaining nutrients, storage of indigestible materials, and removal of waste products, known as *fecal matter*, or *stool*, from the body. The wall of the large intestine does not contain villi; however, the colon does harbor certain kinds of bacteria that, if not contained within the intestines, can produce a massive infection throughout the body.

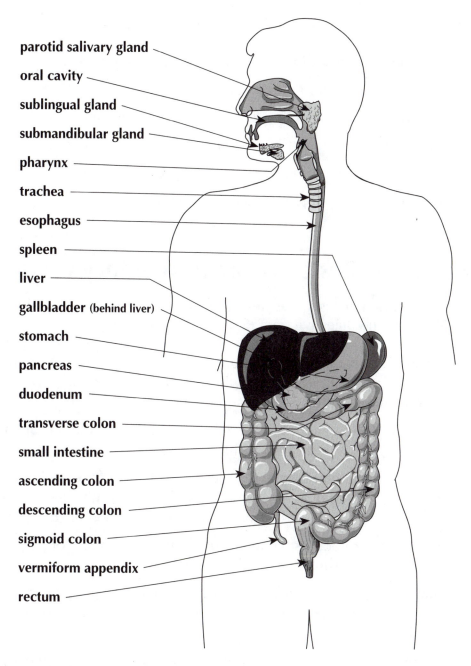

parotid salivary gland

oral cavity

sublingual gland

submandibular gland

pharynx

trachea

esophagus

spleen

liver

gallbladder (behind liver)

stomach

pancreas

duodenum

transverse colon

small intestine

ascending colon

descending colon

sigmoid colon

vermiform appendix

rectum

Figure 16-4: The Digestive System

The **descending colon** empties directly into the S-shaped **sigmoid colon**, which is connected to the rectum. The sigmoid colon is 6 to 8 inches long and acts as a temporary storage for waste products. The rectum is directly connected to a distal, narrow opening of the large intestine known as the **anal canal**. The stool is then expelled through the opening of the anal canal called the **anus**. The entire journey through the alimentary canal can take as long as 36 hours.

The following are disorders that may affect the intestines.

- **appendicitis:** inflammation of the vermiform appendix.

- **colitis:** inflammation of the colon.

- **constipation:** the inability to have a bowel movement; hard stool.

- **diarrhea:** abnormally frequent, watery bowel movements.

- **enteritis:** inflammation and infection of the intestine.

- **hemorrhoids:** enlarged veins in the anal area.

Diagnostic Tests for the Alimentary Canal

There are particular tests that are used to assist in diagnosing abnormal functioning of the digestive tract. Some are listed below.

- **barium enema:** the introduction of a barium sulfate solution into the rectum and colon prior to the fluoroscopic and radiographic examination of the large intestine.

- **barium swallow:** fluoroscopic exam of the pharynx and esophagus following the ingestion of barium.

- **computerized tomography (CT) scan:** a technique for examining transverse planes of internal structures of the body in which x-rays are used to construct a precise image and show the relationship of structures.

- **endoscopy:** direct inspection of the lining of a hollow organ through an instrument called an endoscope.

- **magnetic resonance imaging (MRI):** a diagnostic procedure in which parts of the body are exposed to an electromagnetic field to produce an image.

- **occult blood:** blood, usually found in the stool or gastric contents, that is in such minute quantities that it must be examined microscopically.

- **small bowel series:** fluoroscopy of the intestines following the ingestion of barium.

- **upper GI (gastrointestinal) series:** radiography and fluoroscopy of the esophagus, stomach, and small intestine following the ingestion of barium.

The Accessory Organs

There are several accessory organs in the body that are associated with the process of digestion. One of them, the **liver**, is the largest gland in the body. It is located in the right upper quadrant of the abdomen and has a large right lobe and a smaller left lobe. The liver plays an important role in the digestive system by performing the following functions.

1. The liver produces bile which helps break down fats and makes them **soluble** (able to be dissolved) in water.

2. It stores simple sugar in the form of glycogen, which is released according to the needs of the body as glucose.

3. The liver stores certain vitamins such as A, D, and some of the B vitamins.

4. It produces heparin (a protein that keeps blood from clotting) as well as other proteins, such as fibrinogen and prothrombin which help the blood clot.

5. It **detoxifies** the blood by removing harmful substances such as alcohol, pesticides, or pathogens that may have entered the blood from the intestine.

Several diseases may affect the liver. These diseases are very serious because a person cannot live without a liver that functions properly. The following are the most common of these diseases.

- **cirrhosis:** inflammation of the liver, which is often caused by chronic alcohol ingestion.
- **hepatitis:** inflammation of the liver.

Inferior to the liver is a muscular sac called the **gallbladder**. The main function of this accessory organ is to receive bile from the liver, remove the water, and store the bile until it is needed by the small intestine. Two diseases that directly affect the gallbladder are listed below.

- **cholecystitis:** inflammation and infection of the gallbladder.

- **cholelithiasis:** the formation of calculi or stones in the gallbladder or bile duct.

pancreas:
the organ in the abdominal cavity that produces insulin and aids in digestion

metabolism:
the sum of all physical and chemical processes that take place in the body; the conversion of food to energy

insulin:
a hormone secreted by the pancreas that causes glucose, or sugar, to leave the bloodstream and enter the cell

The **pancreas**, located in the left upper quadrant, posterior to the stomach, is a gland that produces pancreatic juice. This juice, or fluid, contains the following enzymes: **amylopsin**, which is responsible for breaking down sugars; **lipase**, which breaks down the fats; and **trypsin**, which breaks down the **proteins**. These enzymes are essential to proper **metabolism** (the conversion of food to energy). The other function of the pancreas is to produce **insulin**. Insulin is a hormone that is produced by the islets of Langerhans within the pancreas and then released into the bloodstream in response to the amount of circulating blood sugar, or glucose. A delicate balance between the amount of insulin and glucose in the blood must be maintained at all times. Any imbalance in these levels will lead to a blood sugar level that is either too high or too low.

There are two common disorders associated with the pancreas.

- **diabetes:** a metabolic disease that causes an increase in blood sugar and failure of the body to produce insulin.

- **pancreatitis:** inflammation of the pancreas.

Diagnostic Tests for the Accessory Organs

The tests that are commonly used to diagnose health problems in the liver, gallbladder, and pancreas are listed below.

- **amylase blood test:** a blood test in which the level of amylase enzymes in the patient's blood is evaluated. Abnormal levels can be indicative of a disease process.

- **biopsy:** the removal of a small piece of living tissue for examination under a microscope.

- **computerized tomography (CT) scan:** a technique for examining transverse planes of internal structures of the body in which x-rays are used to construct a precise image and show the relationship of structures.

- **liver function tests:** diagnostic blood tests that evaluate the level of the liver enzymes.

- **magnetic resonance imaging (MRI):** a diagnostic procedure in which parts of the body are exposed to an electromagnetic field to produce an image.

- **paracentesis:** a needle puncture of the abdominal cavity followed by the **aspiration** of fluid for analysis.

- **ultrasound of each organ:** inaudible sound waves that can be used to create visual images of the internal structures.

The digestive system is composed of many different organs, all of which must function together for proper digestion to occur.

The Urinary System

The urinary system is one of the excretory systems of the body. Its primary function is to rid the body of waste products that have been filtered from the blood by the kidneys and excrete them in the form of urine. **Urine** contains about 95% water, but it also contains substances such as urea, chloride, sodium, potassium, phosphate, sulfate, creatinine, protein, and various pigments. Sometimes dextrose is excreted in the urine too; but this is usually an indication of a disease process such as diabetes. Approximately 150 quarts (150,000 cc) of liquid are filtered through the kidneys every day, producing 1½ to 2 quarts (1500 cc - 2000 cc) of urine a day.

kidneys:
organs located in the dorsal cavity of the body that are responsible for filtering blood and producing urine

There are several organs included in the urinary system: the two kidneys, the two ureters, a bladder, and the urethra. The **kidneys** resemble the shape of a bean (hence the name *kidney bean*) and are located in the dorsal cavity of the body, against the muscles of the back in the upper abdomen. They are secured in place by connective tissue. The kidneys are very delicate organs and are protected by the ribs, cartilage, and a large layer of fat. They have three primary functions.

1. Excrete waste products, the chief product being urea, in the form of urine.

2. Provide assistance in maintaining the water balance of the body. The average man ingests approximately 2500 cc (2½ quarts) of water daily.

3. Provide assistance in regulating the acid-base balance of the body.

There are two main sections in each kidney. The outer section, called the **cortex**, contains the majority of the nephrons. The inner section, called the **medulla**, contains the collecting tubules.

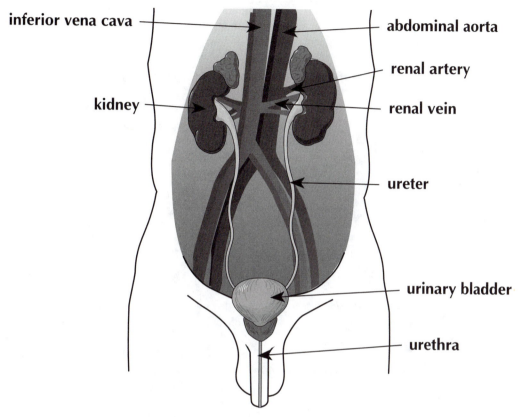

inferior vena cava

abdominal aorta

renal artery

kidney

renal vein

ureter

urinary bladder

urethra

Figure 16-5: The Urinary System (Male)

The kidney is composed of **nephrons**, the functional units of the kidney. It is inside of these nephrons that the blood is filtered free of waste products. Each kidney contains over one million of these nephrons; if they were laid end to end, they would cover a length of approximately 75 miles!

Each nephron contains a tubule with a bulb on one end called the **Bowman's capsule**. This bulb contains a cluster of capillaries called the **glomerulus**, and is the beginning of the built-in filtering system. Blood enters the glomerulus through an arteriole, and water and dissolved materials are filtered from the blood through the capillary walls of the glomerulus and the inner layer of the Bowman's capsule. However, blood cells and large proteins that can be used by the body are retained in the capillaries. At this point the material that has collected in the Bowman's capsule passes through the **convoluted tubule** to the collecting tubule.

nephrons:
the functional units of the kidney that act as the basic filtering units of the kidney

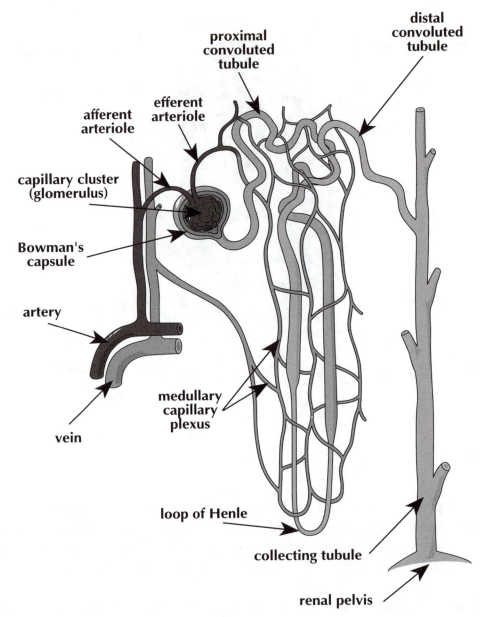

Figure 16-6: A Simplified Nephron

To get to the collecting tubule, the material, also known as the glomerular filtrate, passes through the **proximal** convoluted portion of the renal tubule, the loop of Henle, and the **distal** convoluted portion of the renal tubule. (See Figure 16-6.) On the way, the sugar and some of the salts, water, and other substances from the glomerular filtrate are reabsorbed through the walls of the renal tubule into the blood stream via the capillaries surrounding the tubule. The water that is retained in the nephron is concentrated with waste products; this forms urine. Don't forget—this process takes place over one million times simultaneously; all of this happens in every nephron!

After forming in the nephrons, the urine enters large straight collecting tubules via smaller collecting tubules. The large collecting tubules, located in the medulla of the kidney, empty into the **renal basin** (pelvis), which acts as a collecting area for the urine. This basin is the first section of the ureter. The **ureters** are long, slender, muscular tubes that extend from the kidney basin down through the lower part of the **urinary bladder**. The ureters, like the digestive tract, are capable of peristalsis. The urine travels down the ureters at frequent, rhythmic intervals and empties into the urinary bladder.

The urinary bladder is a hollow, muscular sac contained within the pelvic cavity. The bladder is composed of three layers of involuntary muscle that prevent backflow of the urine into the ureters when the bladder becomes full. The urge to urinate, or void, occurs when the bladder contains about 250 cc (slightly more than 1 cup) of urine. The opening of the bladder is kept closed by a series of circular sphincter muscles. Once the bladder has reached its capacity, receptors in the bladder wall open the sphincters and allow the urine to pass into the urethra. In young children the emptying of the bladder is automatic; but usually, sometime around the age of five, children begin to develop more control over this reflexive response and eventually they are able to delay voiding until an appropriate time presents itself.

The **urethra** is the tube that extends from the bladder to the outside of the body. The urethra in a male is much longer than it is in a female because it is also part of the male reproductive system. The urethra in the female is approximately 1½ inches long, and in the male it is about 8 inches long. The external opening of the urethra is the **urinary meatus**.

ureters: the long, slender, muscular tubes that extend from the kidney basin down through the lower part of the urinary bladder

urinary bladder: the hollow, muscular sac contained within the pelvic cavity that stores urine until it is excreted from the body

Conditions Affecting the Urinary System

Kidney failure results in the accumulation of waste products in the blood, which leads to death. Fortunately, a procedure known as **dialysis** can prolong the life of a person whose kidneys have failed until a kidney transplant is possible. However, in order for a transplant to be possible, the patient's overall health must be strong enough so that he or she will be able to survive both the extensive surgery and the recovery period that follows. Dialysis involves diffusing blood across a semipermeable membrane to remove the toxic wastes that have accumulated. A person may have to be subjected to this procedure every other day until a kidney donor is found or death occurs.

The following are health conditions related to the urinary system.

- **anuria:** the failure to produce urine.

- **calculi:** stones made up of uric acid and calcium salts that precipitate out of the urine instead of remaining in solution; kidney stones.

- **cystitis:** the inflammation of the urinary bladder.

- **dysuria:** painful or difficult urination.

- **hematuria:** the presence of blood in urine.

- **incontinence:** the loss of bladder (or bowel) control.

- **nephritis:** inflammation of the kidney.

- **oliguria:** reduced urine production.

- **polyuria:** excessive urination.

- **pyelonephritis:** inflammation of the kidney and pelvis of the kidney, caused by pathogens.

- **urinary tract infection:** a cluster of symptoms characterized by dysuria, frequent urination, urgency, and white blood cells in the urine.

Diagnostic Tests for the Urinary System

The following tests are used for diagnosing disorders of the urinary tract system.

- **biopsy:** the removal of a small piece of living tissue for examination under a microscope.

- **computerized tomography (CT) scan:** a technique for examining transverse planes of internal structures of the body in which x-rays are used to construct a precise image and show the relationship of structures.

- **cystogram:** a diagnostic test for the urinary bladder, which involves the use of x-rays taken after the instillation of contrast medium.

- **IVP (Intravenous Pyelogram):** a diagnostic test of the kidneys, ureters, and bladder using x-rays following the injection of radiopaque iodine dye; helps in the diagnosis of renal calculi (kidney stones).

- **ultrasound:** inaudible sound waves that can be used to create visual images of the internal structures.

Chapter Summary

The respiratory, digestive, and urinary systems are excretory systems. The respiratory system is concerned with providing the body with oxygen through the breathing process; it excretes carbon dioxide through exhalation. Through the process of gas exchange the respiratory system assists in maintaining the body's delicate acid-base balance.

The digestive system allows the body to use food and fluids as a source of energy. Throughout the alimentary canal (digestive tract), nutrients and fluids are converted into a useful form and absorbed into the bloodstream. Waste products are excreted from the body via the digestive system in the form of stool.

The urinary system is also very important in helping the body maintain its intricate acid-base balance. Approximately 150 quarts of fluid are transported through the kidneys daily and, because of its complex filtering system, about $1\frac{1}{2}$ to 2 quarts of urine are excreted daily.

These three systems are composed of many different organs. If a disease attacks any part of a system, the entire system can be affected severely.

Name _____

Date _____

Student Enrichment Activities

Complete the following statements.

1. The body stores enough oxygen for _____ minutes.

2. Name the parts of the respiratory system: _____,

    _____, _____, _____,

    _____, _____, and the _____.

3. The voice box, or _____, is made up of _____ layers of cartilage.

4. The largest organs of the respiratory system are the _____.

5. The thoracic cavity is separated from the abdominal cavity by the _____.

6. The term _____ means respiration.

7. The respiratory center is located in the _____ _____.

8. A lung disease characterized by wheezing is known as _____.

9. _____ is the enzyme contained in saliva.

10. The stomach is capable of holding a _____ _____ of food and liquid.

11. The main components of the digestive secretions in the stomach are

    _____ _____ and _____.

12. Food generally remains in the stomach for _____ minutes to _____ hours.

13. The small intestine is about _____ _____ long when uncoiled.

14. The large intestine is approximately _____ _____ long.

15. The vermiform appendix is attached to the _____.

16. List four functions of the large intestine:

    A. _____

    B. _____

    C. _____

    D. _____

17. Four functions of the liver are:

    _____

    _____.

18. Produced by the pancreas, _____ is released into the bloodstream according to the amount of circulating glucose.

19. A _____ is a needle puncture of the abdominal cavity followed by aspiration of fluid.

20. The primary component of urine is _____.

21. The kidneys produce about _____ of urine daily.

22. List the three main functions of the kidneys:

    A. _____

    B. _____

    C. _____

Name _____

Date _____

23. The urge to urinate occurs when the bladder contains approximately _____
_____ of urine.

Unscramble the following terms.

24. SHRIOCRIS   _____

25. TENCICONNIEN   _____

26. SLAMYEA   _____

27. LANAS STUMEP   _____ _____

28. SLAISPREITS   _____

29. VENATRSERS LONCO   _____ _____

30. MIGDIOS LONCO   _____ _____

31. SLATECAL   _____

32. SPRANCEA   _____

33. SPAILE   _____

34. TIEXISASP   _____

35. NYDSEAP   _____

Chapter Seventeen
The Specialties: The Sensory, Endocrine, and Reproductive Systems

Objectives

After completing this chapter you should be able to do the following:

1. Define and correctly spell each of the key terms.

2. Identify the five major senses.

3. Explain how sound waves are transmitted, received, and interpreted.

4. Explain how the process of smelling occurs.

5. Identify the four kinds of taste receptors.

6. Name the two types of glands and their secretions.

7. Identify the glands within the endocrine system.

8. Explain the function of insulin.

9. Explain the function of estrogen.

10. Explain the function of testosterone.

11. Name the parts of the female and male reproductive systems.

12. Name four sexually transmitted diseases.

Key Terms

- auditory nerve
- circumcision
- endocrine
- estrogen
- exocrine
- gland
- menstruation

- sexually transmitted diseases
- taste receptors
- testes
- testosterone
- uterus
- vulva

The Special Systems

This chapter introduces some of the body's unique systems such as the sensory, endocrine, and reproductive systems. The **sensory system** includes sight, hearing, smell, taste, and touch. The **endocrine system** involves glands and hormones. The **reproductive system** also involves glands and hormones as well as structures that are designed for the reproduction of a human being.

The Sensory System

The sensory system consists of structures that allow the body to react to the environment through sight, smell, hearing, taste, balance, touch, pressure, temperature, etc. The body responds because of the complex relationship between structures such as the eyes, ears, nose, taste buds, and nerves that carry specific messages to the brain. The brain responds to these messages by transmitting another message to a specific area of the body, causing it to react. For example, if you smell a bad odor, the message that is transmitted to your brain includes information regarding the fact that you are smelling something unpleasant. The brain will then respond by sending a message via the nerves to breathe through your mouth instead of your nose. Your mouth will open, allowing you to receive enough oxygen and reducing the amount of the odor that is assaulting your nose. All of this happens very quickly; you don't even have to think about it. Your sensory system takes care of the problem for you.

The five senses of sight, hearing, taste, smell, and touch are called the **major senses**. Therefore, these senses are particularly worthy of detailed study in any discussion of the sensory system.

The Eye

The eye is a very delicate and detailed organ. The eyeball is spherical in shape and is protected anteriorly by the skull bones and inferiorly by facial bones that form the eye socket, or orbit. The eyelid and eyelashes offer protection to the anterior portion by helping to keep out foreign bodies such as dust, dirt, and pathogens.

The eye is made up of many different parts, each one playing a significant role in a person's ability to see. The eyeball is surrounded by three layers of protective tissue. The outer layer, called the **sclera**, is made from firm, tough, connective tissue and is white in color. The middle layer, called the **choroid coat**, is a delicate network of connective tissue that contains many blood vessels. The inner layer, which is called the **retina**, contains the nerve receptors for vision and approximately 10 different layers of nerve cells. There are two kinds of nerve cells contained within the retina: **cones**, which are used mainly for light vision; and **rods**, which are used when it is dark or dim.

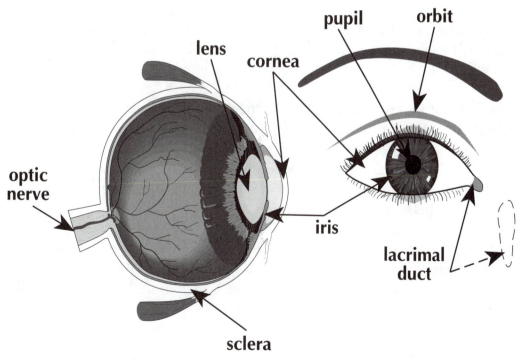

Figure 17-1: The Eye

There are several other important structures contained in the eye. The **cornea** is the clear front portion of the eye. The cornea is very sensitive to injury; visual problems can result if it becomes scarred. The main function of the cornea is to permit light rays to pass through to the retina. This allows the image to be relayed to the brain. **Lacrimal glands** are located within the orbit. They constantly produce tears, which lubricate the eye and allow it to glide smoothly within the socket and under the eyelid. A clear, mucous membrane, called the **conjunctiva**, covers the inner eyelids and the front of the eyeball—except for the cornea. Both the lacrimal glands and the conjunctiva serve to protect the eye.

A person's eye color is determined by the color of the **iris**. This muscular structure is at the front of the eyeball and allows the pupil to adjust its size, depending on the amount of light entering the eye. The **pupil** is the black circle in the middle of the iris. It **constricts** (becomes smaller) when bright light enters it and when focusing on something at close range. The pupil **dilates** (becomes larger) when the light is dim and when focusing on distant objects. Certain drugs, injuries to the head, eye surgeries, and neurological disorders also can effect pupil size.

Behind the iris is the **lens**. It is circular in shape, made of a jelly-like substance, and is suspended in place by ligaments. As light enters the iris, it passes through to the lens. The lens then refracts, or bends, the light rays directly to the retina.

The shape of the eyeball depends on the **aqueous humor** and the **vitreous humor**. The aqueous humor is a clear, watery fluid found in the anterior and posterior chambers of the eye. It helps maintain the forward curvature of the eyeball and helps refract the light rays to the retina. The vitreous humor is necessary to keep the eye in its spherical shape. It fills the entire cavity behind the lens and helps in light ray refraction.

Each eye has six extraocular muscles that coordinate eye movement. Five nerves also serve each eye: two sensory nerves and three motor nerves. Sensory nerves detect pain, temperature, burning, etc., while motor nerves actually transmit messages that result in movement.

Many different injuries and illnesses can affect the clarity of a person's vision. Some of the more common ailments are listed below.

- **astigmatism:** blurred vision and severe eyestrain due to irregularity in the curvature of the cornea or lens.

- **cataract:** a disease in which the lens becomes cloudy and obstructs the passage of light.

- **conjunctivitis:** inflammation of the white of the eye, characterized by redness and a sticky discharge; pink eye.

- **glaucoma:** an eye disorder caused by an increase in intraocular pressure.

- **hyperopia:** farsightedness; a condition in which the rays of light entering the eye come to a focus behind the retina, causing objects that are close to appear blurry.

- **myopia:** nearsightedness; a condition in which the rays of light entering the eye come to a focus in front of the retina, causing objects that are at a distance to appear blurry.

- **strabismus:** a condition in which the muscles of the eyeballs fail to coordinate movement; commonly seen as *cross eyes.*

Diagnosing Problems of the Eye

The following instruments and tests may aid in the diagnosis of eye disorders.

- **ophthalmoscope:** an instrument with a light used to view the internal structures of the eye, especially the retina and the blood vessels.

- **slit lamp:** a microscope used to view the eye under high magnification.

- **Snellen Eye Test:** a test in which the visual acuity is tested by reading the Snellen eye chart from 20 feet away.

- **tonometer:** an instrument used to measure intraocular pressure of the eye.

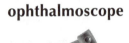

ophthalmoscope

Schiotz tonometer

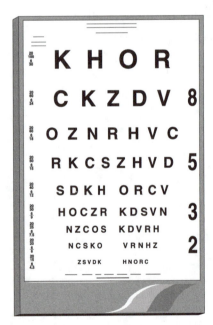

Snellen eye chart

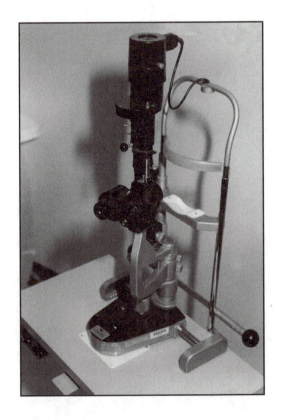

slit lamp

Figure 17-2: Instruments used in diagnosing problems with the eye

The Ear

The ear makes it possible for us to hear and maintain our balance, or **equilibrium**. It is divided into three sections: the outer ear, the middle ear, and the inner ear. The outer ear, known as the **auricle** or **pinna**, is made of cartilage that projects from the head. The pinna leads into the **external auditory canal** and ends at the tympanic membrane (the eardrum). The outer portion of the pinna secretes a special wax, called **cerumen**, which along with hair, traps small particles and foreign bodies and keeps them from entering the middle and inner parts of the ear. The middle ear, or tympanic cavity, is between the eardrum and the inner ear, and leads to the internal auditory canal, called the **eustachian tube**. It conducts sound to the inner ear by passing sound vibrations from the air outside to the fluid in the inner ear via a chain of three tiny bones called **ossicles**. The anterior of the inner ear contains the **cochlea**, which holds the sensory receptors for hearing; and the posterior contains the **semicircular canals** and the **vestibule**, which include the receptors for equilibrium and the sense of position.

Hearing begins when sound waves enter the external ear, and travel into the external auditory canal to the tympanic membrane, which separates the external auditory canal from the middle ear. The sound waves cause the tympanic membrane to vibrate and transmit the sound to the three ossicles of the middle ear: the **malleus**, the **incus**, and the **stapes**. These three ossicles are small bones that are connected in such a way that sound waves are amplified and then transmitted to the fluid contained in the inner ear. The tympanic membrane and the ossicles are extremely delicate and may be injured by the violent movement of air waves (eg, explosions, loud music, or shouting directly into the ear).

Air enters and leaves the middle ear through the eustachian tube. This tube is directly connected to the upper part of the throat, making the ear and throat susceptible to infection. The eustachian tube allows the air pressure in the middle ear to equal the air pressure entering the external auditory canal. This actually keeps the air pressure on both sides of the tympanic membrane equal. When there is unequal pressure in the ear, a *popping* sound can often be heard. Blowing the nose can cause secretions to enter into the middle ear via the eustachian tube, thereby increasing a person's chance of contracting an ear infection.

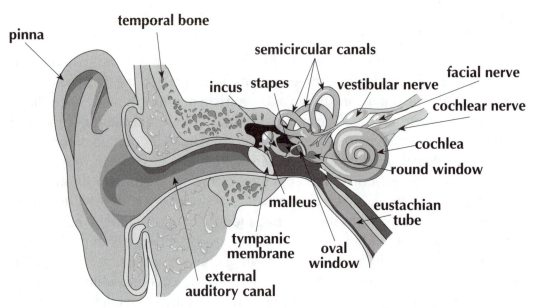

Figure 17-3: The Ear

The inner ear is the most important and complex structure of the ear. It is connected to the middle ear by the attachment of the stapes to the **oval window**. The oval window is a membrane that vibrates with each sound wave transmitted. The cochlea, which resembles a snail in shape, contains the **organ of Corti**, which transmits the sound waves to the brain for interpretation via the **auditory nerve**. The inner ear also contains the centers for equilibrium, or balance: the vestibule and semicircular canals. These canals contain fluid that moves in response to head and body movements. The movement of the fluid is sensed by tiny hair cells that line the canals. These special cells convey messages about the movements to the brain via nerve fibers, forming our sense of balance and equilibrium.

A summary of how hearing occurs is illustrated in Figure 17-4.

auditory nerve: the nerve, contained within the organ of Corti, which conducts sound waves to the brain for interpretation

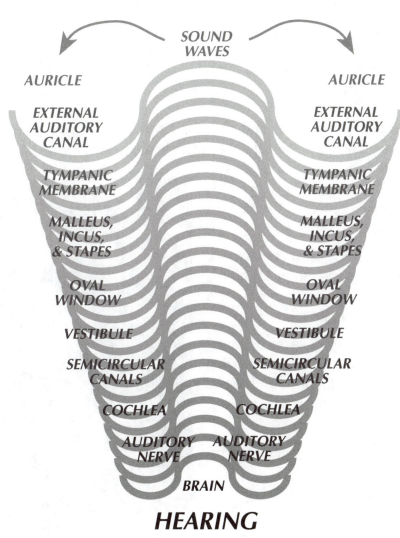

Figure 17-4: How Sound is Heard

Certain problems are specific to the ear and its structures. Some are listed below.

- **cerumen impaction:** an abnormal accumulation of cerumen (wax) in the external auditory canal.

- **deafness:** the partial or complete inability to hear; may be caused by problems in conducting sound waves or in sensing the sound waves.

- **otitis externa:** inflammation of the external ear canal.

- **otitis media:** inflammation of the middle ear.

Diagnostic Tests for the Inner Ear

Special instruments and tests are intended for the diagnosis of ear disorders. Some are listed below.

- **audiometry:** a method of evaluating hearing by introducing sounds at different pitches to the patient through headphones. As the patient hears a sound, he or she indicates in which ear the sound was detected by holding up either the right or left hand.

- **otoscope:** an instrument with a light that is used to examine the external auditory canal and tympanic membrane.

- **Rinne test:** the use of a tuning fork to assess a person's hearing via air conduction and bone conduction of the sound waves.

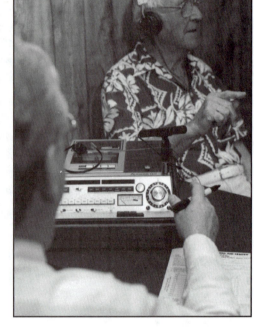

audiometry

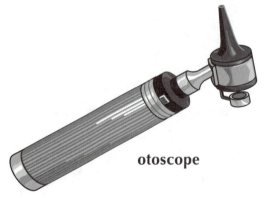

otoscope

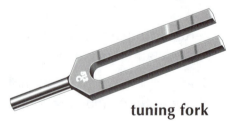

tuning fork

Figure 17-5: Diagnostic Tools for Problems Associated With the Inner Ear

Taste, Smell, and Touch

Taste receptors (taste buds) are located in various areas on the surface of the tongue, but they are only stimulated if the substance to be tasted is in liquid form. Of course, not everything we eat is in liquid form, but saliva mixes with the food in the mouth and moistens it enough to stimulate the taste buds. There are four kinds of taste buds on the tongue: sweet, which are located on the tip of the tongue; sour, located on the lateral aspects of the tongue; salty, also located on the tip of the tongue; and bitter, detected on the posterior aspect. Once taste is detected by the receptors, the lingual and the glossopharyngeal nerves (cranial nerves) carry the taste impulses to the brain.

taste receptors: taste buds; the oval structures located in various areas on the surface of the tongue that transmit the sensation of taste

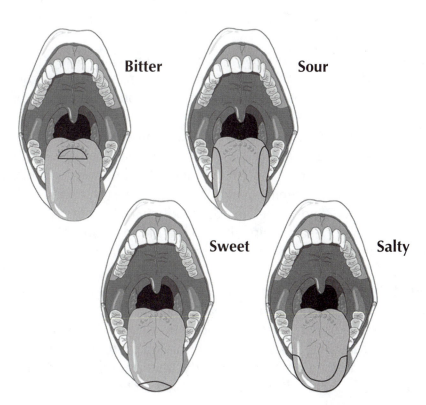

Figure 17-6: The Tastebuds

The sense of taste is closely related to the sense of smell. Receptors located in the upper part of the nasal cavity, the **olfactory epithelium**, are stimulated by scents. On stimulation, the **olfactory nerve**, one of the twelve cranial nerves, transmits the message to the brain. If there is inflammation in the nasal passages, as with a cold, the sense of smell diminishes which, in turn, causes the sense of taste to decrease.

The sense of touch includes perceptions regarding surface texture, shape, size, pressure, pain, and temperature. This sense is produced by numerous receptors located throughout the body. There are two basic types of receptors. The first is simply a nerve fiber that is wrapped around the hair bulbs beneath the surface of the skin. When the hairs move, the receptors respond by sending a message to the brain. The other type of receptor is more complex. They consist of specialized structures that surround the nerve endings. All receptors pass signals through sensory nerves to the spinal cord, which carries the signals to the brain. Once these messages are transmitted to the brain, the body reacts to the stimulus in an appropriate way.

The Endocrine System

gland:
a structure within the body that secretes a substance used elsewhere in the body

The body is regulated by a unique system of **glands**. Glands are divided into two groups: **exocrine**, which have ducts (tubes) to transport the secretion from the gland to another organ or part of the body; and **endocrine**, which are ductless and must depend on the blood or lymph systems to transport their secretion to the different body tissues. The exocrine glands produce the digestive juices, the secretions from the sebaceous glands of the skin, tears from the lacrimal glands, and urine. The endocrine system includes the following glands: pituitary, thyroid, parathyroid, adrenals, pancreas, ovaries, testes, thymus, pineal body, and the placenta. Endocrine glands produce only internal secretions, or hormones that are released directly into the bloodstream. The pancreas is an organ that contains both exocrine and endocrine gland tissue.

exocrine:
describes glands that transport secretions to another part of the body via ducts

endocrine:
pertaining to a gland that secretes chemicals (hormones) directly into the bloodstream

The **pituitary gland** is about the size of a cherry and is located at the base of the brain, posterior to the nose, in an area called the **sella turcica**. It is commonly referred to as the *master gland* of the body because it can control the secretion of hormones from other glands. The anterior and posterior lobes of the pituitary gland secrete hormones that regulate body functions concerned with reproduction, growth, and **metabolism**. The abnormal functioning of the pituitary gland can result in the following diseases.

- **acromegaly:** a chronic disease of the endocrine system, characterized by elongation and enlargement of the bones, especially of the face; caused by excessive production of pituitary hormones.

- **dwarfism:** a condition in which one is abnormally small in size; sometimes the result of inadequate production of the pituitary hormones.

- **gigantism:** a condition in which a person grows to be excessively large in size; sometimes the result of overproduction of pituitary hormones.

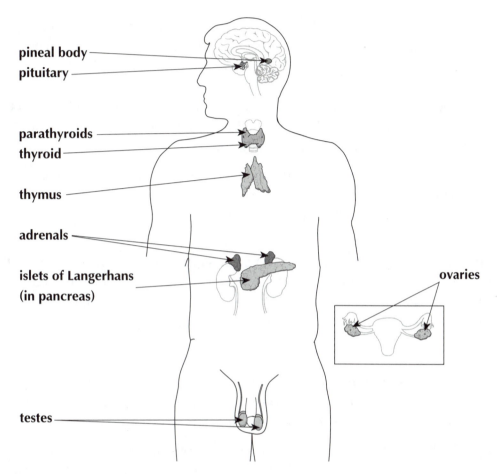

Figure 17-7: The Endocrine System

The **thyroid gland** is located on the anterior portion of the trachea. It is responsible for regulating the body's metabolism, or use of energy. The thyroid gland has two lobes that are located on either side of the larynx. The lobes are attached to one another by a piece of tissue called the **isthmus**. In order to produce its hormones, the thyroid gland must receive iodine. Iodine is obtained from different food sources such as halibut, cod, iodized salt, and vegetables. There are three common disorders involving the thyroid gland.

- **goiter:** the abnormal enlargement of the thyroid gland.

- **hyperthyroidism:** the excessive production of thyroid hormones resulting in irritability, nervousness, and restlessness.

- **hypothyroidism:** underproduction of thyroid hormones resulting in fatigue and weight gain.

The amount of calcium in the blood is regulated by the **parathyroid** glands. These four glands are posterior to the thyroid gland and are attached to it. There are two common conditions that can affect the parathyroid glands.

- **hyperparathyroidism:** overactivity of the parathyroid glands resulting in elevated calcium levels in the blood; leads to the formation of renal calculi and the decalcification of bones.

- **hypoparathyroidism:** underproduction of the parathyroid glands, which results in a decreased level of calcium in the blood; causes tetany of the muscles (spasmodic movement).

Located superior to each kidney is an **adrenal gland**. These glands resemble the kidneys in that each adrenal gland is composed of two parts: the cortex (the outer part), and the medulla (the inner part). Each part produces specific hormones that have specific functions. The following are common health disorders associated with the functioning of the adrenal glands.

- **Addison's disease:** a life-threatening disease of the endocrine system resulting from underproduction of adrenocortical hormones. Symptoms include fatigue, hypotension, vomiting, anorexia, nausea, and others.

- **Cushing's disease:** the excessive secretion of adrenocortical hormones resulting in hypertension, diabetes, obesity, moon-shaped face, edema, osteoporosis, skin discoloration, loss of protein, and other symptoms.

The **pancreas** is a gland located in the left upper abdominal quadrant, posterior to the stomach. Within the digestive system it functions as an exocrine gland, but it is also part of the endocrine system. **Insulin** is an endocrine hormone produced by the pancreas. Insulin regulates the level of blood sugar (**glucose**) in the body through the metabolism of fats and carbohydrates, and is produced in the pancreas within the **islets of Langerhans**.

Like other organs, malfunctions of the pancreas can cause certain diseases. Some are listed below.

- **diabetes mellitus:** a disease caused by the inadequate production of insulin and characterized by excessive thirst (**polydipsia**), excessive urination (**polyuria**), and excessive hunger (**polyphagia**).

- **pancreatitis:** inflammation of the pancreas, usually as a result of alcoholism.

The **thymus gland** is a mass of lymphoid tissue located in the thoracic cavity, superior to the heart. It increases in size rapidly for the first two years of life; however, during puberty it atrophies, or wastes away. The thymus gland is responsible for the formation of the immune system in the newborn. Diseases of the thymus gland are extremely rare and may only involve gland enlargement.

The **pineal body** is located in the brain. Its exact function is not clearly understood; however, evidence indicates that it is involved in the function of the sex glands: the testes and ovaries. Removal of the pineal gland or insufficient secretion of its hormone results in early-onset puberty.

The sex glands will be addressed in detail in the discussion of the reproductive system later in this chapter, but they are also an important part of the endocrine system. The testes are the sex glands of the male. They produce hormones that are responsible for the development of the male's secondary sexual characteristics such as body hair, a low voice, and muscular development, and are also responsible for stimulating the sexual drive. The ovaries are the sex glands of the female. They produce hormones that are responsible for the development of secondary sexual characteristics such as pubic hair, wider hips, and breast enlargement. These hormones also regulate the menstrual cycle. The **placenta** is a unique endocrine gland because it is temporary. It is only present in the pregnant female and is expelled after the birth of the child. It produces hormones that prepare the mother's body for the baby.

Diagnostic Tests for the Endocrine System

The most common form of diagnostic testing for the endocrine system involves hormone-specific blood tests. As with the other body systems, **MRIs** and **CT Scans** may also be used to determine certain conditions.

The Reproductive System

The last body system to be discussed in this text will be the reproductive system. The primary function of this system is to reproduce life. Reproduction is achieved in humans by the fertilization of one ovum (produced by the female) by one sperm (produced by the male). Both the female and the male reproductive systems are extremely intricate.

The Female

The reproductive system of the female is comprised of several parts: the ovaries, the fallopian tubes, the uterus, the Bartholin's gland, the vagina, the vulva, and the breasts. The **ovaries** are the actual sex glands, or gonads, of the female. They are located on either side of the pelvic cavity and are attached to the uterus by ligaments. The almond-shaped ovaries are nourished by a rich blood supply, and contain thousands of sacs called **follicles** that each contain one immature **ovum**, or egg. The ovum is the female sex cell. As it matures, it will enlarge and rupture. This process normally occurs once a month and is called **ovulation**. Several hormones are produced in the ovaries, the primary one being **estrogen**. Estrogen and other hormones produced by the ovaries cause the production of the female's secondary sexual characteristics: the widening of the hip area to accommodate pregnancy and birth, the growth of pubic hair, the enlargement of the breasts, and the preparation of the uterus for possible pregnancy.

estrogen: the female sex hormone, produced by the ovaries, which is responsible for the development of secondary sex characteristics and for the cyclic changes in the lining of the uterus

The **fallopian tubes** extend from the upper part of the uterus. They are about 5 inches in length and contain finger-like projections called **fimbriae**. The fallopian tubes are superior to the ovaries; however, they are not directly attached to them. The fimbriae receive the mature ovum from the ovary. The ovum is transported through the fallopian tube to the uterus by peristalsis. It is in the fallopian tube where **fertilization**, the actual union of a sperm and ovum, occurs.

If each tube is surgically tied off or partially removed, the egg cannot be fertilized. This process, called a **tubal ligation**, is a method some women choose to avoid pregnancy. This procedure makes her *sterile* or *barren.* The term *sterile* does not mean that she is now free of microorganisms; in this case, it refers to the inability to produce children. There are various causes of sterility. Some, such as the one described, are voluntary; and others are congenital, or due to some physiological factor and may or may not be correctable.

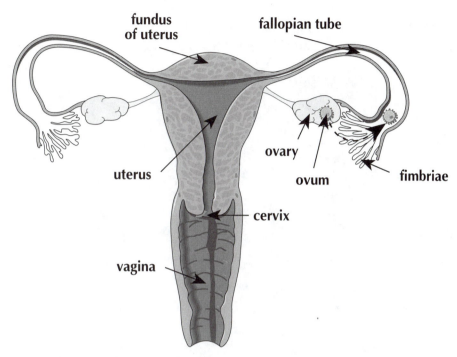

fundus
of uterus

fallopian tube

uterus

ovary

ovum

fimbriae

cervix

vagina

Figure 17-8: The Female Reproductive System (anterior view)

The **uterus** is a hollow, muscular organ that is shaped like a pear. The uterus is located in the abdominal cavity, posterior to the bladder and anterior to the rectum. It is divided into three sections: the top section, called the **fundus**; the middle section, called the body or **corpus**; and the bottom section known as the **cervix**. The uterus is made up of three layers: the inner layer, called the **endometrium**, the middle, muscular layer, called the **myometrium**; and the outer serous layer, called the **parametrium**.

The uterus has two main functions: to provide a place for the growing fetus, and to shed its endometrium every four weeks or so if there is no embryo present. The endometrium provides the area where the fertilized ovum will attach itself and grow. The muscular layer of the uterus thickens throughout pregnancy and, during the birth process, forcibly contracts and delivers the fetus through the **birth canal**, or vagina. If the ovum remains unfertilized, the endometrial layer will slough. This produces the bleeding known as **menstruation**.

Connected to the cervix of the uterus, the **vagina** is a very muscular and highly sensitive tube that receives the penis during sexual intercourse and serves as a passageway for the delivery of the fetus. It enlarges during childbirth and during sexual intercourse. It is supplied by two **Bartholin's glands**, one on either side, which lubricate the vagina with mucus.

uterus:
the organ in the female reproductive system responsible for holding the embryo and fetus from conception until birth

menstruation:
the periodic shedding of the endometrial layer of tissue from the uterus

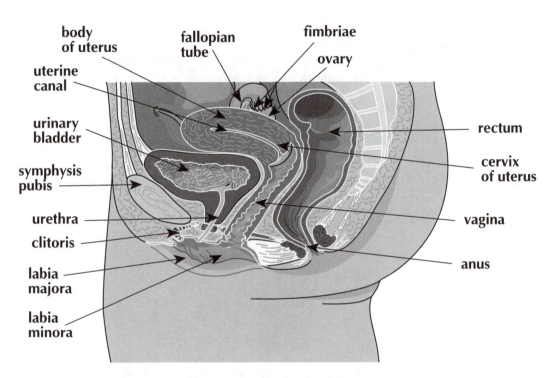

Figure 17-9: The Female Reproductive System (lateral view)

The female's external genitals are known as the **vulva**. The structures contained within the vulva are the **mons veneris**, the fatty pad covered with hair that lies over the pubic area; the **labia majora**, the two large folds of skin that cover and protect the vagina; the **labia minora**, the smaller folds of skin lying within the labia majora; and the **clitoris**, a highly sensitive area located at the junction of the labia minora. Located inferior to the clitoris and superior to the vagina is the external opening of the **urinary meatus**. This is the point at which urine is released from the body. The **perineum** is the area located between the vagina and the anus.

The mammary glands, or the **breasts**, are made up of mostly fatty, or adipose, tissue. They contain milk ducts which exit through the nipples. The main function of the breasts is **lactation** (the formation of milk) following childbirth.

Diseases and Abnormal Conditions of the Female Reproductive System

Like the other systems, the female reproductive system can be affected by specific diseases.

- **amenorrhea:** the absence or suppression of menstruation.

- **ectopic pregnancy:** the growth of a fertilized egg implanted outside the uterus, usually in the fallopian tube.

- **endometriosis:** the presence of endometrial tissue outside of the uterus in various places within the pelvic cavity.

- **gonorrhea:** a **sexually transmitted disease** caused by a specific bacterium.

- **herpes:** a sexually transmitted disease resulting in a chronic viral infection characterized by blister-like vesicles on the genitals.

- **hypermenorrhea:** excessive menstruation.

- **ovarian cyst:** a fluid-filled sac located on the ovary.

- **pelvic inflammatory disease (PID):** an infection that ascends from the vagina or cervix to the uterus, oviducts, and uterine ligaments.

- **syphilis:** a chronic sexually transmitted disease characterized by lesions on an organ or on the skin; may be present without symptoms for years.

sexually transmitted disease: a disease that is acquired during sexual intercourse or other sexually intimate contact with an infected individual

All of the sexually transmitted diseases (STDs) are common to both sexes and include: AIDS, herpes, gonorrhea, syphilis, and chlamydiae. As you have already learned, AIDS is a potentially fatal disease and may also be contracted through infected blood and other body fluids. Early recognition and treatment of sexually transmitted diseases is essential. However, prevention is the best way to avoid the physical and psychological damages these disease can cause.

Diagnostic Procedures for the Female Reproductive System

Some of the most commonly used diagnostic tests for the female reproductive system are listed below.

- **biopsy:** the removal of a small piece of living tissue for examination under a microscope.

- **computerized tomography (CT) scan:** a technique for examining transverse planes of internal structures of the body in which x-rays are used to construct a precise image and show the relationship of structures.

- **conization**: the excision of a cone of tissue, usually of the cervix, for examination.

- **dilation and curettage:** the surgical dilation of the cervix and scraping (curettage) of the uterus.

- **magnetic resonance imaging (MRI):** a diagnostic procedure in which parts of the body are exposed to an electromagnetic field to produce an image.

- **pap smear:** the scraping and examination of cells from the body, especially the cervix and the vaginal walls. This test is used in the detection of cancer. (Papanicolaou test)

- **pelvic ultrasound:** the use of sound waves to detect masses or tumors within the pelvic cavity.

testes:
the male reproductive glands; responsible for producing testosterone

testosterone:
the hormone, produced by the testes, which stimulates the growth of secondary sexual characteristics and is essential for normal sexual behavior in males

The Male

The male reproductive system includes the testes, the epididymis, the vas deferens, the seminal vesicles, the ejaculatory ducts, the urethra, the prostate gland, the Cowper's glands, and the penis.

The primary reproductive organs of the male are the **testes**. There are two testes located within the scrotum, a sac located posterior to the **penis**. The testes produce **spermatozoa**, or sperm, which are the male sex cells. **Testosterone**, a male hormone responsible for producing the secondary sexual characteristics and for assisting in the maturation of the sperm, is also produced in the testes.

The sperm begin their journey to the outside of the body by traveling through the entire length of the **epididymis**. This is a coiled tube that is approximately

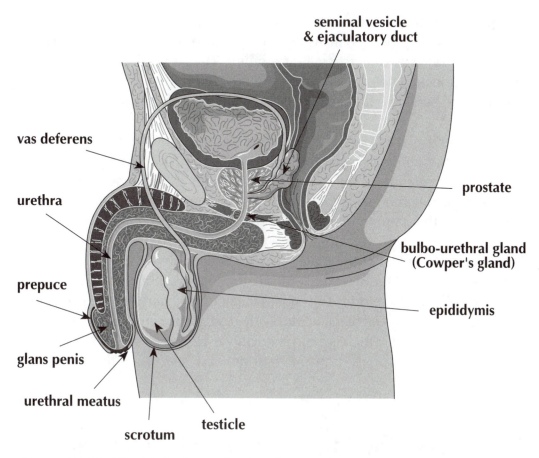

seminal vesicle
& ejaculatory duct

vas deferens

urethra

prepuce

glans penis

urethral meatus

scrotum

testicle

prostate

bulbo-urethral gland
(Cowper's gland)

epididymis

Figure 17-10: The Male Reproductive System (lateral view)

20 feet long when fully extended. It stores the sperm until they are mature and active; it also produces a fluid that is mixed with the sperm. This mixture is called **semen**. The semen then travels up the epididymis to the vas deferens.

The **vas deferens** are the straight extensions of the epididymis. They are located on both sides of the epididymis posterior to the urinary bladder, and are receiving areas for the seminal fluid from the epididymis. During a **vasectomy**, a part of each vas deferens is removed, thus prohibiting the transportation of the seminal fluid through the rest of the reproductive system. This is a method of sterilization that some men choose to undergo to prevent reproduction. Sometimes, a vasectomy can be reversed to restore the ability to reproduce.

Located posterior to the bladder where the vas deferens join the ejaculatory ducts are the **seminal vesicles**. The yellow fluid produced by these vesicles is thick, and contains high amounts of sugar and other nutrients for the sperm. This fluid enters the ejaculatory ducts, which are inside the prostate gland. The seminal fluid flows from the vas deferens to the ejaculatory ducts, where it mixes with the fluid from the prostate gland.

The **prostate gland** is located inferior to the urinary bladder on both sides of the urethra. The fluid produced in the prostate gland helps nourish the sperm in the ejaculatory ducts and increase their motility. The seminal and prostate fluid mixes together and helps neutralize the secretions in the vagina, which allows the sperm to survive once they are ejaculated (expelled) from the body.

The **Cowper's glands** are located inferior to the prostate and are directly attached to the urethra, which serves as a passageway for both urine and semen. The Cowper's glands secrete a mucus-like fluid that functions as a lubricant during sexual intercourse, and helps neutralize the acidity in the urethra from urine so that the sperm remain alive and motile.

The external genitalia of the male include the scrotal sac and the sex organ, which is the **penis**. During sexual arousal, the spaces within the penis become engorged (filled) with blood. This makes the penis stiff and erect. The enlarged structure at the distal end of the penis is called the **glans penis**. It is covered with **prepuce**, or foreskin, which is often surgically removed by an operation called **circumcision**. The penis transports urine and sperm to the outside of the body.

circumcision:
the surgical
removal of the
prepuce, or
foreskin, of
the penis

Diseases of the Male Reproductive System

Some common diseases of the male reproductive system are listed below.

- **cryptorchidism:** a congenital abnormality in which the testes fail to descend into the scrotum. (Also spelled cryptorchism.)

- **gonorrhea:** a sexually transmitted disease caused by a specific bacterium.

- **herpes:** a sexually transmitted disease resulting in a chronic viral infection characterized by blister-like vesicles on the genitals.

- **phimosis:** excessive tightness of the prepuce so that it is unable to be withdrawn.

- **syphilis:** a chronic sexually transmitted disease characterized by lesions on an organ or on the skin; may be present without symptoms for years.

- **tumors:** abnormal growths that may or may not be malignant. These most commonly occur in the prostate gland, but sometimes are found in the testes.

Diagnostic Tests for the Male Reproductive System

The most common diagnostic tests concerning the male reproductive system are listed below.

- **computerized tomography (CT) scan:** a technique for examining transverse planes of internal structures of the body in which x-rays are used to construct a precise image and show the relationship of structures.

- **cystoscopy:** the examination of the urinary bladder using an instrument containing a light and a camera called a cystoscope that is introduced into the bladder through the urethra.

- **magnetic resonance imaging (MRI):** a diagnostic procedure in which parts of the body are exposed to an electromagnetic field to produce an image.

- **radiology studies:** x-ray films; diagnostic tests that use film and radiation to show most of the internal structures.

- **ultrasound:** inaudible sound waves that can be used to create visual images of the internal structures.

Chapter Summary

The systems of the body are highly specialized; however, they all work together. Sight, taste, smell, hearing, and touch are possible through the delicate sensory system; the endocrine system is responsible for the release of hormones that control body changes; and the reproductive system is important for continuing the existence of the human race. All of the body systems, functioning harmoniously together, support the physical aspects of a human being. In order for the body to perform at its optimal level, every part of each system must be in a complete state of wellness. However, it is important to remember that a person also has feelings, emotions, and needs that must be considered. It is the healthcare worker's ethical responsibility to PROVIDE COMPLETE CARE FOR EVERY PATIENT!

Name _____

Date _____

Student Enrichment Activities

Complete the following statements.

1. Name the three layers of the eyeball: the _____, the
   _____ _____, and the _____.

2. There are approximately _____ extraocular muscles that coordinate eye movement.

3. The two types of nerve cells contained within the retina are called
   _____ and _____.

4. The ear is responsible for _____ and _____.

5. The three ossicles are the _____, _____, and
   the _____.

6. List the ten endocrine glands.

   _____

   _____

7. A chronic disease characterized by elongation and enlargement of the bones is
   _____.

8. The body's metabolism is regulated by the _____ gland and the
   hormones secreted by the pituitary gland.

9. _____ is a hormone produced by the pancreas.

10. The sex glands of the female are the _____.

11. The primary hormone produced by the ovaries is _____.

12. The pear-shaped muscular organ located within the female abdominal cavity is the
    _____.

13. Name the parts of the male reproductive system: (Hint: There are nine.)

    _____

    _____

14. The mixture of sperm and other fluid substances is called_____.

Unscramble the following terms.

15. SCRIOMCIUCIN   _____

16. UHCGSINS ISEDSAE   _____ _____

17. STROETOSTENE   _____

18. SNILUIN   _____

19. OOOETSPC   _____

20. CLEANPAT   _____

21. SLIMENA CLEVESIS   _____ _____

22. MENIREPU   _____

Name _____

Date _____

23. LCTTNAAIO

_____

24. SAV SNERFEDE

_____   _____

25. GROESTEN

_____

26. REACON

_____

27. REMUCEN

_____

28. ATRIUMDOEY

_____

29. PECOTIC GRANPENCY

_____   _____

30. CHLEACO

_____

Chapter Eighteen
Basic First Aid

Objectives

After completing this chapter you should be able to
do the following:

1. Define and correctly spell each of the key terms.

2. Describe how to perform the primary survey.

3. Identify the two ways to open an airway.

4. Describe the two ways to control hemorrhage from a
    traumatic injury.

5. Describe the basic procedure for performing a secondary survey.

6. List at least three signs that a person is in shock.

7. List at least three intervention techniques for the management
    of seizures.

8. Identify at least five signs of a possible myocardial infarction.

9. Describe the intervention techniques for a person experiencing
    chest pain.

10. List the two guidelines to be followed for all unconscious patients.

11. Name and describe the four kinds of burns and the interventions
    for each.

12. Describe the three common signs for both a fracture and a sprain
    and the appropriate intervention techniques for each.

Key Terms

- anticoagulant
- antidote
- cardiac arrest
- cardiac compressions
- emetic
- finger sweep
- head-tilt/chin-lift maneuver
- Heimlich maneuver
- hypovolemic shock
- jaw-thrust maneuver
- log roll
- Medic-Alert
- Poison Control
- primary survey
- secondary survey
- seizure
- syncope
- tongue-jaw lift
- toxic

Skilled First Aid: It Saves Lives

Being a healthcare worker involves knowing what to do in case of an unexpected injury or illness. This chapter provides basic information on introductory **first aid**. First aid is the IMMEDIATE care provided to a person who has sustained an injury, sudden illness, or other medical emergency. In the hospital environment, first aid may be required in any department and with any patient. You must be prepared for the unexpected AT ALL TIMES!

First aid must be given promptly and accurately. In cases of severe bleeding, poisoning, or if someone's heart or breathing has stopped, first aid may save a person's life. There also are cases in which first aid has prevented additional injury or medical problems from occurring. Emergency treatment should be provided by the person most qualified and skilled at the scene. In many cases, this will be YOU! First aid intervention must be continued until a more qualified medical professional, or someone at least as qualified as you, arrives or the patient is transported to a location that can provide a higher level of care.

> **Note:** REMEMBER, wear gloves and other protective devices (such as goggles, face masks, etc.) whenever there is the potential for exposure to blood or other body fluids. If you are not wearing them at the time of the incident (sudden hemorrhage, vomiting, etc.), don them immediately.

Guidelines for Administering First Aid

Before rendering assistance, always survey the scene for any hazards. Check for uncontrolled traffic, chemical spills, fire, angry crowds, etc. If the scene is unsafe, DO NOT ENTER! Be sure to request law enforcement along with medical assistance. Remember, a dead hero is no hero! Once you have determined the scene is safe, you can proceed to assist the patient if you have the necessary skills.

Whether you are the only person at the scene or there are others present, YOU MUST REMAIN CALM! Before you do anything, quickly decide if you are skilled enough to help the patient. If you are unsure or confused, do not attempt to offer assistance! There have been many instances when improper treatment increased the problem or resulted in new complications for the patient. Always keep the patient's care first on your mind. DO NOT PLAY HERO WITH A PERSON'S LIFE IN YOUR HANDS! If the situation arises in the hospital, call for help. If you are outside of the hospital, call 911 (if your city uses that system), an ambulance, police, or fire.

Once you have determined you can be of help to the patient, perform a **primary survey** by examining the patient for any life-threatening emergencies. Check for airway obstructions, apnea (absence of breathing), severe hemorrhaging (bleeding), and signs of **shock**. Always remember the ABCs:

primary survey: an examination of the patient to determine the presence of any life-threatening emergencies; the initial assessment of airway, breathing, and circulation on a patient

    A = Airway
      B = Breathing
        C = Circulation

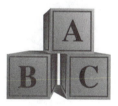

The Primary Survey: Technique and Intervention

The main objective of the primary survey is to detect and correct life-threatening or limb-threatening emergencies. As a healthcare worker you must be knowledgeable and skilled in both performing the assessment and understanding what the data you have collected means. Performing the survey is simple; but interpretation of the data and correct intervention takes consistent practice. The primary survey should be completed in 30 seconds or less. A few seconds can mean the difference between life and death! A number of problems can become life-threatening if they go undetected and uncorrected.

Airway. First check the airway, examining the scene for any clues. The airway assessment includes making sure the airway is not blocked by the patient's tongue, body fluid, or a foreign object.

If the airway is not clear, the airway must be positioned to allow air to enter and escape. The American Heart Association indicates the best and safest method of opening a child's or adult's airway is the **head-tilt/chin-lift maneuver**, which is done by placing one hand on the victim's forehead and applying firm backward pressure to tilt the head back. Place the fingers of the other hand under the lower jaw and lift to bring the chin forward. (Figure 18-1) However, in cases of suspected spinal injury the **jaw-thrust** technique should be used. (Figure 18-2) The jaw-thrust maneuver is done by grasping the angle of the victim's mandible with both hands, one on each side, and lifting it forward. If a patient has fallen or been in an accident, always suspect a spinal injury and treat the patient accordingly. Due to an infant's anatomy, a baby's head should not be hyperextended as an adult's would; instead, it is put into the **sniffing position**, wherein the chin is placed neither too high nor too low. (Figure 18-3) It is the position in which you would hold your head if you were sniffing a baking pie.

head-tilt/chin-lift maneuver: a procedure for opening a blocked airway in which the patient's head is tilted back and the chin is lifted; the most effective method for opening the airway of an unconscious person without a neck or back injury

jaw-thrust maneuver: a method used to open the airway in a neck-injured patient, in which the jaw is lifted up and the neck is not moved

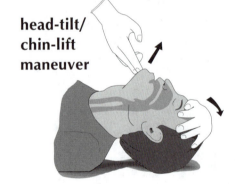

head-tilt/chin-lift maneuver

Figure 18-1

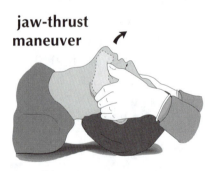

jaw-thrust maneuver

Figure 18-2

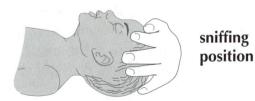

sniffing position

Figure 18-3

IF THE AIRWAY IS NOT CLEAR:

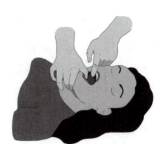

1. PUT ON GLOVES.

2. GRASP THE MOUTH AND OPEN THE JAW WITH YOUR THUMB AND INDEX FINGER.

3. PERFORM A **FINGER SWEEP** TO REMOVE ANY FOREIGN OBJECTS. DO NOT perform a blind finger sweep on a child or infant. This is only done on a child or infant if you can see the object! (The American Heart Association defines a child as from 1 to 8 years of age and an infant as under the age of 1.)

Figure 18-4

finger sweep: a method of removing a foreign object from a choking patient's mouth

4. PERFORM THE HEAD-TILT/CHIN-LIFT MANEUVER (OR JAW-THRUST MANEUVER IF THE PATIENT IS A TRAUMA VICTIM).

Breathing. You can assess the victim's breathing as you check the airway by listening and feeling for the presence of air escaping through the nose or mouth. Look at the chest and watch to see if it rises and falls. Remember, the brain cannot survive without oxygen; irreversible brain damage will occur within 4 to 6 minutes.

1. LOOK for the chest to rise and fall.

2. LISTEN for air escaping through either the mouth or nose by kneeling next to the patient and placing your ear next to the nose and mouth.

3. FEEL for any slight indication of exhalation with your cheek next to the patient's nose and mouth.

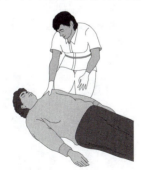

Figure 18-5

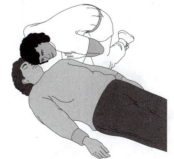

Figure 18-6

If the patient is not breathing and if there is nothing obvious at the scene that indicates an airway obstruction from food or another object, call for help and proceed with rescue breathing. Remember—NOISY BREATHING IS OBSTRUCTED BREATHING!

Rescue breathing is done by inflating the victim's lungs with your own oxygen supply using the mouth-to-mask, mouth-to-mouth, mouth-to-nose, or mouth-to-stoma method. When available, use a pocket mask or bag-valve mask connected to a source of oxygen. Oxygen outlets are found in the wall at each patient unit, and an oxygen tube can be connected to the oxygen inlet of the mask while mouth-to-mask ventilations are performed. This will protect you and provide additional oxygen to the patient. The patient is always given two initial ventilations followed by a pulse check. If a pulse is present, continue rescue breathing by giving one breath every 5 seconds for an adult victim, and one breath every 3 seconds for an infant or child. If no pulse is felt, **cardiac compressions** also must be started. (See the procedure for CPR.)

cardiac compressions: the controlled and repeated application of pressure to the sternum of a cardiac arrest victim to keep the oxygen supply moving throughout the body

Rescue Breathing	
Adult	1 breath every 5 seconds
Child	1 breath every 3 seconds
Infant	1 breath every 3 seconds

To perform mouth-to-mask ventilation, place the mask over the victim's mouth and nose. Press the heel and thumb of each hand along the border of the mask to prevent air from leaking out around the edges. Use your remaining fingers to lift the jaw while performing a head-tilt. Ventilate twice, and watch for the rise and fall of the chest. This should take 1$^1/_2$ to 2 seconds per breath for adult patients and 1 to 1$^1/_2$ seconds per breath for a child or infant. If the victim cannot be ventilated, reposition the head and try again. If ventilation is still unsuccessful, perform the **obstructed airway maneuver**. To perform mouth-to-mouth ventilation on an adult or child, pinch the victim's nostrils, cover his or her mouth with your mouth, and ventilate twice. Proceed with rescue breathing as you would for mouth-to-mask resuscitation.

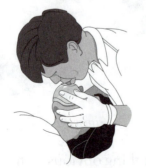

mouth-to-mask resuscitation

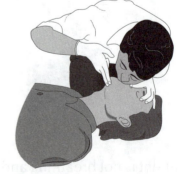

mouth-to-mouth resuscitation

Figure 18-7: The Most Common Methods of Artificial Ventilation

Mouth-to-nose **ventilation** is used when the mouth cannot be opened or there is extensive facial trauma. The head is tilted back and the mouth closed while air is blown into the victim's nose. Mouth-to-stoma ventilation is performed on patients who have undergone a **laryngectomy** or **tracheostomy**. These people have an opening in the front of the neck through which they breathe. To perform this procedure, seal the area around the stoma with your mouth and blow air into the opening. If you can feel air escaping from the nose and mouth, close the mouth and pinch the nostrils as you perform the ventilations.

Remember, if you must begin ventilating a patient without a mask, obtain a mask as soon as possible. Pocket masks are carried in the pockets of staff members and are found at the bedside near the disposable gloves. Typically, they are mounted on the wall in the patient care unit.

A **bag-valve device** can be used with a face mask. (Figure 18-8) Stay at the top of the victim's head and maintain the airway position and an airtight seal between the mask and the patient's face with one hand while squeezing the bag with the other hand. These devices are used for rescue breathing and in conjunction with two-person CPR. Bag-valve masks are found on the crash cart and in the Critical Care and Intensive Care Departments, operating rooms, and Emergency Departments. As soon as the physician, respiratory therapist, or paramedic has intubated the patient, the mask is removed and the bag-valve device is used with a **universal adapter** to ventilate the patient through an **endotracheal tube** or **esophageal airway**.

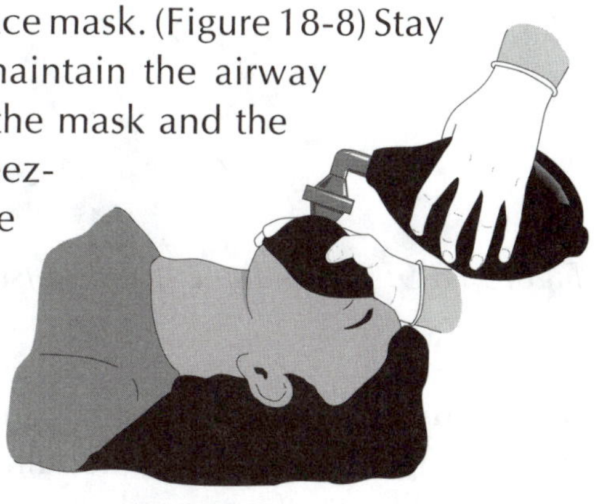

Figure 18-8

In the hospital, respiratory therapists respond to all code situations. They are specially trained in the use of equipment and ventilators (breathing machines) that can be used to **reoxygenate** the patient. Either a nurse, physician, respiratory therapist, or laboratory technician will do special blood tests to measure oxygen levels and take blood from an artery. This test is called an **arterial blood gas (ABG)**. After the blood is drawn, a gloved hand and a cotton ball or gauze are used to apply pressure to the puncture site for at least 6 to 10 minutes. When the bleeding stops, a pressure bandage is applied.

cardiac arrest:
asystole; the
absence of a
heartbeat

Circulation. The last step in the primary survey is to check the circulation. Sometimes when respirations stop, or shortly thereafter, the heart stops beating too. When **cardiac arrest** occurs the heart stops pumping blood through the body, robbing the tissues of vital oxygen and nutrients. Always feel for an adult patient's pulse by locating the carotid artery. This artery is located on either side of the Adam's apple (thyroid cartilage). Keep your fingers in place on the carotid artery for at least 5 to 10 seconds. If there is no pulse present, the proper intervention is to begin CPR.

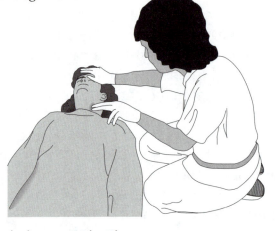

Figure 18-9: Check the carotid pulse.

Management of respiratory arrest, full arrest, and foreign body airway obstruction is taught through a cardiopulmonary resuscitation (CPR) course offered through organizations such as the American Heart Association or the American Red Cross. All hospital employees MUST maintain recognition or certification in this procedure!

CPR for Adults

Cardiopulmonary resuscitation is a procedure that combines rescue breathing and chest compressions. Cardiac compressions provide circulation to the heart, lungs, brain, and other organs. When accompanied by rescue breathing, chest compressions can circulate sufficient oxygen to these vital organs to sustain life. The victim must be **supine**, and a board is placed under the back for effective compressions. You can assure proper hand placement by placing your middle and index fingers over the lower margin of the victim's rib cage and tracing the bony structure to the bottom of the **sternum**. With the middle finger in this notch, place the index finger next to it on the lower end of the sternum. The heel of the hand is placed between the middle and the lower third of the sternum. The long axis of your hand should be placed on the long axis of the sternum. (See Figure 18-10.)

The first hand is removed from the notch and placed on top of the hand on the sternum so that both hands are parallel to each other. Keeping the fingers off of the chest and the elbows locked in position, straighten the arms and thrust the hands straight down, depressing the sternum 1$\frac{1}{2}$ to 2 inches. Then release the pressure, keeping the hands in position on the chest. (See Figure 18-11.) The compression rate should be 80 to 100 per minute. For one-person CPR, the ratio of compressions to ventilations is 15:2. This means that for every 15 compressions there should be two ventilations. For two-person CPR, the ratio of compressions to ventilations is 5:1.

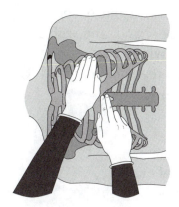

Figure 18-10

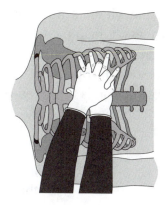

Figure 18-11

After four cycles (four sets of fifteen compressions and two ventilations) of compressions and ventilations or 1 minute of CPR, the pulse and breathing are reevaluated. If there still is no pulse or ventilations, continue CPR and reevaluate the patient every few minutes.

Foreign Body Airway Obstruction in the Adult Patient

An unconscious person can have an obstructed airway due to the position of the airway. For example, the tongue can fall back and block the airway, or the tongue and/or **epiglottis** can be **edematous** and cause obstruction. Making an airway using the head-tilt/chin-lift maneuver can correct this problem.

A foreign body obstruction or choking emergency can occur in a conscious or unconscious person. Choking results in a partial or complete airway obstruction. If there only is a partial obstruction the victim will be able to cough, whisper, and breathe because of being able to exchange some air. In this case, encourage the victim to cough and do not interfere. If the airway is completely obstructed the victim won't be able to cough, speak, or breathe. Usually the victim's hands grasp his or her neck. This is the universal sign for choking.

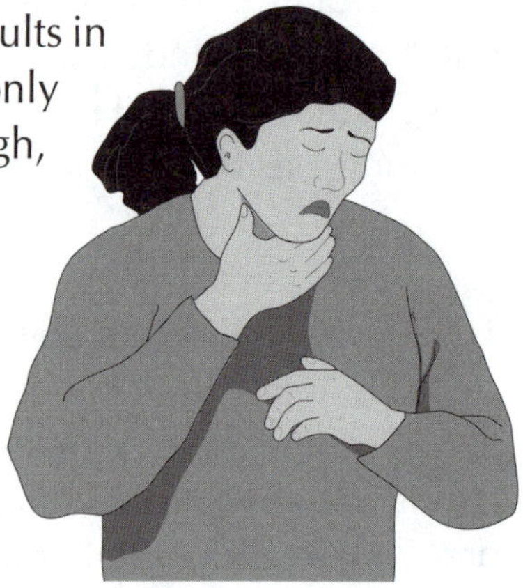

Heimlich maneuver: an obstructed airway maneuver in which a fist is thrust against the abdomen and subdiaphragmatic pressure is applied to remove a foreign body in the airway

Ask the victim if he or she is choking, and then perform the **Heimlich maneuver**. (Figure 18-12) This maneuver is performed with you, the rescuer, standing behind the CONSCIOUS victim. Wrap your hands around the victim's waist and make a fist with one hand. Place the thumb side of the fist against the victim's abdomen directly above the navel, but below the **xiphoid process**. Grasp the fist with your other hand, and with a quick upward thrust, attempt to knock the wind out of the person to remove the obstruction. This is done repeatedly until the obstruction is removed or the victim becomes unconscious.

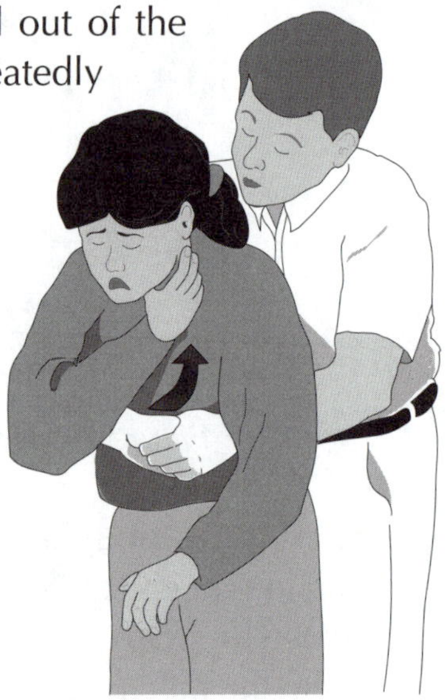

Repeat until the object is removed or the victim becomes unconscious.

Figure 18-12: The Heimlich Maneuver

If the victim becomes UNCONSCIOUS, lay him or her in a supine position and kneel astride the victim's thighs. Place the heel of one hand against the victim's abdomen above the navel, but below the xiphoid process. Place your other hand on top of the first hand and deliver upward abdominal thrusts five times. Open the victim's mouth using the tongue-jaw lift and do a finger sweep. To do a **tongue-jaw lift**, lift the victim's jaw up and forward by placing your thumb inside the victim's mouth just behind the front teeth, and grasp the victim's chin with your fingers. While you are doing this, do a finger sweep using your index finger to search for a foreign object. (Figure 18-13) Remove the object if you can see or feel it, but it is preferable to use the suction machine if it is available.

tongue-jaw lift: a method of opening the mouth of a choking victim to help ensure that the tongue is not part of the obstruction

If the victim is pregnant or obese, an alternate chest thrust can be used. (Figure 18-14) Stand behind the victim, place your arms under the victim's armpits, and encircle his or her chest. Place the thumb side of your fist in the middle of the victim's chest, grab your other hand, and with a quick upward thrust, attempt to knock the wind out of the person to remove the obstruction. Do this repeatedly until the obstruction is removed or the victim becomes unconscious.

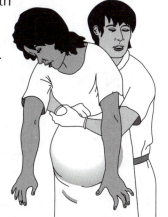

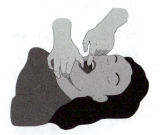

Figure 18-13: Tongue-Jaw Lift   *Figure 18-14: Alternate Chest Thrust*

Pediatric Basic Life Support

Emergencies involving children are due more often to airway problems than to cardiac problems. Children are more likely to choke, drown, suffocate, poison themselves, or have an accident than to have a heart attack. If the respiratory arrest is dealt with immediately, a cardiac arrest may be prevented.

The procedure for CPR in infants and children is the same as with adults except for a few modifications due to the size of the individual. For the purpose of CPR, the word *child* is used to describe an individual 1 to 8 years of age, or the physical size of an average 1- year-old to 8-year-old. The term *infant* is used for babies up to 1 year of age.

CPR for Children and Infants

1. DETERMINE UNRESPONSIVENESS. Gently shake the child or tap the infant's feet and shout, "Are you OK?"

2. CALL FOR HELP.

3. POSITION THE VICTIM. The infant or child must be supine on a firm surface. If an injury is suspected, **log roll** the victim onto his or her back.

log roll: the method used to turn a victim with a spinal injury, in which the patient is moved to the side in one motion

4. OPEN THE AIRWAY. Use the head-tilt/chin-lift method. Avoid overextending the neck in infants. For traumatic injuries, use the jaw-thrust maneuver.

5. DETERMINE BREATHLESSNESS. Look, listen, and feel for ventilations.

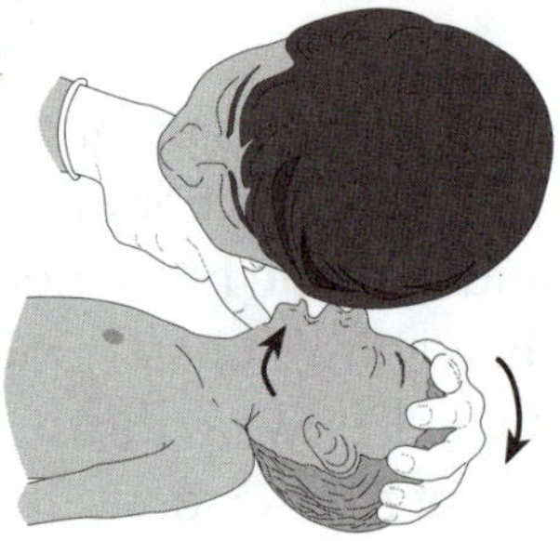

Figure 18-15: Determine breathlessness.

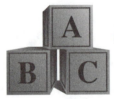

6. BEGIN RESCUE BREATHING. If the victim is not breathing, and the patient is a child, pinch the nose and give two mouth-to-mask or mouth-to-mouth ventilations that are 1 to 1¹/₂ seconds each in duration. (See the procedure for mouth-to-mask ventilation on page 18-6.) Pocket masks can be used for children, but they are too large for infants. Bag-valve masks can be used for both infants and children, but they must be the appropriate size. Follow the two initial ventilations with a pulse check.

   If the patient is an infant, cover the baby's nose and mouth with your mouth, or use a pediatric bag-valve mask, and deliver enough air to make the infant's chest rise and fall. Give two initial ventilations that are 1 to 1¹/₂ seconds each in duration, followed by a pulse check.

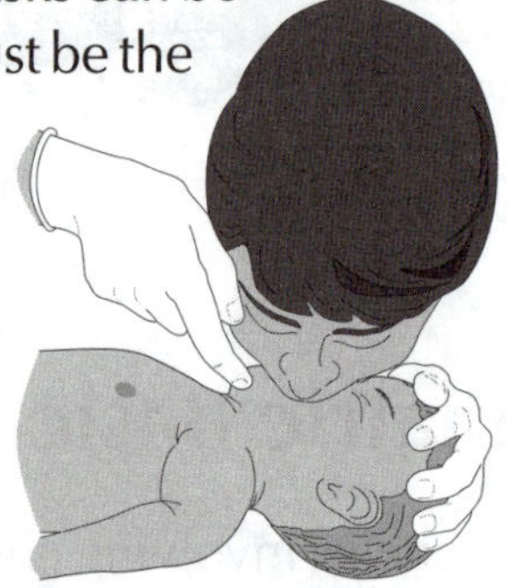

Figure 18-16: If a pediatric bag-valve mask is not available, mouth-to-nose ventilations must be performed on infants.

7. CHECK THE PULSE. In an older child, the carotid pulse is monitored, but the best pulse to monitor on an infant is the brachial pulse. This pulse is found on the inside of the upper arm, between the elbow and the shoulder. If a pulse is present, continue rescue breathing by giving a breath every 3 seconds.

8. BEGIN CHEST COMPRESSIONS: If no pulse is found, perform chest compressions. Chest compressions are done with rescue breathing. Place the infant or child supine on a firm surface. If necessary, you can transport the infant while doing CPR using the football position. Lay the infant supine on the palm of your hand and cradle the baby's head with your fingers to maintain the airway position. (Figure 18-18)

To begin chest compressions on an infant, locate an imaginary line horizontally between the nipples over the sternum. The index finger of your hand closest to the infant's feet is placed one finger's width below this imaginary line. Use two fingers and compress the sternum ½ to 1 inch at a rate of at least 100 times a minute. The compression to ventilation ratio is 5:1. (See Figures 18-17 and 18-18.)

Chest Compressions for Infants

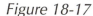

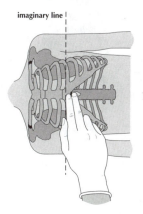

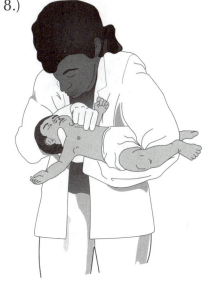

Figure 18-17   *Figure 18-18*

CPR	INFANT ONE PERSON	CHILD (1 - 8 yrs) ONE PERSON	TWO PERSON	ADULT (over 8 yrs) ONE PERSON	TWO PERSON
INITIAL BREATHS	2	2	2	2	2
COMPRESSIONS to BREATHS	5 to 1	5 to 1	5 to 1	15 to 2	5 to 1
COMPRESSIONS PER MINUTE	at least 100	at least 100	at least 100	at least 80	at least 80
COMPRESS THE STERNUM	½ - 1 inches	1 - 1½ inches	1 - 1½ inches	1½ - 2 inches	1½ - 2 inches
APPLICATIONS	two fingers	one hand	one hand	two hands	two hands

To do chest compressions on a child, locate the lower margin of the victim's rib cage with your middle and index fingers. Trace this margin up the rib cage to the sternal notch. With the middle finger on the notch and the index finger placed next to the middle finger, note the location of your index finger. (See Figure 18-19.) Now place the heel of the same hand in that spot. The long axis of the heel of your hand should align with the long axis of the sternum. (See Figure 18-20.) The chest is compressed 1 inch with the heel of one hand at a rate of 80 to 100 times a minute. The compression to ventilation ratio is 5:1. Remember to keep your fingers off of the chest. (See Figure 18-21.)

Chest Compressions for Children

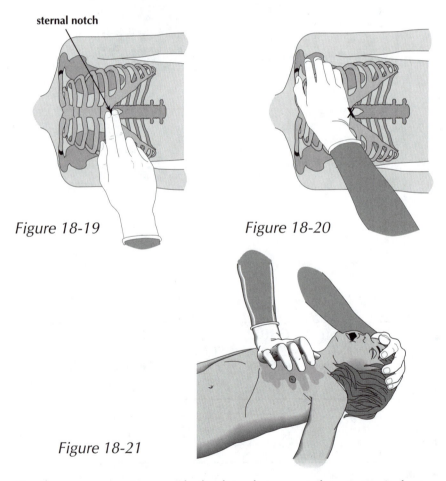

sternal notch

Figure 18-19   *Figure 18-20*

Figure 18-21

Do the compressions with the hand nearest the victim's feet, and maintain the airway position with your other hand. MAINTAIN THE AIRWAY POSITION AT ALL TIMES! If you move your hand from the patient's head at any time, you will lose the airway position. If this happens, you must reposition the airway and recheck it.

Airway Obstruction in Children and Infants

The Heimlich maneuver is the same for children as it is for adults. However, the procedure for infants is quite different: abdominal thrusts are not performed on infants; chest thrusts are done instead. If a child is choking and still CONSCIOUS, stand behind the victim. (Figure 18-22) Wrap your hands around the child's waist and make a fist with one hand. Place the thumb side of the fist against his or her abdomen directly above the navel, but below the xiphoid process. Grasp the fist with your other hand, and with a quick upward thrust, attempt to remove the obstruction as if knocking the breath out of the child. Repeat this multiple times until the obstruction is removed or the victim becomes unconscious.

If the child becomes UNCONSCIOUS, lay him or her in a supine position and kneel astride the victim's thighs. Place the heel of one hand against the child's abdomen above the navel, but below the xiphoid process. Place your other hand on top of the first hand and deliver upward abdominal thrusts five times. (Figure 18-23) Open the child's mouth, visually examine for a foreign object, and, if present, do a finger sweep using your index finger or a suction device to remove the object. Reassess the child's breathing and attempt to ventilate. Repeat the procedure if ventilation is unsuccessful.

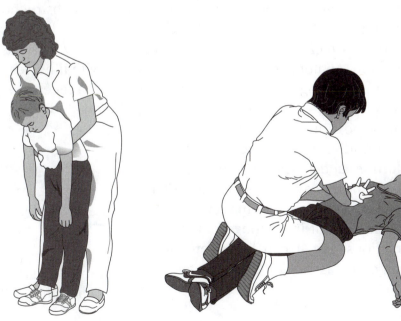

Figure 18-22   Figure 18-23

If the victim is an infant, straddle the infant over your arm, positioning the head lower than the trunk. Supporting the infant's head by firmly holding the jaw, deliver five back blows with the heel of one hand between the infant's shoulder blades. (See Figure 18-24.)

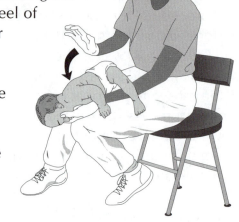

Support the infant with one hand on the back and one hand on the chest. Turn the infant over, and perform five chest thrusts. To perform chest thrusts, locate an imaginary line between the nipples over the sternum (the same imaginary line you used for chest compressions), and place your index finger just below this line. Place the middle and fourth fingers on the sternum, and compress

Figure 18-24: Deliver five back blows.

the sternum with a downward and forward motion to a depth of $\frac{1}{2}$ inch. Check the infant's mouth and remove any objects that you find. Reassess the infant's breathing and attempt to ventilate the baby. Repeat the procedure if ventilation is unsuccessful.

Extra caution must be used when dealing with airway obstructions in infants and children. The airway can become obstructed by a foreign body (a marble, hard candy, a button, food, etc.), or by an anatomical obstruction. Anatomical obstructions can occur with illnesses that cause swelling in the air passages. A history of a recent illness, fever, sore throat, or noisy breathing should alert you to the possibility of an anatomical obstruction. Many childhood diseases like **croup**, **epiglottitis**, and **tonsillitis** can cause the tissues in the airway to swell and obstruct the airway. The Heimlich maneuver will not be successful in treating anatomical obstructions, but it can be helpful if a foreign object is blocking the airway.

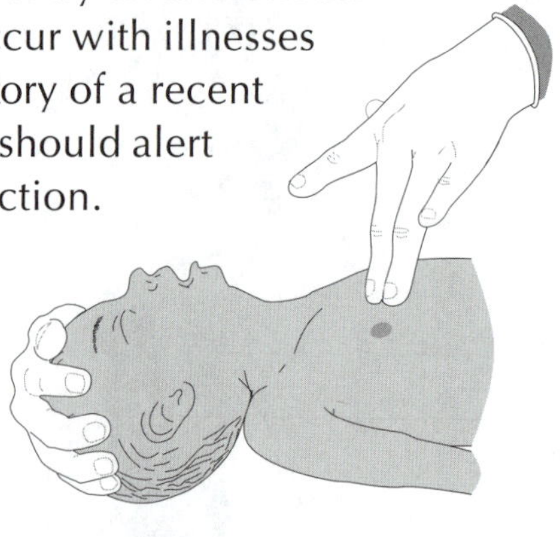

Figure 18-25: Perform five chest thrusts.

Controlling Bleeding

Since the body does not have an excess supply of blood, all bleeding must be controlled. Profuse bleeding, or a **hemorrhage**, is a serious life-threatening condition that can lead to **shock**. Bleeding can result from **lacerations**, **amputations**, **fractures**, or severe **trauma**.

Internal bleeding can result from blunt trauma or a catastrophic medical condition (eg, ulcers or ectopic pregnancy), and can only be controlled through surgery. External bleeding can occur from **capillaries**, **veins**, or arteries. Capillary bleeding is the most common type of external bleeding, and occurs with most injuries. Applying a sterile pad and ice will usually control the capillary bleeding found in minor cuts, scratches, and **abrasions**; however, if a vein or artery is punctured or severed by a cutting instrument, the blood will flow steadily. The amount of blood loss depends on the size of the vessel.

To control venous or arterial bleeding, apply **direct pressure** over the wound and elevate the extremity if possible. WEAR GLOVES and place sterile gauze directly on the wound. It takes normal blood 4-6 minutes to clot, so pressure should be applied for at least 6 minutes. If a person has a bleeding condition such as **hemophilia** or takes anticoagulants (blood thinning medications such as Coumadin, heparin, or aspirin), the pressure will have to be continually applied until the patient is seen by the doctor. If the blood seeps through the bandage, leave it in place and put more gauze on top of it. Call out for help. DO NOT LEAVE THE PATIENT UNATTENDED!

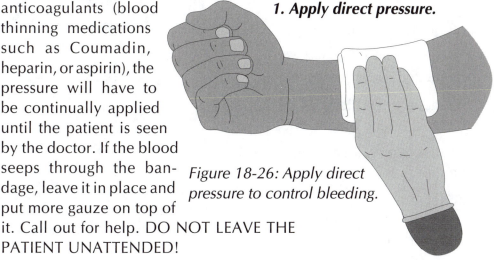

1. Apply direct pressure.

Figure 18-26: Apply direct pressure to control bleeding.

If direct pressure is not successful, the second method is to use indirect pressure, or **pressure points**. To apply indirect pressure, locate the pressure point SUPERIOR to the injury and apply pressure to that artery until the pulsation in the artery stops, or the bleeding from the wound is controlled. Pressure points exist at the following arteries:

- the temporal artery, located **anterior** to the ear.

- the carotid artery, located **laterally** to the thyroid cartilage, just **inferior** to the mandible.

- the subclavian artery, located deep in the hollow **proximal** to the clavicle.

- the brachial artery, located on the **medial** aspect of the upper arm, about 3 inches inferior to the axilla.

- the ulnar artery, located on the **medial** aspect of the elbow.

- the radial artery, located in the wrist on the thumb side.

- the iliac artery, located in the groin.

- the **femoral** artery, located in the groove between the groin and the hip.

- the popliteal artery, located **posterior** to the patella.

- the dorsalis pedis artery, located on anterior of the foot at the angle in the ankle.

2. Apply indirect pressure.

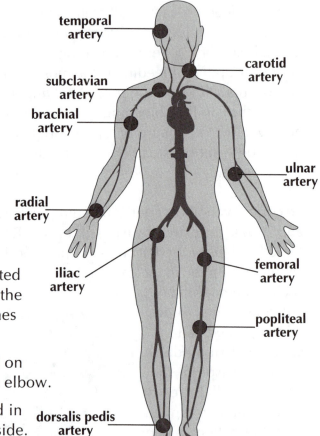

temporal artery
carotid artery
subclavian artery
brachial artery
ulnar artery
radial artery
iliac artery
femoral artery
popliteal artery
dorsalis pedis artery

Figure 18-27: If bleeding cannot be controlled through direct pressure, apply indirect pressure.

Once the life-threatening emergencies have been identified and assistance provided, perform the **secondary survey**. The secondary survey is another assessment of the patient; however, this survey is a complete head-to-toe check for any additional problems the patient may have.

The Secondary Survey: Patient Re-Assessment

Once the primary survey has been completed and the appropriate interventions performed, the patient should be re-examined for additional injuries in a secondary survey. Since the secondary survey is typically done in an Emergency Department, this procedure is detailed in *The Emergency Department Technician* textbook in this series; however, general guidelines for this procedure are summarized in the following paragraphs.

Call out for help—DO NOT LEAVE THE PATIENT UNATTENDED! Keep the victim in the position found until help arrives to move the patient. Ask the patient how he or she feels. Is there any pain or limited movement? If the patient has sustained a fall, check his or her head for any **lacerations** or **contusions** (bruises). Intervention techniques for lacerations include the following.

1. Notify your supervisor and the primary healthcare provider of the patient's injuries.

2. Cover any lacerations with sterile gauze and secure in place.

3. Complete the appropriate documentation on the appropriate form.

If the patient you are treating is a child, remember the following rules.

- Always hold his or her hand.
- Keep sharp objects out of his or her reach.
- Place all solutions and medications out of his or her reach.

Remember—children are naturally curious and very fast. Don't be caught off guard!

secondary survey: a head-to-toe physical assessment; an additional assessment of a patient to determine the existence of any injuries other than those found in the primary survey

Management of Shock

The common definition for shock is the failure of blood to circulate, but there are many different kinds of shock. This chapter will only provide information on **hypovolemic shock**, shock due to severe blood loss, because it is the most common form.

hypovolemic shock: shock caused by severe blood loss

A patient may experience severe blood or fluid loss from many different causes. Sudden and severe blood loss can result from incisions opening after a surgical procedure, wound drainage, vomiting blood due to internal bleeding, and rectal bleeding from a bleeding area in the intestines. Interventions include having the patient lay down and elevating his feet above the level of his heart; applying direct pressure; and surgery.

A patient exhibiting the following signs and symptoms may be experiencing hypovolemic shock:

- a change in mental status (ie, slow at answering questions, giving inappropriate answers, or failing to respond verbally at all).

- staring of the eyes and dilated pupils.

- pale, cool, and **diaphoretic** (profusely sweating) skin.

- a weak, rapid pulse.

- rapid and shallow respirations.

- hypotension (systolic blood pressure less than 90 in an adult or child, or less than 70 in infants and children under 6 years old). This is a late sign, indicating shock.

Vital sign changes, such as increased pulse and respiratory rates may provide early indications of hypovolemic shock in adults; however, children's vital signs may not reflect a hypovolemic problem until it is severe. It takes longer for children's bodies to compensate, or adapt, to changes than it does adults' bodies; therefore, when a pediatric patient's vital signs reflect changes indicative of shock, immediate action must be taken or the child may not survive. For example, an adult's vital signs may not change until there has been a blood loss of 1000 to 1500 cc (1 to 1$^1/_2$ quarts); an infant may be unable to tolerate a blood loss of 30 cc (1 ounce).

Intervention techniques for hypovolemic shock include the following:

1. In all cases of hypovolemic shock, position the patient with his feet elevated above the level of his heart (approximately 8 to 12 inches). This position, called the **Trendelenburg position**, directs the flow of blood toward the brain. If the patient is on a bed or a gurney, use the controls to raise and lower the various parts to position the patient. Be sure to gently remove the pillow from beneath the patient's head.

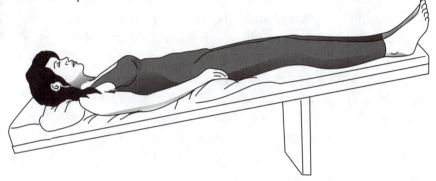

Figure 18-28: Trendelenburg Position

2. If the patient is hemorrhaging, apply direct pressure or pressure proximal to the bleeding point. A tourniquet is only used in a *controlled* setting in the hospital. If the bleeding is uncontrollable, surgery may be necessary.

3. If the patient is vomiting blood, or bleeding from his or her rectum, surgery may be required.

4. Keep the patient comfortably warm.

5. Do not move the patient unnecessarily.

6. Patients who are in shock will require careful monitoring.

Seizures

Another common emergency you might encounter is a patient who is having a **seizure**. A seizure is usually characterized by loss of consciousness and involuntary, spasmodic muscle twitching. Most people who are aware of their seizure disorder will be wearing a **Medic-Alert** identification tag. These are silver or gold with a red medical caduceus on the upper side. The side next to the patient's skin contains important medical information such as the type of medical problem, allergies, and any medications they may take. The tags are attached to either a necklace or bracelet.

There are many underlying causes of seizures; however, **epilepsy**, drug poisoning, brain tumors, fever (in children), and head injuries are the most common. Epilepsy is a recurrent, chronic disorder involving disturbed rhythms of the electrical impulses that sporadically fire throughout the cerebrum, causing seizures. There are approximately 1 million people in the United States with some form of epilepsy.

Seizure intervention involves the following steps.

1. Make sure the airway is open.

2. Protect the patient from harm. Move any objects that the patient may accidentally strike with either his head or extremities.

3. Make the patient comfortable by placing a soft object behind his or her head and loosening tight clothing. (Do not expose the patient more than necessary.)

4. Protect yourself. NEVER put your fingers in the patient's mouth!

Seizures usually last between 1 and 2 minutes; however, there are rare instances when a seizure could last quite a bit longer. NEVER LEAVE THE PATIENT UNATTENDED IN ORDER TO GET HELP! When the seizure activity has stopped, carefully roll the patient to one side in case he or she vomits. This will help prevent the patient from aspirating (inhaling the vomitus into the lungs).

It is important to note and chart the time the seizure started, how long it lasted, whether it began in a certain part of the body or seemed generalized from the beginning, and whether the patient lost control of the bowel or bladder.

---

seizure:
a neurological dysfunction caused by a sudden episode of uncontrolled electrical activity in the brain that may result in involuntary, uncontrolled muscle contractions

Medic-Alert:
a symbol that indicates important medical information, usually found on a bracelet or pendant provided by the nonprofit organization which bears its name

Chest Pain

There are millions of people who suffer from various degrees of chest pain resulting from coronary vascular disease (CVD). Coronary vascular disease includes all aspects of heart and blood vessel disease, including chest pain, angina, stroke (CVA), hypertension (HTN), deep vein thrombosis (DVT), and acute myocardial infarction (AMI). According to the Department of Health and Human Resources, approximately 2,600 Americans die daily from one form or another of coronary vascular disease. This means that in the United States, approximately 949,000 people die from CVD each year. Despite these alarming statistics, this section will limit discussion to chest pain presumed to be cardiac in origin, possibly resulting in a myocardial infarction. Cardiac chest pain occurs when there is decreased blood flow through the coronary arteries, causing the vessels to spasm (resulting in pain). This usually happens because a blood clot has formed in the vessel, either partially or completely blocking blood flow to the myocardium. Blood carries oxygen to all of the body's cells; if there is inadequate blood flow, the cells do not receive enough oxygen to survive. The death of tissue is called **necrosis**. Death of cardiac tissue is known as a **myocardial infarction**. Although not everyone complaining of chest pain is experiencing a myocardial infarction, you should watch for these warning signals of AMI.

- Chest pain that began either while resting or during exercise.

- The pain is usually a tight, squeezing type of pain and may be described as a "big band around my chest." In rare cases, the pain may be sharp or stabbing. The patient may complain of "indigestion" or chest pressure.

- Pain may be located in the middle of the chest, directly behind the sternum. It also may be felt in one or both upper extremities (usually the left), or it also may be felt in the jaw, the neck, or in the back.

- The patient's skin color may be pale, gray, cool, and **diaphoretic**.

- The patient will usually be anxious and uneasy.

- The patient may complain of nausea or vomit.

- The patient may be short of breath. (People over the age of 65 or who have diabetes may not have chest pain; they may only experience shortness of breath.)

Any complaint of chest pain should be taken seriously. Perform the following intervention techniques if a patient complains of chest pain.

1. Put the patient in a comfortable position; usually with his head elevated to assist breathing.

2. If oxygen is set up at the bedside, or available in your department, give oxygen to the patient.

3. Call out for help; DO NOT LEAVE THE PATIENT UNATTENDED!

4. Do not give any food or liquids.

5. In all cases, REMAIN CALM and offer reassuring words; but never tell a patient that everything is going to be fine. There are instances when this may not be true. Use phrases such as, "We are doing everything possible to help you."

Shortness of Breath

Throughout the United States, there are increasing numbers of people with some type of respiratory problem such as asthma, emphysema, and bronchitis. Recent studies indicate many reasons for this increase including smoking, air pollution, and different allergies. If a patient complains of feeling short of breath, there are a few basic first aid interventions that should be undertaken.

1. REMAIN CALM and reassure the patient.

2. Position the patient in either a sitting position, or with his or her head elevated to at least a 45° angle (if NOT contraindicated by the patient's condition). This 45° position is called **Fowler's position** or **semi-Fowler's position**; if the patient is sitting at a 90° angle, it is called **high Fowler's position.**

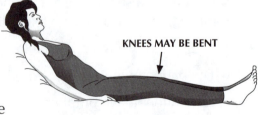

KNEES MAY BE BENT

3. Call for help by dialing the operator on the bedside telephone and/or call out for help.

Figure 18-29: Semi-Fowler's Position

4. If there is oxygen at the bedside or available in the department, administer it to the patient.

5. DO NOT LEAVE THE PATIENT UNATTENDED.

Shortness of breath is a very frightening experience. People who are suffering from it often express a fear of dying. Patients may be agitated and restless due to the decreased level of oxygen to the brain. Be very compassionate and caring!

Syncope

The medical term for fainting is **syncope**. It is characterized by a sudden, brief, and temporary loss of consciousness. There are many reasons a syncopal episode may occur, but the physiological cause is always the same: the blood pressure decreases and does not transport enough oxygen to the brain. Syncope most often occurs while the patient is standing. A patient who is about to faint may exhibit some of the following signs and/or symptoms.

syncope: fainting; sudden, brief, and temporary loss of consciousness; passing out

- The patient may not verbally respond to questions.
- He or she may complain of ringing in the ears.
- The patient's skin may be pale, and slightly diaphoretic.
- He or she may yawn excessively. (This is an effort by the body to receive more oxygen.)
- The patient may complain of feeling warm, hot, and/or nauseous.

Syncopal interventions include the following.

1. If the patient has not lost consciousness, have him or her lay down with feet elevated above the level of the heart; or have the patient sit down and lower the head between the knees.

2. If the patient has lost consciousness, help the patient to the floor to prevent injury if possible.

3. Check the ABCs, and intervene if necessary.

4. If the patient starts to vomit, gently turn the patient to one side to help prevent aspiration.

5. Call out for help—NEVER leave the patient alone.

The Unconscious Patient

Loss of consciousness can be caused by many things. For all unconscious patients, use the following guidelines:

1. NEVER give liquids or food to an unconscious person.

2. Always suspect a spinal injury if the patient is on the floor. Be sure to log roll the patient when moving him or her to prevent additional injuries. See the following pages for the procedures for three-person and four-person log rolls.

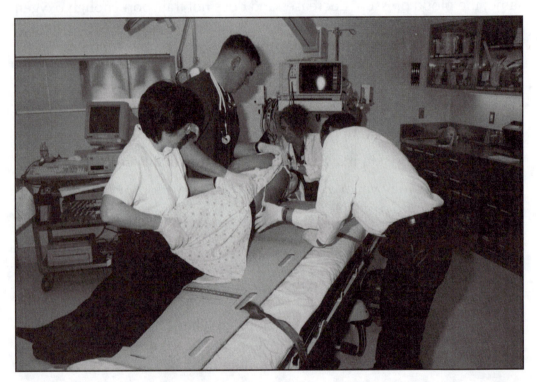

Figure 18-30: If you must move a patient with a suspected spinal injury, log roll the patient to prevent additional injury.

Interventions include checking the patient's airway, breathing, and circulation. If necessary, begin CPR.

Performing a Three-Person Log Roll

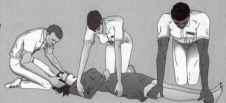

Materials needed:

✓ gloves and other appropriate protective wear (if blood or other body fluids are present)

✓ a cervical collar

✓ two rolled towels

1. Procedural Step: Call for help.
   Reason: A properly performed log roll requires the assistance of at least two other healthcare workers, one of whom should be a licensed nurse.

2. Procedural Step: Wash your hands.
   Reason: Standard Precaution.

3. Procedural Step: Put on gloves if any blood or other body fluid is present. (Or other protective wear as indicated. See Chapter Nine.)
   Reason: Standard Precaution.

4. Procedural Step: Establish verbal contact with the patient. If the patient does not verbally respond, continue to assess the ABCs (airway, breathing, and circulation).
   Reason: To determine if other life-saving interventions are required.

5. Procedural Step: After the patient is secured, kneel at the head of the patient. You are positioner #1.

6. Procedural Step: Gently but firmly stabilize the head and neck of the patient by applying in-line manual immobilization.

Reason: By placing the head and neck in a neutral, in-line, "eyes forward" position, the risk of causing further injury to the spinal cord from unnecessary movement is greatly reduced.

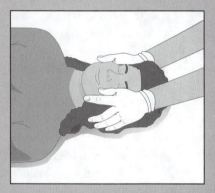

7. Procedural Step: Continue to maintain manual in-line immobilization until at least two other healthcare workers have arrived to provide assistance. Once help has arrived, you will direct the positioning of those who are providing assistance.
   Reason: In-line immobilization must be continuously maintained throughout the log roll procedure until the patient is completely immobilized with a cervical collar and a cervical immobilization device (such as two rolled towels— one placed on each side of the patient's head), and secured onto a long, firm backboard.

Performing a Three-Person Log Roll (Cont.)

8. Procedural Step: Positioner #2 should apply the appropriately sized cervical collar to the patient, but only if he or she has been properly trained in this procedure. If positioner #2 has not been properly trained in this procedure, find someone who has been.
Reason: An individual must never perform a procedure that is not within the legal scope of practice for which he or she has been trained, nor should anyone do anything that is against the hospital's policy.

9. Procedural Step: Once the cervical collar has been properly applied to the patient, positioner #2 should kneel next to the patient's mid-torso. Positioner #3 should kneel next to positioner #2 by the patient's knees, and you should continue to direct the others while maintaining in-line immobilization.
Reason: The positioner at the head of the patient is in charge of the procedure in order to prevent movement of the patient before everyone is properly positioned. In-line immobilization must be maintained throughout the procedure until the patient has been completely immobilized.

10. Procedural Step: Positioner #2 must assure that the patient's arms are straightened by his or her side. The palms are placed next to the patient's torso. Positioner #3 must extend the patient's lower extremities and bring them together in natural alignment.
Reason: Raising the upper extremities causes unnecessary movement of the spine. Bringing the lower extremities together properly aligns them to avoid lateral movement of the spine.

11. Procedural Step: Positioners #2 and #3 should place their hands on the far side of the patient.
Reason: This position will provide more leverage and reduce the risk of injury to the positioners.

12. Procedural Step: You (positioner #1) should direct positioner #2 to place one hand on the upper torso and the other hand on the pelvis of the patient.
Reason: This position allows the spine and pelvis to be moved as a unit.

13. Procedural Step: Next, you should direct positioner #3 to place one hand on the upper thigh of the patient and the other hand under the ankle or lower calf of the patient.
Reason: This position allows the lower extremities to be moved as a unit. The ankles must be elevated during the log roll in order to maintain lateral alignment of the lower extremities. Positioners #2 and #3 are now in correct position to properly align, stabilize, and immobilize the patient's torso, pelvis, and lower extremities.

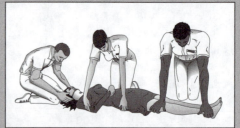

14. Procedural Step: Once positioners #2 and #3 are in proper position, you will direct the team to turn the patient as a unit (as if the patient were a log).
Reason: To prevent further spinal injury.

Performing a Three-Person Log Roll (Cont.)

15. Procedural Step: You (positioner #1) must watch the torso turn, and maintain in-line immobilization of the head and neck by rotating the head and neck simultaneously with the torso and lower extremities. Do not allow any flexion or hyperextension of the head and neck, and do not release manual in-line immobilization until the patient has been secured with a cervical immobilization device onto a long, firm backboard, or the patient is positioned according to the nurse's or physician's instructions. If the patient is not already on a backboard, one can be placed under the patient as he or she is being log rolled.
Reason: To prevent further injury to the patient's spine.

16. Procedural Step: In the hospital setting, a cervical immobilization device can be constructed using two rolled towels. Positioner #2 or #3 should place a rolled towel on either side of the patient's head while in-line immobilization continues to be maintained by positioner #1.

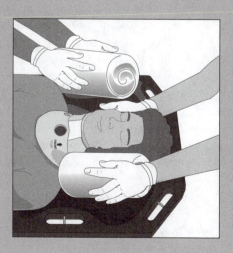

The patient's head, along with the rolled towels, are then secured to the backboard with tape. The first strip of tape should begin at one edge of the backboard near the patient's head, and extend across the first rolled towel, over the patient's forehead, across the second rolled towel, and end at the opposite edge of the backboard. Another strip of tape should extend from the edge of the backboard near the patient's head, across the cervical collar (under the patient's chin), and end at the opposite edge of the backboard near the patient's head.
Reason: To prevent further injury to the patient's spine.

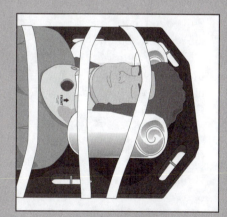

17. Procedural Step: Once you have finished providing care to the patient, and before providing care to another patient, remove your protective wear and wash your hands.
Reason: Standard Precautions.

Performing a Four-Person Log Roll

Materials needed:
✓ gloves and other appropriate protective wear (if blood or other body fluids are present)
✓ a cervical collar
✓ two rolled towels

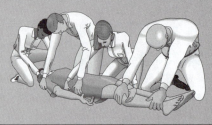

1. Procedural Step: Call for help.
   Reason: Ideally, a properly performed log roll requires the assistance of three other healthcare workers, one of which should be a licensed nurse.

2. Procedural Step: Wash your hands.
   Reason: Standard Precaution.

3. Procedural Step: Put on gloves if any blood or other body fluid is present. (Or other protective wear as indicated. See Chapter Nine.)
   Reason: Standard Precaution.

4. Procedural Step: Establish verbal contact with the patient. If the patient does not verbally respond, continue to assess the ABCs (airway, breathing, and circulation).
   Reason: To determine if other life-saving interventions are required.

5. Procedural Step: After the patient is secured, kneel at the head of the patient. You are positioner #1.

6. Procedural Step: Gently but firmly stabilize the head and neck of the patient by applying in-line manual immobilization.

Reason: By placing the head and neck in a neutral, in-line, "eyes forward" position, the risk of causing further injury to the spinal cord from unnecessary movement is greatly reduced.

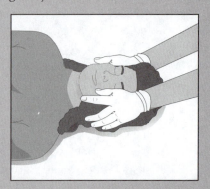

7. Procedural Step: Continue to maintain manual in-line immobilization until at least two other healthcare workers have arrived to provide assistance. Once help has arrived, you will direct the positioning of those who are providing assistance.
   Reason: In-line immobilization must be continuously maintained throughout the log roll procedure until the patient is completely immobilized with a cervical collar and a cervical immobilization device (such as two rolled towels–one placed on each side of the patient's head), and secured onto a long, firm backboard.

Performing a Four-Person Log Roll (Cont.)

8. Procedural Step: Positioner #2 should apply the appropriately sized cervical collar to the patient, but only if he or she has been properly trained in this procedure. If positioner #2 has not been properly trained in this procedure, find someone who has been.
Reason: An individual must never perform a procedure that is not within the legal scope of practice for which he or she has been trained, nor should anyone do anything that is against the hospital's policy.

9. Procedural Step: Once the cervical collar has been properly applied to the patient, positioner #2 should kneel next to the patient's shoulder and place one hand on the patient's far upper arm and the other hand on the patient's far upper thigh. Positioner #3 should kneel by the patient's pelvis and place one hand on the patient's far lower torso and the other hand on the patient's far knee. Positioner #4 should kneel by the patient's calf and place one hand on the patient's far pelvis and one hand under the patient's ankles or under the lower part of the calf. You (positioner #1) should continue to direct the others while maintaining in-line immobilization.
Reason: The positioner at the head of the patient is in charge of the procedure in order to prevent movement of the patient before everyone is properly positioned. In-line immobilization must be maintained throughout the procedure until the patient has been completely immobilized.

10. Procedural Step: Positioner #2 must assure that the patient's arms are straightened by his or her side. The palms are placed next to the patient's torso. Positioner #4 must extend the patient's lower extremities and bring them together in natural alignment.
Reason: Raising the upper extremities causes unnecessary movement of the spine. Bringing the lower extremities together properly aligns them to avoid lateral movement of the spine.

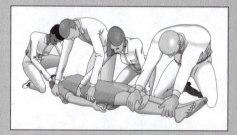

11. Procedural Step: Once all the positioners are in proper position, you will direct the team to turn the patient as a unit (as if the patient were a log).
Reason: This prevents further injury to the spine.

Performing a Four-Person Log Roll (Cont.)

12. <u>Procedural Step:</u> You (positioner #1) must watch the torso turn, and maintain in-line immobilization of the head and neck by rotating the head and neck simultaneously with the torso and lower extremities. Do not allow any flexion or hyperextension of the head and neck, and do not release manual in-line immobilization until the patient has been secured with a cervical immobilization device onto a long, firm backboard, or the patient is positioned according to the nurse's or physician's instructions. If the patient is not already on a backboard, one can be placed under the patient as he or she is being log rolled.
<u>Reason:</u> *To prevent further injury to the patient's spine.*

13. <u>Procedural Step:</u> In the hospital setting, a cervical immobilization device can be constructed using two rolled towels. Positioner #2, #3, or #4 should place a rolled towel on either side of the patient's head while in-line immobilization continues to be maintained by positioner #1.

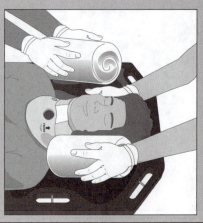

The patient's head, along with the rolled towels, are then secured to the backboard with tape. The first strip of tape should begin at one edge of the backboard near the patient's head, and extend across the first rolled towel, over the patient's forehead, across the second rolled towel, and end at the opposite edge of the backboard. Another strip of tape should extend from the edge of the backboard near the patient's head, across the cervical collar (under the patient's chin), and end at the opposite edge of the backboard near the patient's head.
<u>Reason:</u> *To prevent further injury to the patient's spine.*

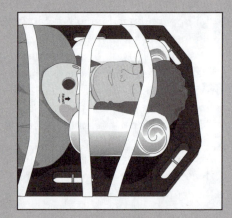

14. <u>Procedural Step:</u> Once you have finished providing care to the patient, and before providing care to another patient, remove your protective wear and wash your hands.
<u>Reason:</u> *Standard Precautions.*

Poisoning

A poison is any substance that, when introduced into the body, impairs health or results in death. Often, as with pesticides, caustics, alcohol-based products, or substances with iron, even very low doses can be harmful or even fatal to the patient. Poisonings can occur in many ways: medications, chemicals, or household cleaners can be **ingested**; **toxic** fumes, gases, dusts, or mists can be **inhaled**; poisonous substances from plants or toxic liquids can be **absorbed** through the skin; or poisons can be **injected** through the skin by needles or as a result of a bite or a sting.

toxic: poisonous

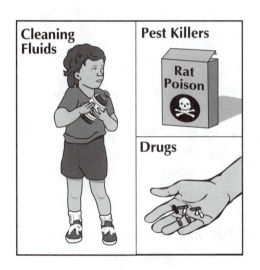

ingestion

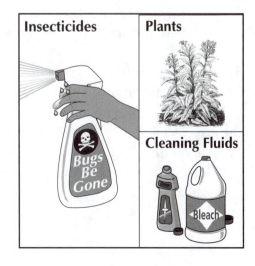

inhalation

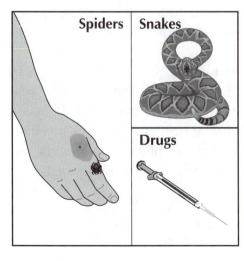

injection

absorption

Figure 18-31: Various Methods in Which Poisonings May Occur

antidote:
a substance that neutralizes a poison

Poisonings can occur either accidentally or intentionally. In both instances, treatment requires either the removal of the toxic (poisonous) substance or neutralization of the toxin. The method used depends on the type of poison involved. Sometimes a poison can be neutralized by administering an **antidote**. However, if the recommended antidote is not available, diluting the poison is accomplished by having the CONSCIOUS person drink either milk or water.

The following are general intervention guidelines for all types of poison.

1. Make sure the airway is open and the patient is breathing. If not, intervene as indicated.

2. Call for help.

3. Retrieve the container or label identifying the substance ingested.

4. If the label indicates the appropriate antidote, administer it if possible, or dilute with milk or water. NEVER GIVE LIQUIDS TO AN UNCONSCIOUS PATIENT OR A PATIENT WHO IS HAVING A SEIZURE! The patient might aspirate the liquid.

Poison Control:
an agency for both the general public and professional healthcare providers that provides information and first aid instructions for every poison available

5. If there is no antidote identified, call **Poison Control**. This service, which is available 24 hours a day will provide first aid instructions and definitive care instructions.

6. If not already in a hospital, call 911 or an ambulance and have the patient transported to the emergency department.

emetic:
an agent that induces vomiting

Syrup of ipecac is the an oral **emetic** used to induce (cause) vomiting. This can be purchased at any drug store; however, as with all medications, it must be kept out of reach of children. Most accidental poisonings occur in children between the ages of 1 and 5 years old. Most poisonings that occur on purpose are either threatened suicides or intentional suicide attempts. Habitual drug abusers also may have an accidental overdose. In all cases, the patient must be treated by a physician!

Burns

Burns can occur in any age group and at all times of the year. They are classified into three categories according to the amount of tissue damage:

1. **superficial:** a thermal or chemical burn in which only the outer layer of the epidermis is affected. The skin will be red and very tender. Superficial burns used to be described as first degree burns.

2. **partial thickness:** an extremely painful burn in which damage extends through the epidermis and into the dermis, but not so seriously that it permanently impairs the regeneration of the epidermis. Characterized by blisters, these burns usually are accompanied by superficial burns. Partial thickness burns used to be described as second degree burns.

3. **full thickness:** a burn in which all layers of the skin, and the nerves in it, are destroyed down to the bone. Superficial and partial thickness burns usually are present as well. Full thickness burns themselves are NOT painful because the nerves have been destroyed. Full thickness burns used to be described as third degree burns.

Due to the large numbers of chemicals available in the hospital environment, patients and employees often are exposed to chemicals that may cause superficial and partial thickness chemical burns. Labels on all chemicals must be read and gloves must be worn.

Intervention techniques differ according to the specific type of burn.

- **chemical burns:** flush CONTINUOUSLY with large amounts of water for at least 20 minutes; seek medical attention.

- **superficial burns:** immerse the burn in cold water for at least 20 minutes; apply a **sterile** dressing.

- **partial thickness burns:** immerse the burn in cold water for at least 20 minutes; apply a sterile dressing. DO NOT OPEN ANY BLISTERS.

- **full thickness burns:** the skin will be white or charred. Immediately cover with a large sterile dressing and seek medical attention.

Never put any ointment or greasy substance, such as butter or an antibiotic ointment, on any kind of burn. Monitor the patient's airway and breathing if there are burns to the face or chest. All burns that involve the face, hands, feet, or genitals must be immediately treated by a physician.

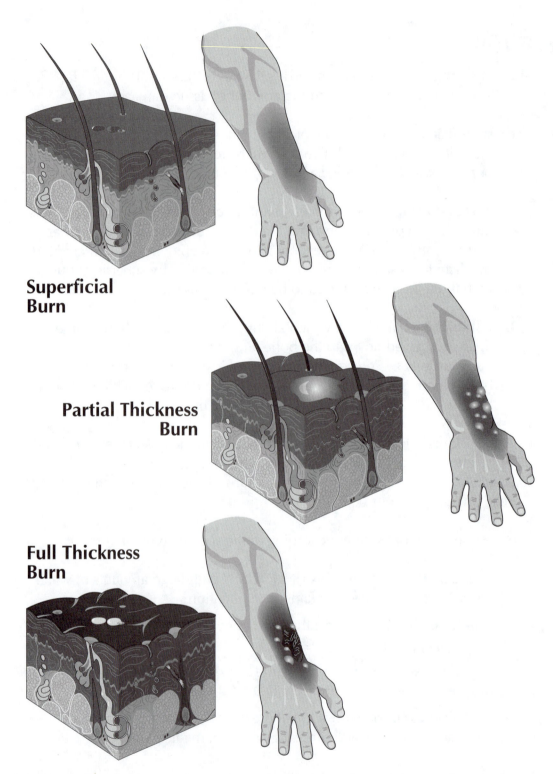

Superficial Burn

Partial Thickness Burn

Full Thickness Burn

Figure 18-32: The category of burn is determined according to the number of tissue layers damaged.

Sprains and Fractures

A **fracture** is a break in the continuity of a bone. Although there are different types of fractures, first aid intervention is the same for all of them. A **sprain** is an injury to ligaments and tendons. At times it will be difficult for the physician to diagnose a sprain or a fracture without an x-ray because the signs and symptoms exhibited by the patient are usually the same. These signs and symptoms include the following:

- pain and swelling at the affected area.

- **deformity** at the site.

- possible loss of use of the affected part.

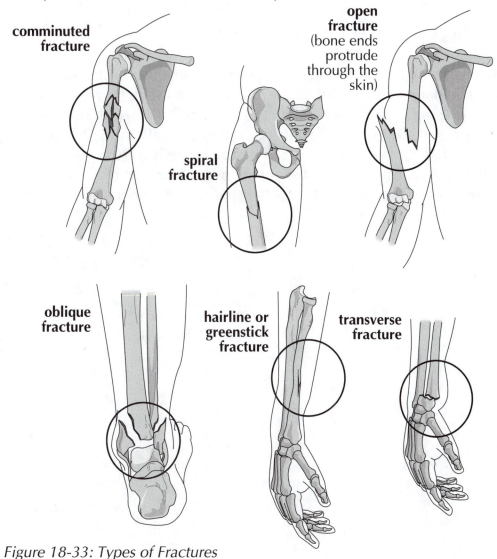

Figure 18-33: Types of Fractures

First aid intervention is the same for either type of injury.

1. Do not attempt to move the affected part back into its natural position.

2. Immobilize the area EXACTLY as it is before moving the patient. Splinting the area involves immobilizing the joint superior and inferior to the injury.

3. Elevate the affected part above the level of the heart to reduce swelling.

4. Call out for assistance and seek medical attention for the patient.

5. NEVER LEAVE THE PATIENT ALONE.

Patients who fall, striking their head, should also be suspected of having a spinal cord injury. If this is the case, the patient must be moved to a supine position (lying on their back). To do this properly, however, the patient must be log rolled. DO NOT attempt to position the patient by yourself. The procedure for three-person and four-person log rolls were provided earlier in this chapter. This maneuver should only be attempted by ONE person if no other help is available and the patient needs CPR. Otherwise, a minimum of three people is required!

Epistaxis: Nosebleeds

The medical term for a nosebleed is **epistaxis**. Degrees of bleeding may vary from a trickle to a nasal hemorrhage. Patients with hypertension and those taking particular medications, such as **anticoagulants** are prone to spontaneous epistaxis. There are usually no warning signs; the flow of blood is spontaneous.

anticoagulants: medications that thin the blood and prevent or delay blood coagulation

The nurse in charge of the patient must be notified whenever epistaxis occurs. Regardless of the cause, immediate intervention is the same.

1. If there is no suspected neck injury, have the patient sit up. This will reduce the chance of blood flowing down the esophagus and into the stomach or the trachea, causing the patient to vomit or cough.

2. Apply pressure by tightly pinching the soft part of nostrils with GLOVED fingers for at least 15 to 20 minutes.

3. Apply ice or a cold cloth over the nose if the bleeding does not stop with the application of pressure.

4. Seek assistance if the bleeding continues or recurs.

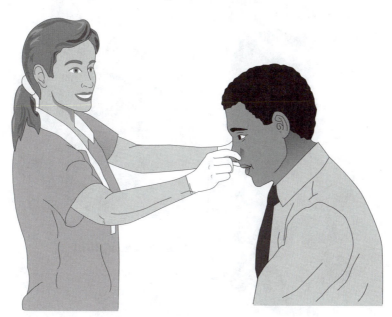

Figure 18-34: Apply pressure by tightly pinching the patient's nostrils with gloved fingers for at least 15 to 20 minutes.

Soft Tissue Injuries

There are several types of soft tissue injuries that can occur. These injuries are usually considered to be minor; however, they also can occur with episodes of severe trauma.

Soft tissue injuries can be grouped into the following categories.

- **abrasions:** open wounds, road burns, or rug burns in which the outer layer of skin has been scraped off. These injuries are very painful due to the exposed nerve endings.
- **incisions:** clean, straight, knife-like cuts.
- **puncture wounds:** soft tissue injuries caused by the penetration of a sharp object.

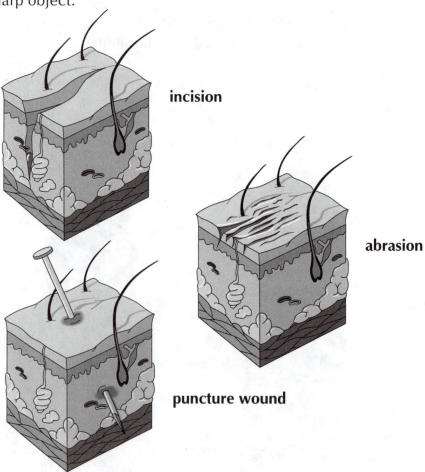

incision

abrasion

puncture wound

Figure 18-35a: Types of Wounds

- **avulsions:** painful soft tissue injuries in which a flap of tissue is torn loose or pulled off completely.

- **contusions:** (commonly called bruises) soft tissue injuries caused by the seepage of blood into tissue, and characterized by ecchymosis (black and blue marks). A large contusion may be indicative of a large amount of blood loss.

- **lacerations:** jagged tears in the flesh like those received from glass, broken bottles, or blunt trauma.

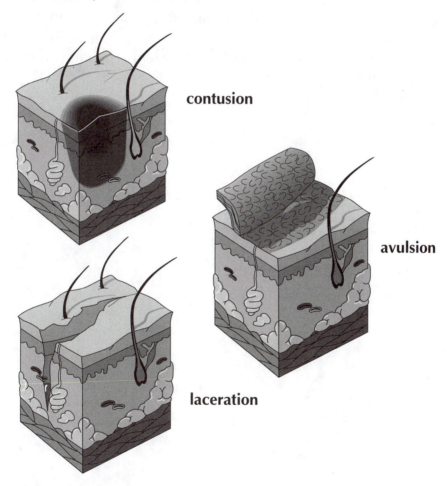

contusion

avulsion

laceration

Figure 18-35b: Types of Wounds (cont.)

Appropriate interventions for soft tissue injuries include prevention of infection; the application of ice to all closed, soft tissue injuries; and the application of a clean, sterile dressing to all open wounds.

Chapter Summary

The administration of first aid involves proper assessment and rapid intervention. First aid may be needed by any patient, at any time, in any hospital department. If you are unsure of what to do for the patient or if you are confused, DO NOT DO ANYTHING! Incorrect procedures can cause additional injury to the patient.

This chapter has provided information on some of the common emergencies hospital workers may face. Additional information on these and other emergencies is available in *The Emergency Department Technician* textbook in this series. Learn CPR and keep current. The life you save may be someone you love.

Name _____

Date _____

Student Enrichment Activities

Complete the following statements.

1. _____ _____ is the immediate care provided to a person who has sustained an unexpected injury, sudden illness, or other medical emergency.

2. The _____ _____ involves assessing the patient for any life-threatening emergencies.

3. The primary survey should be completed in _____ _____ or less.

4. The three parts of the primary survey are: A for _____, B for _____, and C for _____.

5. The two recommended ways of opening an airway are the _____ _____ and the _____ _____.

6. _____ _____ is the method that should be applied first when attempting to control bleeding.

7. Reassessment of the patient is called the _____ _____.

8. Severe shock due to extreme blood loss is called _____ shock.

9. Two causes of seizures are _____ and _____ _____.

10. List four warning signs of a possible myocardial infarction.

A. _____

B. _____

C. _____

D. _____

11. List three respiratory diseases: _____,

_____, and _____.

12. Sudden, brief, and temporary loss of consciousness is called _____.

13. Four possible warning signs of impending syncope include:

A. _____   C. _____

B. _____   D. _____

14. Poisonings can be _____, or they can be

_____.

15. An oral emetic used for poisoning is _____ _____ _____.

16. List the four types of burns:

A. _____   C. _____

B. _____   D. _____

17. A _____ is an injury to ligaments and tendons.

18. Patients who have hypertension may experience spontaneous

_____.

Name _____

Date _____

Unscramble the following terms.

19. NOSIPO CTNOOLR   _____   _____

20. CRADICA STARRE   _____   _____

21. SRIFT AID   _____   _____

22. SNOBARIA   _____

23. GLO ORLL   _____   _____

24. SLAUVION   _____

25. ZIERUSE   _____

26. XIOCT   _____

27. SCOPENY   _____

28. SCRIESON   _____

29. MYPLHVOOEIC SCKHO   _____   _____

30. SHOCCIMESY   _____

Chapter Nineteen
Healthful Living

Objectives

After completing this chapter you should be able to do the following:

1. Define and correctly spell each of the key terms.

2. Describe the concept of preventive healthcare.

3. Identify the health risks associated with the inhalation of tobacco smoke.

4. Identify the difference between essential and secondary hypertension.

5. Describe the health risks associated with untreated hypertension.

6. Identify measures for maintaining ideal blood pressure.

7. List the health problems often seen in patients who chronically abuse alcohol and drugs.

8. Understand the concepts of stress and coping mechanisms.

9. Identify the nutritional and energy values of carbohydrates, fats, and proteins.

10. Explain the function of each type of cholesterol carrier.

11. Identify health risks for those who are overweight.

Key Terms

- aerobic

- basal metabolic rate

- calorie

- carbohydrate

- cholesterol

- fat

- high-density lipoprotein

- low-density lipoprotein

- minerals

- preventive healthcare

- protein

- vitamins

A Longer and Healthier Life

The quest for better and more affordable healthcare has prompted an increasing number of businesses to contract with Health Maintenance Organizations (HMOs) to provide insurance coverage to employees and their families. HMOs typically try to promote the maintenance of proper health by encouraging a comprehensive approach to healthcare as a means of preventing more serious health problems in the future. As a result of this trend, healthcare providers everywhere now place additional emphasis on **preventive healthcare**. This type of healthcare focuses on patient instruction in areas such as proper eating habits, weight control, stress management, exercise, cholesterol reduction, and eliminating smoking. The goal of this approach is to help the patient avoid complications that can result from a destructive lifestyle.

preventive healthcare: healthcare that focuses on patient education that emphasizes the promotion of health and the prevention of disease

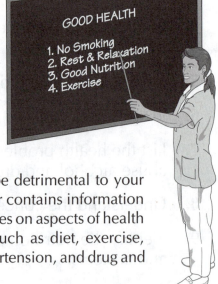

As a healthcare worker, it is important for you to understand how certain habits can influence a person's health. It is vital not only to your ability to understand the factors that may affect patients, but also to your ability to identify aspects of your own life that may be detrimental to your mental and physical well-being. This chapter contains information that is important for optimal wellness. It focuses on aspects of health and wellness that the patient can control such as diet, exercise, smoking, and the management of stress, hypertension, and drug and alcohol use.

Figure 19-1: Preventive healthcare can help people live longer and healthier lives.

Smoking: It Takes Our Breath Away!

The respiratory system is very delicate and fragile. Research has revealed a great deal of evidence relating to the many health hazards associated with smoking. The American Cancer Society and the Surgeon General have released numerous studies that show a direct correlation between cigarette smoking and the development of lung cancer. The American Cancer Society has compiled statistics which show at least 85% of lung cancer cases among men and at least 75% of lung cancer cases among women are caused by cigarette smoking. Approximately 30% of all cancer deaths are due to smoking. The risk of developing lung cancer increases 25 times for those who smoke two or more packs of cigarettes daily or who have a 20-year history of smoking.

Tobacco smoke has long been recognized as a major cause of death and disease. According to the Environmental Protection Agency (EPA), tobacco smoke is responsible for an estimated 434,000 deaths annually in the United States. It contains a mixture of 4,000 chemical compounds. At least 43 are known to be carcinogens. A **carcinogen** is a substance that has been proven to cause cancer. **Nicotine** is a poison that is found in all parts of the tobacco plant, especially the leaves. It is an extremely addicting and toxic substance that acts very swiftly. It also constricts the blood vessels, especially those of the heart. Nicotine is a powerful and potentially lethal poison. Second hand smoke is the only source of nicotine in the air.

Second hand smoke, or environmental tobacco smoke (ETS), is responsible for approximately 3,000 nonsmoker deaths in the United States annually. ETS has been classified as a Group A carcinogen under the EPA's Carcinogen Assessment Guidelines. According to the CDC, second hand smoke causes 30 times as many lung cancer deaths as all regulated air pollutants combined.

Due to the systemic effects of nicotine and the central effects of cigarette smoke on the lungs, patients with diseases such as asthma, emphysema, bronchitis, upper respiratory infections, circulation deficiencies in the extremities, cardiac problems, and hypertension must be discouraged from smoking. This can be a difficult task, however, because nicotine is both physically and psychologically addicting. Therefore, patients who have smoked most of their lives will present the biggest challenge. Be supportive and encouraging to the patient.

Although the best cure for smoking is to never start, many programs are available for people who want to stop smoking. Provide the patient with literature available through the hospital's education department concerning the devastating effects smoking can have on the body. Keep your patients educated and keep them healthy!

Hypertension

Hypertension (high blood pressure) is often called the *silent killer* because it often does not exhibit any signs or symptoms to the patient until it has reached a dangerously high level. Untreated, this may result in a cerebrovascular accident (CVA), or stroke. High blood pressure can have devastating effects on various parts of the body and on one's lifestyle.

Research has identified two specific kinds of hypertension: primary (or essential) and secondary. **Essential hypertension** is defined as hypertension without an apparent medical cause. **Secondary hypertension** is directly caused by an underlying disease process.

The control of essential hypertension is often attempted through reducing the intake of sodium, managing stress, exercising, reducing weight, and eating a healthy diet. If these therapies are unsuccessful, oral medication may have to be prescribed by a physician. The control of secondary hypertension is attempted through therapy that is coordinated with the treatment of the primary disease. For example, people who retain excess fluid are frequently prescribed medication that removes the fluid through the kidneys, reducing the blood pressure.

The chronic, or long-lasting, effects will be the same for both kinds of hypertension. Eyesight may become worse and diabetes may develop. The heart will not pump as effectively, causing a fluid overload in the lungs and other areas of the body. In addition, the heart will become enlarged, and the kidneys will be damaged.

Measures for maintaining the ideal blood pressure are as follows:

1. Develop a regular exercise program.

2. Manage stress effectively.

3. Maintain the recommended weight for one's height.

4. Follow a healthy diet, which may include reducing the intake of fats and sodium.

There are thousands of Americans walking around with undiagnosed hypertension. Warning signals, such as waking up with a headache over a period of time (3 days or longer), blurred vision, or general weakness, should not be ignored!

The Use of Drugs and Alcohol

There are many people who habitually use drugs (both prescription and nonprescription, including alcohol). Any drug taken in excessive amounts can result in addiction or death. When someone becomes addicted to a drug, he or she is physically and/or psychologically dependent on the substance; without using the drug, he or she is unable to function. If someone is addicted to a drug, the sudden cessation of its use often results in **withdrawal** symptoms such as seizures and hallucinations. These symptoms also may occur when an alcoholic is admitted to the hospital for another health problem and alcohol consumption suddenly is stopped. These symptoms usually appear within 48 to 72 hours. It is important to note that with some drugs, any amount is too much. Sometimes only a single experience with a drug will result in addiction or death.

Many hospitals have a Chemical Dependency Department that assists patients in stopping drug abuse. In fact, there are hospitals that provide only those services. There, both the physical and psychological changes the patient will experience can be monitored and managed. The healthcare professionals in these facilities are specially trained to deal with the psychological and emotional side of chemical dependency as well as the physical effects. Crisis intervention involves particular communication skills that require special training. If you find yourself in a difficult situation with a patient who has a drug or alcohol dependence, call for help! Never attempt to handle a psychological crisis alone!

Patients who have a drug or alcohol addiction often have other health problems too. Some addicts get frequent infections due to the fact that their dependency weakens the immune system; and because drugs and alcohol create additional stress on the liver, damage to this essential organ is another side effect of chemical dependency. Furthermore, many addicts are malnourished because the majority of their money is spent on drugs and alcohol instead of food.

Patients who are addicted to a substance should be managed with kindness and tact. Remember, they have an illness and they need help—just like your other patients. Once again, prevention is the key to success!

Effective Stress Management

Stress is present in everyone's life. It occurs in both our work and home environments; it also is a part of our social life, and even affects our sleep. The American Academy of Family Physicians estimates that symptoms linked to stress account for about 66% of all visits to a family physician.

A general definition of stress is the perception that a person has of events or circumstances that have challenged, or exceeded, the individual's ability to cope. Not all stress is negative. In fact, some stress is positive in that it stimulates us to overcome some sort of perceived challenge. A person's **coping mechanisms** and how he or she responds to stress determine whether the stress will have a positive or negative effect. A coping mechanism is a method by which a person manages perceived stress. This explains why a circumstance such as hospitalization, can overwhelm one person and merely *inconvenience* another.

Some people actually thrive on stress; however, most people function at their optimal level with a moderate amount of stress in their life. There are both psychological and physiological aspects of stress. Too much stress in a person's life may cause the patient to have essential hypertension, chest pain, shortness of breath, headaches, insomnia, mood swings, and even a myocardial infarction.

There are several ways to reduce or relieve stress. Reducing the level of stress in one's life will, in turn, help reduce the risk of developing many of the symptoms mentioned above. The following guidelines can be effective in managing stress:

1. Eat a healthy diet. Studies have shown that a high intake of the B vitamins help people cope with an increased level of stress.

2. Develop and implement a regular exercise program.

3. Know your limits and effective coping mechanisms.

4. Take vacations.

5. Make time for yourself!

Stress is an inherent part of the American lifestyle. Through education, people can be trained to recognize the warning signs and symptoms of stress and take action before they become a problem. Working in healthcare can be very stressful. Learn to recognize the signs of stress in yourself and take appropriate measures to reduce the level. A healthcare worker who cannot effectively cope with stress is of very little benefit to patients!

The Healthy Diet

Eating a well-balanced diet will give a person enough energy to get through each day and still have reserves left over. The American Heart Association, the National Academy of Sciences, and the National Institutes of Health recommend a diet in which 30% of the total calories consumed come from fats, 55% are derived from carbohydrates, and 15% come from proteins. The body also needs about eight 8 oz glasses of water each day. Eating a healthy diet may require making some changes in the way one currently eats.

Food consists of fats, carbohydrates, proteins, vitamins, and minerals. The chemical composition of food determines how easily it is converted by the body into energy. Fats, carbohydrates, and proteins are used for energy and to maintain, repair, and rebuild the different parts of the body. Most of the **vitamins** and some **minerals** regulate many of the chemical processes that occur within the body. Other minerals help form the tissues, including the blood, bones, and teeth. Water is vitally important to provide fluid for the blood.

Carbohydrates are the principle source of energy for the body. The digestive system converts carbohydrates in food into **glucose**. Glucose is a simple sugar and is transported in the blood to the tissues. The cells use the glucose as energy. At the cellular level, glucose is further broken down into carbon dioxide and water. The excess glucose is converted into **glycogen**, which is stored in the muscles and liver. Since the body can only store about ³/₄ of a pound of glucose; the excess is stored in the body as fat. A **calorie** is a unit of heat. This, in simple terms, is a measurement of the amount of energy each type of food produces. If a person ingests more calories per day than he or she *burns* off, weight will be gained.

vitamins: organic compounds, other than proteins, carbohydrates, fats, and organic salts that are essential in small quantities for normal body function

minerals: inorganic compounds that are essential to body function

carbohydrate: a complex sugar that is a basic source of energy for the body

calorie: a unit of heat

Carbohydrates are made of carbon, hydrogen, and oxygen. They are classified as **complex sugars**; that is, they are chemically arranged to form long chains of simple sugars (sucrose) in the form of starches. The simple sugars are contained in candy, cookies, jams, and many soft drinks. These sugars are high in calories and do not offer much nutritional value. When these foods are consumed in high levels, the body is unable to burn up all of the calories, so the excess is stored as fat. Complex sugars are found in foods such as breads, pasta, rice, corn, and a variety of vegetables and legumes. These carbohydrates are saturated with vitamins, minerals, fiber, and water. Fruits contain a simple sugar, fructose, as well as vitamins, minerals, and fiber.

fat:
a substance made up of lipids or fatty acids that is a source of energy and is vital to growth and development

Fats are also an important source of energy. They too are made from carbon, hydrogen, and oxygen; however, they are combined in a different form than a carbohydrate. In order to convert to energy, fats need oxygen and the by-products formed when carbohydrates release energy. It is very difficult for muscles to use fat for energy without the presence of carbohydrates in the diet. One of the main differences between carbohydrates and fats is that carbohydrates can produce energy for short periods of time without the use of oxygen. This often occurs when you are not inhaling enough oxygen. During exercise for endurance, carbohydrates provide about half of the body's energy, while fat, and to a lesser degree, protein, supply the other half. Contrary to the popular myth, fat is necessary in the diet. Fat transports many of the important vitamins such as Vitamins A, D, E, and K. It is necessary to maintain healthy skin and hair and for the body to manufacture certain hormones. There are two kinds of fat: saturated and unsaturated. Saturated fats form a solid at room temperature and are mainly responsible for forming plaque on the walls of the arteries; unsaturated fats remain liquid and do not lead to the formation of plaque.

protein:
any of a class of complex, nitrogenous, organic compounds that function as the primary building blocks of the body

Protein is the primary building block of the body. It makes up the skin, muscles, tendons, ligaments, blood cells, and the brain cells, but it provides the body with very little energy. Protein should account for 15% of the total calories in the diet. The preferred sources of protein are found in lean meats, chicken, turkey, and fish. Red meat contains mostly saturated fat and more protein than the body can convert to energy. Remember, any excess is stored in the body as fat!

The energy value of both carbohydrates and protein is the same: 4 calories per gram. The energy value for fat is 9 calories per gram. Therefore, the body requires more than twice the amount of physical exercise to burn a gram of fat than it does to burn a gram of carbohydrates or protein. Approximately 3,500 calories equals 1 pound of fat! That means you must not only eat right, you also must exercise!

Recommended Dietary Allowances[1]

FAT SOLUBLE VITAMINS
Adults (Age 25-50)[2]

	Food Sources[3]	Function[3]	Results of Deficiency[3]	Results of Excessive Consumption[3]
A **male** 1000 μg RE[4] **female** 800 μg RE[4]	Liver; fishliver oils; carrots; eggs; whole milk products; dark green leafy vegetables; sweet potatoes	Prevents night blindness; helps keep skin & mucous membrane linings healthy; promotes resistance to certain infectious diseases.	Frequent infections; night blindness; dry skin; retarded growth; respiratory, gastrointestinal & genitourinary problems.	Nausea; headache; liver & spleen damage; joint pain; hair loss dry, peeling skin.
D **male** 5 μg[5] **female** 5 μg[5]	Fortified milk; fish liver oils; oysters; butter; liver; egg yolk; salmon; sardines (Also produced in the body in response to sunlight.)	Promotes strong bones & teeth; regulates calcium & phosphorus absorption.	Inadequate mineralization of bones.	Nausea; fatigue, bone pains; calcium deposits in soft tissues such as the kidney; loss of appetite; constipation.
E **male** 10 mg α-TE[6] **female** 8 mg α-TE[6]	Margarine; nuts; vegetable oils; green leafy vegetables; & wheat germ	Prevents oxidation of unsaturated fatty acids.	Lethargy; apathy; loss of concentration; loss of balance; anemia.	Generally nontoxic with doses up to 800 mg.
K **male** 80 μg **female** 65 μg	Spinach, broccoli & other green leafy vegetables; milk; eggs; and cereals.	Assists in regulation of blood clots.	Impaired clotting; bruises; & frequent nosebleeds.	Possible clot formation.

Note: Endnotes and sources appear on page 19-13.

Figure 19-2: Nutrient Needs of a Healthy Body—Fat Soluble Vitamins

Recommended Dietary Allowances (Cont.)[1]

WATER SOLUBLE VITAMINS[2]
Adults (Age 25-50)

	Food Sources[3]	Function[3]	Results of Deficiency[3]	Results of Excessive Consumption[3]
B$_1$ (Thiamine) **male** 1.5 mg **female** 1.1 mg	Whole grains; dried beans; organ meats; yeast; seeds & nuts	Assists in energy release from carbohydrates; necessary for efficient digestive & nervous systems.	Confusion; anorexia; weakness; peripheral paralysis; tachycardia; loss of coordination.	Generally nontoxic.
B$_2$ (Riboflavin) **male** 1.7 mg **female** 1.3 mg	Cheese, milk, green vegetables, ice cream, enriched bread, cereals, fish, poultry & meats	Essential for metabolism of carbohydrates, amino acids, & fats; Maintains nerves & blood cells.	Mouth lesions; seborrheic-dermatitis; scrotal & vulval skin changes; anemia.	Generally nontoxic.
B$_3$ (Niacin) **male** 19 mg NE[7] **female** 15 mg NE[7]	Meat, poultry, fish, peanuts, whole grains, enriched cereals & breads	Important in glycolysis, tissue respiration, & fat synthesis; necessary for cell reproduction & repair.	Irritability; depression; anxiety; sore mouth & tongue; gastrointestinal problems; pellagra.	Heartburn, nausea, burning, itching skin, & flushing of the face.
B$_6$ (Pyridoxine) **male** 2 mg **female** 1.6 mg	Poultry, fish, kidney, liver, pork, whole grains, soy beans & peanuts	Necessary for tryptophan metabolism; assists in utilization of other amino acids.	Anemia; nausea; convulsions; dermatitis around eyes & mouth.	Loss of muscular coordination & nerve sensation.
B$_{12}$ **male** 2 µg **female** 2 µg	Animal foods, such as meat, fish, eggs, cheese, milk & chicken	Helps develop red blood cells & maintain nervous system.	Pernicious anemia; fatigue; sore tongue; memory loss; & neurological symptoms.	Generally nontoxic.
Folate (Folic acid) **male** 200 µg **female** 180 µg	Liver, brewer's yeast, leafy vegetables, dried beans & peas, fresh oranges & whole wheat products.	Involved in synthesis of nucleic acid; prevents blood disorders; essential for growth.	Anemia; impaired cell division; alterations in protein synthesis; diarrhea; fatigue.	May interfere with anti-seizure drugs; stomach & sleep disturbances.
C (Ascorbic Acid) **male** 60 mg **female** 60 mg	Citrus fruits & juices, spinach, broccoli, green & red peppers, potatoes & tomatoes	Important to skin, tooth & bone formation; promotes iron absorption; helps heal wounds.	Scurvy; bleeding gums; tender joints; nosebleeds; increased susceptibility to infections.	Diarrhea; possible kidney stones.

Note: Endnotes and sources appear on page 19-13.

Figure 19-3: Nutrient Needs of a Healthy Body—Water Soluble Vitamins

Recommended Dietary Allowances (Cont.)[1]

MINERALS
Adults (Age 25-50)[2]

	Food Sources[3]	Function[3]	Results of Deficiency[3]	Results of Excessive Consumption[3]
Calcium **male** 800 mg **female** 800 mg	Milk & milk products; leafy, green vegetables; salmon & sardines (with bones)	Essential to healthy bones and teeth; assists in nerve conduction & muscle contraction.	Abnormal heartbeat; muscle cramps; numbness & tingling of hands & feet; dementia.	Possible constipation or increased risk of kidney stones; possible kidney damage.
Phosphorus **male** 800 mg **female** 800 mg	Milk, fish, poultry, meat, eggs, cereal products, nuts, dried beans & peas	Necessary for normal muscle metabolism, skeletal growth & tooth development.	Bone loss; weakness; anorexia; malaise; bone pain.	Unknown.
Magnesium **male** 350 mg **female** 280 mg	Whole grain cereal, bananas, nuts, peas, beans, & green leafy vegetables	Important to bone structure; assists in nerve & muscle functioning; regulates heart rhythm.	Loss of appetite; nausea; diarrhea; muscle weakness; irritability; confusion.	Low blood pressure; fatigue, weakness, fluid retention; nausea; vomiting.
Iron **male** 10 mg **female** 15 mg	Red meat, fish, poultry, egg yolk, whole grain products, dark green vegetables	Promotes formation of hemoglobin; contributes to energy release during metabolism.	Anemia; fatigue; impaired concentration; impaired immune function.	Constipation; possible increased risk of heart disease.
Zinc **male** 15 mg **female** 12 mg	Shellfish, beef, liver, lamb, pork, eggs, wheat germ, dry beans & peas	Maintains senses of taste & smell; aids in healing.	Loss of appetite; slow healing of wounds; frequent infections; retarded growth; skin changes.	Depressed immunity; gastrointestinal distress; vomiting.
Iodine **male** 150 µg **female** 150 µg	Iodized salt, seafood, vegetable oil, seaweed	Necessary for production of hormones that regulate growth, reproduction, & nerve & bone formation.	Fatigue; apathy; enlarged thyroid; weight gain; dry skin; intolerance to cold.	Thyroid problems; inflammation of salivary glands; elemental form can be fatal.
Selenium **male** 70 µg **female** 55 µg	Seafoods, kidney, liver, some whole grains & seeds	Enhances immune function; helps prevent cancer & buildup of fatty deposits in arteries.	Muscular discomfort or weakness; predisposition to development of Keshan disease; heart problems.	Nausea; diarrhea; fatigue; hair loss; irritability; fingernail tenderness & loss.

Note: Endnotes and sources appear on page 19-13.

Figure 19-4: Nutrient Needs of a Healthy Body—Minerals

Estimated Safe and Adequate Dietary Intakes of Selected Vitamins and Trace Elements[8]

Vitamins/Adults (Age 25-50)[2]

	Food Sources[3]	Function[3]	Results of Deficiency[3]	Results of Excessive Consumption[3]
Pantothenic Acid No specific RDA (safe range may be 4-7 mg)	Liver, wheat germ, dried beans, eggs, nuts, lean meats, broccoli, milk	Involved in proper skin growth & nerve function; maintains health of adrenal glands.	Headache; fatigue; nausea; muscle cramps; immune problems; mood changes; loss of coordination & sleep.	Generally nontoxic.
Biotin No specific RDA (safe range may be 30-100 µg)	Yeast, liver, egg yolks nuts, soy flour, whole grains	Assists in metabolism of fats & carbohydrates; essential for making protein and nucleic acid.	Anorexia; nausea; vomiting; pallor; hair loss; depression; inflamed tongue; dermatitis.	Generally nontoxic.

Trace Elements/Adults (Age 25-50)[9]

	Food Sources[3]	Function[3]	Results of Deficiency[3]	Results of Excessive Consumption[3]
Copper No specific RDA (safe range may be 1.5 to 3 mg)	Liver, kidney, crab, oysters, fruit, nuts, whole grain cereals	Helps form red blood cells; acts as an antioxidant.	Anemia; skeletal defects; nerve degeneration; altered hair texture.	Unknown.
Manganese No specific RDA (safe range may be 2 to 5 mg)	Nuts, whole grain cereals, peas, beans & tea	Normal bone growth; activation of enzymes used in carbohydrate & protein metabolism.	Retarded growth; poor reproductive performance; impaired glucose tolerance; bone & cartilage malformations	"Manganese madness" (hysterical laughter, impulsiveness & sleeplessness, depression, muscle spasms & rigidity).
Fluorine (Fluoride) No specific RDA (safe range may be 1.5 to 4 mg)	Fish, tea, fluoridated water	Increases resistance of teeth to disease; may help prevent osteoporosis.	Tooth decay; possible decreased bone growth.	Mottled tooth enamel; kidney damage; muscle & nerve damage; death.
Chromium No specific RDA (safe range may be 50 to 200 µg)	Liver, beef, poultry, wheat germ, thyme, broccoli, brewer's yeast	Maintains normal glucose metabolism.	Nerve degeneration; diabetes-like symptoms; glucose intolerance.	Unknown.
Molybdenum No specific RDA (safe range may be 75 to 250 µg)	Milk, beans, breads & cereals	Detoxifies sulfites; may also act as an antioxidant.	Rapid pulse; headache; rapid breathing; nausea; vomiting; night blindness.	Possible gout-like symptoms; loss of copper.

Note: Endnotes and sources appear on page 19-13.

Figure 19-5: Nutrient Needs of a Healthy Body—Additional Vitamins and Trace Elements

Estimated Sodium, Chloride, and Potassium Minimum Requirements of Healthy Persons

Adults (Age 18 and Over)[10]

	Food Sources[3]	Function[3]	Results of Deficiency[3]	Results of Excessive Consumption[3]
Sodium[11, 12] No specific RDA (safe amount may be 500 mg)	Table salt & processed foods	Regulates the body's fluid balance & acid-base balance; aids in the transmission of nerve impulses.	Loss of weight; loss of thirst; muscle cramping & weakness; nerve disorders; digestive disorders.	Edema & increased blood pressure.
Chloride[11, 12] No specific RDA (safe amount may be 750 mg)	Table salt & processed foods	Helps transport electrical charges through body; activates nerve impulses.	Constipation; inability to gain weight; electrolyte abnormalities.	Dehydration; Increased blood pressure.
Potassium[13] No specific RDA (safe amount may be 2000 mg)	Shellfish, most fruits & vegetables, beans & peanuts	Promotes regular heartbeat; controls nerve conduction, muscle contraction & energy production.	Fatigue; weakness; abnormal heartbeat; drowsiness; muscle pain.	Muscle weakness; cold, pale skin; confusion; numbness & tingling of extremities; heart failure.

1. The allowances, expressed as average daily intakes over time, are intended to provide for individual variations among most normal persons as they live in the United States under usual environmental stresses. Diets should be based on a variety of common foods in order to provide other nutrients for which human requirements have been less well defined.

2. Amounts shown are not for pregnant or lactating females, or for individuals outside the range of 25 to 50 years. Recommended amounts for pregnant or lactating females or for individuals outside the range of 25 to 50 years may or may not be different than those shown above. These recommended ranges can be found in *Recommended Dietary Allowances, 10th Edition*, Food and Nutrition Board, Commission on Life Sciences, National Research Council, National Academy Press, Washington, DC, 1989.

3. May or may not be complete listings.

4. Retinol equivalents. 1 retinol equivalent = 1µg retinol or 6 µg β-carotene.

5. As cholecalciferol. 10 µg cholecalciferol = 400 IU of vitamin D.

6. α-Tocopherol equivalents. 1 mg d-α tocopherol = 1 α-TE.

7. 1 NE (niacin equivalent) is equal to 1 mg of niacin or 60 mg of dietary tryptophan.

8. Because there is less information on which to base allowances, these figures are not given in the main table of RDA and are provided here in the form of ranges of recommended intakes.

9. Since the toxic levels for many trace elements may be only several times usual intakes, the upper levels for the trace elements given in this table should not be habitually exceeded.

10. Values have been averaged for males and females. Values for pregnant or lactating females may be different.

11. No allowance has been included for large, prolonged losses from the skin through sweat.

12. There is no evidence that higher intakes confer any health benefit.

13. Desirable intakes of potassium may considerable exceed these values (~3500 mg for adults).

Source: Printed with permission from *Recommended Dietary Allowances: 10th Edition*. Copyright 1989 by the National Academy of Sciences. Courtesy of the National Academy Press, Washington, DC.

Additional information obtained from: *Taber's Cyclopedic Medical Dictionary*, 18th Edition, F.A. Davis Company, Philadelphia, PA, 1997; Ellen Moyer, *Vitamins and Minerals: Questions You Have... Answers You Need*, Wings Books, Avenel, NJ, 1993; Stanley Gershoff, PhD, *The Tufts University Guide to Total Nutrition*, Harper & Row Publishers, New York, NY, 1990.

Figure 19-6: Nutrient Needs of a Healthy Body—Electrolytes

A Word About Cholesterol

cholesterol:
a waxy, white substance that humans and animals make from fat

Cholesterol is a waxy, white substance that humans and animals make from fat. Plants do not make cholesterol; therefore, cholesterol is not present in vegetarian foods. Cholesterol is contained in all meats, poultry, fish, dairy products, and egg yolks. It assists in forming the outer membrane of cells and provides an insulating sheath around nerve fibers. It is not necessary to consume cholesterol because the liver can manufacture enough as long as the recommended amount of fat, 30% of the calories, is consumed on a daily basis.

low-density lipoprotein (LDL):
a cholesterol carrier that delivers cholesterol to all the cells of the body

Cholesterol, in excessive quantities, can form deposits on the walls of the arteries. This forms a condition known as **atherosclerosis**. The blood contains two cholesterol-carriers known as **lipoproteins**. **Low-density lipoproteins** (**LDLs**) deliver cholesterol to all the cells of the body. Throughout this process, some of the cholesterol becomes attached to the arterial wall. The **high-density lipoproteins** (**HDLs**) appear to remove some of the cholesterol from the bloodstream and transport it to the liver where it can be broken down and excreted. Rather than the overall level of cholesterol, it is the level of the cholesterol in the form of LDLs versus HDLs that is important in determining if a person is at risk for developing vascular and/or cardiac disease.

high-density lipoprotein (HDL):
a cholesterol carrier that functions to remove excess cholesterol from the bloodstream and transport it to the liver where it is broken down and excreted

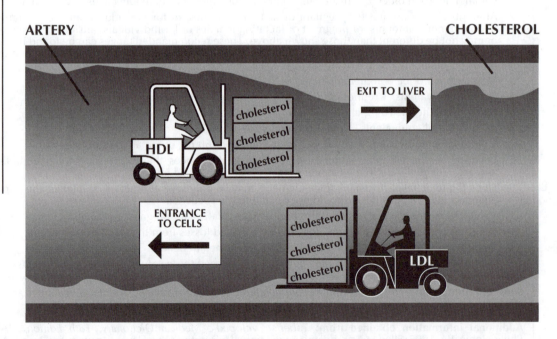

Figure 19-7: Cholesterol is carried to the cells by LDLs and is removed from the bloodstream via the liver by HDLs.

The Value of Exercise

The value of exercise cannot be overemphasized! Performed consistently, exercise will burn off extra calories. The more vigorous the exercise, the deeper the inhalations. The deeper the inhalations, the more oxygen is consumed to help burn calories. Exercise not only improves one's physical appearance, it also is an excellent way to release stress.

Before anyone begins an exercise program, a medical examination is recommended. An exercise program should include a variety of exercises to help eliminate boredom. The exercises should be vigorous so that deep inhalations will occur and transport oxygen to the cells. This form of exercise is called **aerobic**.

aerobic: requiring oxygen; a form of exercise that raises the pulse, thereby transporting more oxygen to the cells

It is easy to overdo a new exercise routine by being overly enthusiastic about getting into shape. To prevent overexertion, always start slowly and work up to more difficult levels of exercise and longer periods of aerobic activity as time goes on. During all phases of aerobic exercise, you should be able to carry on a conversation without getting short of breath. The diet should be high in carbohydrates for endurance. The most valuable nutrient lost during exercise is water. Drink at least one glass of water 20 minutes prior to beginning to exercise, every 20 minutes during exercise, and immediately after. Do not wait until you are thirsty; by then, the muscles are beginning to dehydrate and will fatigue faster.

As mentioned before, one pound of fat is equal to 3,500 calories. This means that you must burn off 3,500 EXTRA calories in order to remove 1 pound of fat. As a person gets older, the **basal metabolic rate** decreases. This is the rate at which the body normally burns calories. It is controlled and determined by the thyroid gland. The more active a person is, the higher his metabolic rate is. This is why it is more difficult for people over the age of 35 to burn calories—their metabolic rate has decreased. Encourage those who express a desire to change their eating habits or want to start an exercise program—it takes a lot of determination and perseverance!

basal metabolic rate: the rate at which the body normally burns calories while at rest

People who are overweight are at a higher risk for a number of health conditions: joint and bone problems (arthritis and pain), adult-onset diabetes, asthma, cardiovascular diseases, varicose veins, hypertension, myocardial infarctions, depression, low self-esteem, and cerebrovascular accidents. Be very sensitive to the physical and psychological needs of these patients. Admitting they have a weight problem and need help is the most important step to solving the problem!

Suggested Weights for Men (Age 25-29)

Height	Small Frame	Medium Frame	Large Frame
5'2"	128-134	131-141	138-150
5'3"	130-136	133-143	140-153
5'4"	132-138	135-145	142-156
5'5"	134-140	137-148	144-160
5'6"	136-142	139-151	146-164
5'7"	138-145	142-154	149-168
5'8"	140-148	145-157	152-172
5'9"	142-151	148-160	155-176
5'10"	144-154	151-163	158-180
5'11"	146-157	154-166	161-184
6'0"	149-160	157-170	164-188
6'1"	152-164	160-174	168-192
6'2"	155-168	164-178	172-197
6'3"	158-172	167-182	176-202
6'4"	162-176	171-187	181-207

* Weight is in pounds with clothing weighing five (5) pounds.
  Height is with shoes with one (1) inch heel.

Suggested Weights for Women (Age 25-29)

Height	Small Frame	Medium Frame	Large Frame
4'10"	102-111	109-121	118-131
4'11"	103-113	111-123	120-134
5'0"	104-115	113-126	122-137
5'1"	106-118	115-129	125-140
5'2"	108-121	118-132	128-143
5'3"	111-124	121-135	131-147
5'4"	114-127	124-138	134-151
5'5"	117-130	127-141	137-155
5'6"	120-133	130-144	140-159
5'7"	123-136	133-147	143-163
5'8"	126-139	136-150	146-167
5'9"	129-142	139-153	149-170
5'10"	132-145	142-156	152-173
5'11"	135-148	145-159	155-176
6'0"	138-151	148-162	158-179

* Weight is in pounds with clothing weighing three (3) pounds.
  Height is with shoes with one (1) inch heel.

Figure 19-9: Suggested Weights for Adults, Age 25 to 29

Although many people are familiar with the height and weight charts such as the one on the preceding page, there is much disagreement over which is the best one to use. Some tables consider frame size, age and sex, while others do not. Furthermore, none of the tables distinguish excess fat from muscle. This means that a person with a lot of muscle may appear to be obese when, in fact, he is not. Body Mass Index (BMI) has been the medical standard for obesity measurement since the early 1980s. Government researchers developed it to take height into account in weight measurement. However, many of the same problems that exist with the height and weight tables apply to BMIs as well.

Generally speaking, recommended BMI's are in the range of 20 to 26 for those over the age of 35. People who are in the 26 to 27 range are usually considered to be overweight. In general, a person age 35 or older is obese if he or she has a BMI of 27 or more. Those who are under the age of 35, a BMI of 25 or more indicates obesity. Most authorities agree that anyone with a BMI over 30 is moderately to severely obese. Although the term *obese* often carries a negative connotation in normal usage, in the field of healthcare it is a non-judgemental term that simply indicates a body mass index within a certain range.

A person's BMI is calculated using a mathematical formula in which BMI equals a person's weight in kilograms divided by the height in meters squared. (BMI = kg ÷ m^2). For example, is a woman who weighs 155 lbs obese? It depends on her height. The answer is different for a woman who is 61″ tall than it is for a woman who is 70″.

1. Convert weight to kilograms: (Use the formula from Chapter 10.)

    155 lbs ÷ 2.2 = 70.45 kg

2. Convert height to meters: (Divide the height inches by 39.37.)

    Example 1   Example 2
    61 in ÷ 39.37 = 1.54 m   70 in ÷ 39.37 = 1.77 m

3. Use the formula: (BMI = kg ÷ m^2)

    Example 1   Example 2
    BMI = 70.45 kg ÷ (1.54 x 1.54)   BMI = 70.45 kg ÷ (1.77 x 1.77)
    BMI = 70.45 kg ÷ 2.37   BMI = 70.45 kg ÷ 3.13
    BMI = 29.72   BMI = 22.5

Therefore, the woman who is 61" tall and weighs 155 lbs has a BMI of 29.72, and is generally considered obese. The woman who is 70" and weighs 155 lbs has a BMI of 22.5 and is in the healthy range.

Chapter Summary

There are a number of health conditions people may be at risk to develop through poor health habits. Cigarette smoking, drug and alcohol abuse, elevated levels of low-density lipoproteins, hypertension, poor management of stress, and being overweight are some of the conditions that may lead to health problems.

Conditions such as asthma, emphysema, bronchitis, chest pain, shortness of breath, bone and joint disorders, diabetes, cerebrovascular accidents, chronic infections, and depression are all common in those who have poor health practices. Prevention is the key to minimizing the risk of acquiring one or more of these health problems.

As a healthcare worker, learning to help patients who may be experiencing one or more of these diseases is a challenge. These are very sensitive subjects for patients and all members of the healthcare team must communicate with one another. Sensitivity and privacy are important aspects in communicating ideas and programs to the patient and the family. Patients and family members will ask you questions as they look for assistance and encouragement. You can help your patients best by being informed and helping them to become informed. Most hospitals provide classes on many of these topics. Hospital departments such as the dietary and patient education departments provide literature, video tapes, and verbal information for patients and their families. Show compassion to your patients and their families by helping them in their search for information that can help them.

Name _____

Date _____

Student Enrichment Activities

Complete the following statements.

1. A substance that causes cancer is called a _____.

2. A toxic substance that is found in all parts of the tobacco plant is _____.

3. Hypertension without an apparent medical cause is _____ _____.

4. One's _____ _____ often determine whether stress will be positive or negative.

5. Five ways to effectively manage stress include the following:
   A. _____   D. _____
   B. _____   E. _____
   C. _____

6. A healthy diet should be made up of _____ % carbohydrates, _____ % fats, and _____ % protein.

7. The principal source of energy for the body is provided by _____.

8. Carbohydrates are broken down into _____.

9. Fats are needed in order to transport vitamins _____, _____, _____, and _____.

10. The primary building block of any body part is _____.

11. A waxy, white substance made from fat is _____.

12. Cholesterol-carriers contained in the body are _____.

13. The rate at which the body normally burns calories is the _____

_____ _____.

Unscramble the following terms.

14. ASALB CIMETBOLA TERA   _____ _____ _____

15. YGLONCEG   _____

16. TINCIONE   _____

17. SLENTI KRELLI   _____ _____

18. WALWITHARD   _____

19. SSSTER   _____

20. TRIPONE   _____

21. TRIOPLEPION   _____

22. GARCIONCEN   _____

23. EROACIL   _____

24. BROAICE   _____

Chapter Twenty
Career Planning

Objectives

After completing this chapter you should be able to
do the following:

1. Define and correctly spell each of the key terms.

2. Identify and describe at least four resources for locating
   job openings.

3. Explain the difference between a job and a career.

4. Identify at least five areas to evaluate during a self-assessment
   prior to writing your resumé.

5. Write your resumé.

6. Write a cover letter.

7. Identify at least six guidelines to consider when preparing for
   an interview.

8. Identify the four aspects of being a positive influence on the
   healthcare team.

9. List the Ten Commandments of Human Relations.

Key Terms

- career
- cover letter
- job
- resumé

Planning for Success

career:
a profession for which one trains and that is undertaken as one's lifelong work

job:
a specific duty, role, or function that is performed regularly for compensation

Choosing a fulfilling **career** requires careful thought and continuous planning. Career satisfaction comes from proper career selection and identification of your career goals. A career is not just a **job**. A career involves a steady progression and the realization of financial and personal goals through diligent planning and work. Usually a job is less rewarding than a career because it involves working for pay without any sense of progression beyond getting the task done; there is little or no personal reward. Only you can make the decision. Do you want a career or just a job? Since adults typically spend about 30% of their time at work, proper planning is very important. This chapter will provide you with some practical guidelines concerning finding a position and keeping it, selling yourself to potential employers, and surviving interviews.

Where Do I Start?

Getting started in anything is often the most difficult thing to do, and beginning the search for that *perfect job* is no exception. There are several things to think about when you are beginning your career. Deciding on a career is not easy; careers affect all aspects of life. They affect our **activities of daily living**, our children, our relationship with a significant other, and our self-fulfillment. Sometimes as we grow older our goals and priorities change; therefore, keep in mind that what is important now may not be so vital in 5 years.

Searching for an entry-level position in your chosen career can be very time-consuming. There are many different sources to examine when searching for a position in your field.

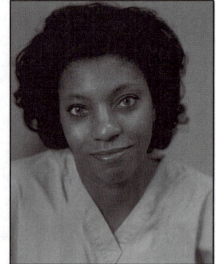

Figure 20-1: Deciding on a career can be difficult.

Medicine, nursing, and allied health careers boast a wide variety of specialties and positions. Through this course, you have been introduced to several different types of healthcare facilities and a variety of specialties. In addition to field trips and interviews with healthcare professionals, there are other sources that may provide information concerning health-oriented positions:

1. Newspaper Classified Advertisements: Many of the available positions in health occupations are listed under Nursing, Laboratory, Rehabilitation, Physical Therapy, and Medical. There is an abundance of positions available in both the medical field and the allied health field. Watch for the large advertisements hospitals often put in the newspapers!

2. Your Instructors: Throughout your course of study, your instructors have watched you grow and mature. They have observed your strengths and know your skill level. They probably have professional contacts who might be interested in your knowledge and skills. If you wish to use an instructor as a reference, be sure to ask permission BEFORE putting his or her name on a job application.

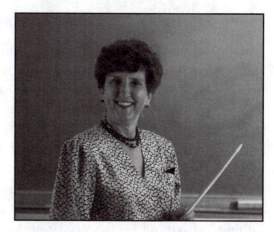

Figure 20-2: Your instructor may be a good source of information regarding potential positions.

3. Job Placement Counselors: Most educational institutions have job counselors on staff. Their main function is to assist students in finding part-time employment during school. The employment may or may not be in the chosen field; however, all employment should be viewed as an education. Job placement counselors are excellent resource people!

4. Employment Agencies: Every state has an agency responsible for assisting people in finding a job that matches their skill level. They interview each applicant, test their abilities, and attempt to match their interests with an appropriate job. Because these are state programs, there is no fee for the applicant. Private employment agencies provide the same services, but these agencies often have the applicant sign a contract and receive a fee for their service. If you choose to go through a private agency, MAKE SURE YOU UNDERSTAND ALL CONTRACTS BEFORE YOU SIGN!

5. Networking: Meeting people who are established in the field in which you are seeking a career may provide opportunities for employment. Use of this powerful tool involves making full use of the people-skills you have developed.

6. Hospital Job-Opportunity Bulletin Boards: Most hospitals have bulletin boards that list current openings in the various departments. These are often located outside of the Personnel or Human Resources Department.

7. Relatives, Friends, and Acquaintances: Do not underestimate family and friends! Ask for their opinions. Word of mouth is a powerful means of advertising.

8. Job Fairs: This is a great opportunity to explore many options by meeting several different potential employers at one event. The informal atmosphere makes it possible for you to ask a wide variety of questions about the companies represented. Bring plenty of **resumés** with you!

resumé:
a brief, written account of personal and professional qualifications and experience that is prepared by an applicant for a position

Setting goals is an important part of making the most of your career. Both short-term and long-term goals should be set and be attainable within a reasonable amount of time. For example, what do you want to be doing in 1 year? What about 5 years? How about 10 years? Your goals should be the driving force behind everything you do: writing your resumé, searching for a position, applying for a position, and interviewing for a position. In order to be effective, goals should be organized and specific. Do not be afraid to set goals. Remember, they are not set in concrete; they can be changed. As your priorities change, so will your goals.

Selling Yourself: The First Impression

"First impressions are lasting ones." This old saying has proven to be true in everything from the first day of school to the first patient contact. An employer's first impression of you may be from a telephone call or from a letter requesting an interview for a position.

Telephones are a very important part of modern communication systems. Business thrives on the use of telephones. If you choose to contact a potential employer by telephone, PRACTICE PROPER TELEPHONE ETIQUETTE! Review the chapter on communication skills. Consider the following guidelines when conducting telephone business.

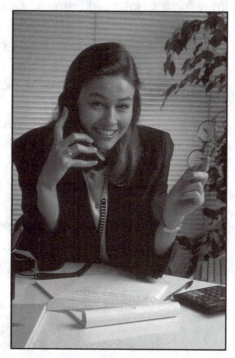

1. Be prepared! Know what questions you want to ask BEFORE you dial the telephone. Write the questions down in advance and keep them in front of you during the call. Mark them off as each one is asked and answered.

2. Practice asking the questions BEFORE you make the telephone call. Stand in front of a mirror and rehearse the questions. Watch your facial expressions.

Figure 20-3: A professional tone and pleasant attitude will enhance your telephone communication.

3. Have a positive frame of mind. Attitude is projected through your voice. Smile while you speak; this will help transmit your smile across the telephone lines!

4. Introduce yourself and ask to speak to someone about the position advertised.

5. Remember your manners!

6. Show consideration for the receptionist's time.

7. Inquire whether it would be all right to follow up the telephone call by bringing in your resumé and/or filling out the job application.

8. Always thank the person for answering your questions and for his or her time.

Positions that are advertised in the newspaper may provide a mailing address for resumés. The following are guidelines to follow whenever written material may form a potential employer's first impression of you.

1. Use a word processor or a typewriter that has a memory. It is much easier to make corrections and/or changes. Use a simple style of type; remember, you want the person to be able to read it!

2. Do not use *white out* or *strike over* an error. Make the correction and print an error-free copy.

3. Use a letter-quality or near-letter quality printer.

4. Use correct grammar and punctuation. If you have a question concerning the proper spelling of a word, LOOK IT UP! Employers notice poor English!

5. Use unlined, white bond paper.

6. Limit the length of the general resumé to no more than one page. Employers like information to be concise and easy to read.

7. Use common terminology and phrases. Employers are not necessarily impressed with advanced vocabulary—especially if the words are used incorrectly or the employer has to look them up!

8. Be specific; avoid the use of vague and general statements.

9. Keep sentences short, specific, and action-packed.

10. NEVER LIE on a resumé!

It is always preferable to make a personal appearance at the hospital in which you would like to work. Picking up an application is often the first impression; and remember, the receptionist will be passing that first impression on to the appropriate person.

Writing the Resumé

A resumé is a summary of you. It is a biographical sketch of your professional work experience and personal attributes. Producing a resumé that entices a potential employer to call you for an interview is a time-consuming project. The most important aspect of achieving this goal is writing the resumé WHEN YOU ARE IN A POSITIVE FRAME OF MIND! If you are not thinking positively about yourself, the resumé will project a negative impression. The goal of the resumé is to spark the interest of the person who is doing the hiring!

Employers have their own methods of evaluating job applicants. For example, some employers place the most emphasis on past work experience, whereas others use the information gathered from the job interviews. Eventually, all areas will be given consideration: education, professional work experience, personal qualities and attributes, career objectives, references, and recommendations.

Before writing the resumé, it may be helpful to perform a self-assessment of the qualities an employer is looking for in an employee. Ask yourself (and honestly answer) the following questions.

1. **Dependability:** Am I punctual? Do I keep my word? Do I go that *extra* mile? Do I finish projects that I start? Do I abuse the allotted time for breaks and meals? Do I have too many commitments that could prevent me from following through on some aspect of my job?

2. **Integrity:** Am I honest? Am I willing to admit I don't know something? Do I exaggerate the facts? Can I accept the blame for something I did or did not do?

3. **Appearance:** Do I look neat and clean, including fingernails, shoes? Do I wear the proper attire? For the women: Does my make-up look fresh and natural? For the men: Are my beard and mustache trimmed and clean? Is their presence appropriate for the position?

4. **Attendance:** Have I been absent from school due to illness or other commitments on a regular basis?

5. **Initiative:** Do I work best by myself or do I need supervision and direction? Do I do extra work and projects without being asked? Do I anticipate needs and take care of them?

6. **Communication Skills:** How is my telephone etiquette? Do I do more listening than speaking? Do I shake hands with a firm handshake? Do I introduce myself well? Do I introduce others well? Do I have good posture when sitting and standing? (This is called body language.) Am I kind, courteous, and helpful?

7. **Cooperation:** Do I function well as a team member? Can I work well on a committee? Am I concerned about what I can contribute to my employer? Am I part of the problem or part of the solution?

SELL YOURSELF as you develop the resumé! You are the marketing department, and you are selling a product—YOU! Focus on all of your positive aspects.

Organizing the Resumé

Resumés may be organized in several different ways. The order in which a resumé presents the information is called the format. Resumés are designed to provide potential employers with selected information. Therefore, only information you choose to reveal about yourself is included. In addition to your qualifications, there are three items that must appear as a heading on every resumé:

1. You must include your first and last name.

2. Use your complete address—avoid the use of a post office box number; employers associate instability with a post office number; use the correct, post office approved state abbreviation.

3. Include your complete telephone number, including the area code. Make sure this is a telephone number where you can be reached easily.

When writing about your qualifications for a job, only include the information that is directly pertinent to the position for which you are applying. This means there may be times when you have to change your resumé. The following categories of information are generally included on every resumé.

1. *Career Goal:* A statement that reflects your career goal. This goal should be attainable in the position for which you are applying.

2. *Summary of Qualifications:* This section highlights your strongest attributes such as integrity, self-motivation, self-initiative, communication skills, etc. If you have held a previous job, your employment history appears here too. Jobs should be listed in reverse chronological order. This means that your current or most recent job is listed first, then the one you held before it, etc. List all applicable experience, and be sure to list your responsibilities and duties as well as the name and address of the business for which you worked. Unless you only worked at these places for a short time, you also should include the dates you started and ended your employment at each job.

3. *Educational Background:* It is generally best to start with your most recent educational experience including seminars and additional training. If you have been out of high school for more than 5 years, it is acceptable to omit high school information from the resumé. Vocational training, college education, and degrees all are important to potential employers.

Additional information that may be included in the resumé is listed below.

1. *Community Activity Involvement:* Membership in professional organizations indicates a desire for continuous self-improvement and to increase professional contacts.

2. *Offices Held:* Official positions can indicate leadership abilities and respect from peers.

3. *References:* Only provide names if they are specifically requested. Otherwise state, "References available upon request."

4. *Miscellaneous:* You may use this heading to indicate your willingness to travel or relocate and the date you would be available for work. This section also should include any professional achievements such as professional certifications and titles.

5. *Salary Range:* NEVER put down a specific salary unless the potential employer requests it. Indicate "Salary negotiable."

Formatting the Document

There are several acceptable formats for resumés. The style and organization of your resumé should reflect your personality. General guidelines to consider for format follow.

1. All margins should be the same size. (If you use 2-inch right and left side margins, use 2-inch top and bottom margins as well.)

2. Strive to make the document look balanced. For example, double-space between the category title and first sentence, single space between the sentences, and either double or triple space between the last sentence in that section and the title of the next category.

3. Proofread the document at least twice. Have someone else proofread it after you have corrected the errors you discovered. NEATNESS COUNTS!

Putting together a resumé takes time. Your career is an extremely important part of your life. Finding the position that will allow you to pursue your career goals and objectives is vital to career satisfaction.

Jennifer Hard Worker
1234 Career Place
Options, CA 00000-0000
Telephone: (123) 555-5678

CAREER OBJECTIVE: An entry level position in health occupations with the potential for advancement to a supervisory level.

SUMMARY OF QUALIFICATIONS: I have developed the following professional and interpersonal skills through my education, work experience, and participation in various community activities.

- Two years experience in operating a word processor
- Proficient in operating a 10-key adding machine
- Manage incoming telephone calls
- Excellent verbal communication skills
- Work well with others
- Prompt and efficient in completing assigned duties
- Follow written and verbal directions well
- Self-motivator
- Excellent organizer

WORK EXPERIENCE: January 19__– Present
Cook County Hospital
1340 Gramacy Place
Evanton, IL

Part-time aide. Duties and responsibilities include transporting patients from one department to another; delivering specimens to the laboratory; picking up expendable items from Central Supply; answering patient call lights; serving meals to patients and picking up empty trays; assisting the nursing staff with procedures such as vital signs, recording intake and output fluid levels, and weighing patients; escorting patients to family vehicles upon discharge; participating with other healthcare workers in fire and other disaster drills.

EDUCATIONAL BACKGROUND: 19__: Honor Graduate of Health Occupations Vocational Training Institute 19__: Honor Graduate of Superior High School

COMMUNITY ACTIVITIES: 19__: Developed Health Student Volunteers Organization at Superior High School 19__: Received Volunteer of the Year Award from Student Volunteers of America 19__

REFERENCES: Available upon request.

Figure 20-4: A Sample Resumé

The Cover Letter

cover letter:
a letter that
accompanies
a resumé to
explain or
introduce its
contents

All resumés should be accompanied by a **cover letter**. The purpose of the cover letter is to introduce yourself. To do this effectively, you must communicate your desire to be considered for a particular position. Keep the letter short and simple. Do not boast about your qualifications or personal attributes; these will be reflected in the resumé. The letter should be formatted in business style, spaced as shown in Figure 20-5, with equal margins.

Jennifer Hard Worker
1234 Career Place
Options, CA 00000-0000
Telephone: (123) 555-5678

November 15, 19__

Mr. Brian Taylor
Director of Human Resources
Healing Hospital
6789 Healthy Lane
Wellness, HI 11223-4567

Dear Mr. Taylor:

I am responding to your advertisement in the _____ on
_____ for the position of _____. I am a
recent honor graduate of _____ and am pursuing
a career in Health Occupations.

Enclosed for your review is my resumé. I would appreciate consideration
for an interview for the above position. As my resumé reflects, I have a year
of part-time experience in a clinical setting as an aide. Now that I have
graduated, I am eager to begin a full-time career in the field of healthcare.

If you desire additional information, or would like to schedule an interview,
please contact me by telephone at (123) 555-5678.

Thank you for considering my application.

Sincerely,

Jennifer Hard Worker

Jennifer Hard Worker

Enclosure

Figure 20-5: A Sample Cover Letter (Full Block Style)

The All-Important Interview

Remember what we said about first impressions? The interview is your chance to shine! People tend to hire those who impress them. This means that just because you are the most qualified person for a certain position, does NOT mean you will be offered the job!

A positive outlook is the most important thing you can bring with you to the interview. Attempt to get a position offered to you at the completion of every interview. The position may not be the one you had your heart set on,

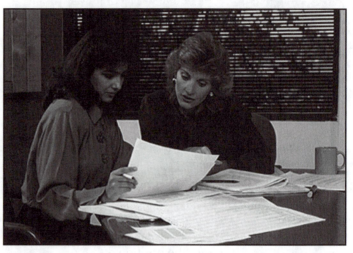

Figure 20-6: Being prepared for the interview will help you present a favorable image to a potential employer.

but receiving an offer for a position is a fantastic way to boost your self-image and self-confidence! Here are some general guidelines that may help you as you prepare for the interview:

1. THINK ABOUT YOURSELF IN A POSITIVE WAY!

2. Review the qualities that are positive selling points about you. Think about answers to the questions in the Writing the Resumé section.

3. Research the hospital's accomplishments and community contributions.

4. Formulate your own questions for the interviewer. This means you do some research concerning the hospital's background.

5. Dress for success! Select clean, well-fitting, business-like clothes.

6. Be prepared to answer the common questions:

    - Why do you want to work here?

    - Why are you interested in this position?

    - What are your strengths?

    - What are your weaknesses?

    - What do you know about the company?

    - Can you describe your current job for me?

    - Why do you want to leave your present job?

    Be sure to answer all questions directly and honestly! Maintain good eye contact with the interviewer!

7. ALWAYS arrive at least 15 minutes early. This will give your nerves time to calm down and let you relax.

8. Be prepared to complete the employer's application. The application will probably ask for the following information: your name, address, and telephone number; the telephone number of your nearest relative; your Social Security Number; the phone numbers and addresses of at least three professional references; and the dates of honors and certificates you have received. Make sure it is completed NEATLY!

9. Be sincerely interested in the company.

10. Follow-up on the interview with a letter or telephone call. The letter should briefly express your appreciation for the interview and the interviewer's time. Repeat your continuing interest in the company (if this is indeed the case), and express the desire to get back in touch with them.

All of the above suggestions can be summarized into four categories: courtesy, self-confidence, common sense, and assertiveness. Sell the positive you!

The Ideal Employee

Throughout this text, emphasis has been placed on education, competency, and the provision of quality care to the patient. The phrase *healthcare team member* has been repeated numerous times. What exactly does it mean to be a member of a team? Being a positive contributor to the healthcare team involves developing the proper attitude concerning your contribution:

1. I make a difference here! I'm part of what the public sees when they judge my department or hospital. How I feel on a given day affects the people with whom I work. I help set the tone here.

2. I take responsibility for what bothers me. I do what I can to change the situation. If it's unchangeable, I look for ways to minimize its effects on me. Most important, I REMEMBER THAT I HAVE CHOSEN TO WORK HERE, AND AS LONG AS I'M HERE, I'LL GIVE MY BEST!

3. I will take an interest in the organization. I'm interested in how this organization got to be what it is today, and how the people in it have grown as they have. I try to see the big picture—to think beyond my particular job to the kind of product or service I'd like to receive as a customer or client.

4. I am proud to be a strong, reliable member of my organization's team. I know that my success, as well as my organization's, depends on it!

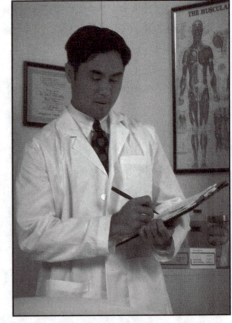

Today's world can be very stressful. The medical field is made up of men and women who have many responsibilities. Many are single parents; some may be caring for elderly parents; others juggle school, work, children, and homelife; and many work more than one job! Treat people as if each and every one of them is special to you; show them consideration and courtesy. This applies to your patients AND your coworkers!

Figure 20-7: The ideal employee is a reliable and knowledgeable member of the healthcare team.

The following is a list of the Ten Commandments of Human Relations that are essential to use when working with people:

1. **SPEAK TO PEOPLE.** There is nothing as nice as a cheerful greeting.

2. **SMILE AT PEOPLE.** It takes 72 muscles to frown, only 14 to smile.

3. **CALL PEOPLE BY NAME.** The sweetest music to anyone's ears is the sound of his or her own name.

4. **BE FRIENDLY AND HELPFUL.** If you want to have friends, be a friend.

5. **BE CORDIAL.** Speak and act as if everything you do is a genuine pleasure.

6. **BE GENUINELY INTERESTED IN PEOPLE.** You can like almost everyone if you try.

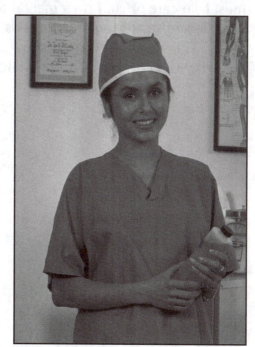

Figure 20-8: The ideal employee is also friendly and helpful.

7. **BE GENEROUS WITH PRAISE;** be cautious with criticism.

8. **BE CONSIDERATE** with the feelings of others. There are usually three sides to a controversy: yours, theirs, and the right side.

9. **BE ALERT TO PROVIDE SERVICE.** What counts most in life is what we do for others.

10. **ADD TO THIS** a good sense of humor, a big dose of patience, and a dash of humility, and you will be rewarded many times over.

Chapter Summary

As you progress in your allied health career, do not forget you are in the *people business*. You render care to patients; however, in order to be effective, you must take care of your own mental and physical health. People need others who sincerely care about their needs, and who are in a position to meet those needs. This means you must show both concern and compassion for your patients, your coworkers, and YOURSELF!

Name _____

Date _____

Student Enrichment Activities

1. Resources available to assist in finding an entry-level position include

   _____, _____, _____,

   _____, and _____.

2. Aspects of proper telephone etiquette include _____,

   _____, _____, and _____.

3. Identify seven areas of self-assessment that all job applicants should honestly evaluate:

   A. _____   **E.** _____

   B. _____   **F.** _____

   C. _____   **G.** _____

   D. _____

4. In addition to the heading, the categories that are generally included on all resumés

   are the _____ _____, the _____ _____

   _____, and the _____ _____.

5. List seven questions that are commonly asked of job applicants during an interview.

   A. _____

   B. _____

   C. _____

   D. _____

   E. _____

   F. _____

   G. _____

6. Write your resumé and a cover letter. Role play in small groups by reviewing each other's documents and assist each other in *polishing* them up.

Glossary

A

a-: absent, deficient, without, not, or a lack of.

ab-: away from, absent.

*abandonment: the termination of supervision of a patient by a physician without adequate written notice or the patient's consent.

abdomin/o: abdominal area.

abdominal: pertaining to the abdomen; respirations using primarily the abdominal muscles while the chest is mostly still.

abdominal cavity: the part of the anterior cavity that contains the pancreas, spleen, liver, gall bladder, lower portion of the esophagus, stomach, ureters, kidneys, appendix and intestines.

abduction: the lateral movement of a body part away from the middle of the body.

*Abraham Maslow: a psychologist who is credited with a theory of motivation that identified five levels of human needs in which the lower levels must be satisfied before attention is given to the higher levels.

abrasion: an open wound, road burn, or rug burn in which the outer layer of skin has been scraped off.

abscess: an infected, pus-filled sac that is swollen, red, and painful.

absorbed: sucked up; taken in.

acceptance: the final stage of the dying process as identified by Elisabeth Kubler-Ross in which the person comes to terms with his or her fate.

Achilles tendon: the tendon located at the distal part of the gastrocnemius muscle (calf), which secures that muscle to the calcaneus (heel).

acne: an inflammatory disease of the skin that involves the sebaceous glands, and that most commonly occurs on the face.

acquired immune deficiency syndrome (AIDS): a viral disease caused by the human immunodeficiency virus (HIV), which destroys the immune system and renders the patient susceptible to other infections. It is contracted through blood and other body fluids and sexual contact.

acromegaly: a chronic disease of the endocrine system characterized by elongation and enlargement of the bones, especially of the face; caused by excessive production of pituitary hormone.

active listening: making a conscious effort to hear what the sender is communicating; an essential element of effective and meaningful communication.

*activities of daily living (ADL): normal, everyday actions, such as self care, communication, and mobility skills, that are required for independent living.

*acute: sudden onset; short duration.

acute care facility: a healthcare facility that provides care to patients requiring short-term healthcare; acute care hospital.

ad-: near; toward.

Addison's Disease: a life-threatening disease of the endocrine system resulting from underproduction of adrenocortical hormones.

adduction: the movement of a body part toward the middle of the body.

aden-, adeno-, aden/o: gland.

adenitis: inflammation of the lymph nodes or a gland.

adenoids: spongy lymphoid tissue that protrudes from the posterior superior wall of the pharynx; pharyngeal tonsils.

adipose: refers to fat, as in fatty tissue.

Admissions Department: the department in a hospital that is responsible for obtaining important patient information including insurance data, patient identification data, and admitting diagnosis.

adolescence: the life stage that generally includes individuals between the ages of 12 and 20 years old, and in which physical, mental, emotional, and social changes occur rapidly.

adrenal gland: one of the triangular glands located above each kidney that secretes hormones from each of its two parts.

*advance directive: a legal document prepared when an individual is alive, competent, and able to make decisions. It provides guidance to the healthcare team if the person is no longer able to make decisions.

*aerobic: requiring oxygen; a form of exercise that raises the pulse, thereby transporting more oxygen to the cells.

afferent neurons: neurons that transmit messages, or impulses, from the sensory organs and the skin to the brain and spinal cord; sensory neurons.

agranulocyte: a leukocyte that does not contain granules in its cytoplasm.

*airborne transmission: a method of transmitting pathogens when a susceptible host is exposed or infected by the nuclei of evaporated, infected droplets. The nuclei remain suspended in the air for longer periods of time than droplets.

*AIDS: acquired immune deficiency syndrome; a viral disease caused by the human immunodeficiency virus (HIV), which damages the immune system leaving the patient susceptible to other infections. It is contracted through infected blood and other body fluids and sexual contact.

airway: a tube (either natural or man-made) that provides a passageway for air to and from the lungs.

-algia: painful.

*alignment: a physical position in which there is no stress or strain on any part of the body; the proper anatomical position; the positioning of parts in a straight line.

*alimentary canal: a general term for the digestive tract.

allergies: acquired, abnormal immune reactions to one or more substances.

alternating pressure mattress: a special mattress that is filled with air that changes pressure on various locations of the body to prevent skin breakdown.

*alveoli: microscopic air sacs within the lungs responsible for the exchange of oxygen and carbon dioxide.

*Alzheimer's disease: a neurological disease that causes irreversible memory loss and physical deterioration, which eventually leads to the complete loss of intellectual and physical functions.

ambi-: both, two-sided.

*ambulation: the process of walking.

ambulatory surgery: an operation that can be performed and completed within a short period of time and that does not require the patient to stay in the healthcare facility overnight.

amenorrhea: the absence or suppression of menstruation.

amniotic fluid: the liquid contained in the amnion, a thin sac that holds the fetus, that protects the fetus from injury.

amputation: the removal of a body part, usually done surgically.

amylase: a class of enzymes produced by the pancreas.

amylase blood test: a blood test in which the level of amylase enzymes in the patient's blood is evaluated.

amylopsin: a pancreatic enzyme that breaks down starch into achroodextrin and maltose.

an-: absent, deficient, without, not, or a lack of.

anaerobic: able to live without oxygen.

anal canal: the terminal end of the long intestine.

*anatomy: the study of the structure of the body.

anemia: a reduction in erythrocytes (red blood cells) or the amount of hemoglobin in the blood.

anesthesia: the partial or complete loss of sensation with or without the loss of consciousness.

anesthesiology: the branch of medicine that practices the science of anesthesia.

aneurysm: a weak section in the wall of a blood vessel that could rupture and cause a hemorrhage.

anger: the second stage of the dying process as identified by Elisabeth Kubler-Ross. Frustration, bitterness, and hostility are often displayed during this stage.

angina: cardiac pain caused by a low blood oxygen level in the coronary arteries that supply the heart muscle.

angi/o: vessel, either blood or lymph.

angiography: x-ray of the blood vessels after the injection of a contrast medium.

anorexia nervosa: an eating disorder that stems from an excessive fear of becoming overweight and that usually requires psychiatric treatment.

anoxia: a lack of oxygen.

ante-: before; preceding.

anter/o: in front of, ahead of, or before.

anterior: front; ventral.

anterior cavity: the space located along the front part of the interior of the body which is separated into three sections: the thoracic, abdominal, and pelvic cavities.

anti-: against.

antibiotic: a drug with the ability to kill or prevent the growth of living organisms and treat infections.

antibodies: molecules produced by the lymphocytes that protect the body from bacteria, viruses, and other antigens.

*anticoagulants: medications that thin the blood and prevent or delay blood coagulation.

*antidote: a substance that neutralizes a poison.

anuria: the failure to produce urine.

anus: the rectal opening that lies in the fold of the buttocks.

aorta: the main artery in the body.

aortic valve: the one-way valve located between the left ventricle of the heart and the aorta.

apex: the pointed tip of a conical structure; the location where the heartbeat is the loudest.

apical: refers to the apex of the heart, located at the left fifth intercostal space, mid-clavicular line; the apex (point or tip) of a cone-shaped structure.

apnea: the temporary cessation of spontaneous breathing.

appearance: the way one looks, including one's clothes, grooming habits, and facial expressions.

appendectomy: the surgical removal of the appendix.

appendicitis: inflammation of the vermiform appendix.

*appendicular skeleton: the part of the skeletal system formed by the extremities, shoulder girdle, and pelvic girdle.

aqua-K pad: a method of providing dry heat to an area of the body via heated water that is electrically circulated through the pad.

aqueous humor: the watery fluid found in the anterior and posterior chambers of the eye.

arachnoid membrane: the delicate middle layer of the meninges that resembles a spider web.

arteri/o: artery.

arterial blood gas: any of the gases that normally occur in the blood, such as oxygen and carbon dioxide, when analyzed from the artery rather than from a vein.

arterial blood gas test: a blood test used to determine acidity or alkalinity as well as the oxygen and carbon dioxide levels in the blood.

arterioles: a tiny artery that joins directly to a capillary.

arteriosclerosis: thickening and hardening of the arterial walls.

*artery: a blood vessel that carries highly oxygenated blood away from the heart to the tissues.

arthr/o: joint.

arthritis: the inflammation of a joint, usually involving pain and swelling.

arthrogram: the injection of dye into a specific joint followed by serial x-rays for diagnostic purposes.

arthroscopy: the visual examination of all aspects of a joint using a special instrument that contains a light and camera.

asbestos: a form of magnesium and calcium silicate formerly used in construction and for fireproofing.

ascending colon: the first portion of the large intestine that extends up from the cecum, along the right side of the abdomen, to the inferior portion of the liver.

-ase: enzyme.

*asepsis: a condition in which no pathogens, infection, or any form of life is present.

*aseptic: sterile; preventing infection.

aspirate: to inhale vomit or other substances into the lungs; the removal of fluid using suction.

aspiration: removal or drawing in by suction.

assault: the threat of an immediate harmful or offensive contact, without actual commission of the act.

assessment: an evaluation of a patient's condition.

asthma: a lung disorder that causes breathing difficulty, wheezing, and coughing, and that can lead to airway obstruction.

astigmatism: blurred vision and severe eyestrain due to irregularity in the curvature of the cornea or the lens.

astride: straddled; sitting or standing on something with one leg on each side.

*asymptomatic: not showing any signs of disease.

atelectasis: a condition in which the lung tissue is airless; a collapsed lung.

atherosclerosis: an accumulation of fat or cholesterol that forms a blockage in the arteries.

attendance: the number of times a person is present or available to perform certain obligations, as in at work.

*atrium: either the upper right or left chamber of the heart, also known as a receiving chamber.

atrophy: wasting away; a decrease in size usually due to lack of use (eg, muscle atrophy from strict bed rest).

audi/o: sound.

audiometry: a method of evaluating hearing by introducing different sounds at different pitches to the patient through headphones.

auditory: pertaining to the sense of hearing.

*auditory nerve: the nerve, contained within the Organ of Corti, which conducts sound waves to the brain for interpretation.

auricle: the outer or external portion of the ear.

auscultate: to hear.

auto-: self.

autoclave: a device that is used to sterilize items by steam under pressure.

*autonomic nervous system: a division of the peripheral nervous system that regulates the balance between the involuntary functions of the body and causes the body to react in emergency situations.

avulsion: a painful soft tissue injury in which a flap of tissue is torn loose or pulled off completely.

*axial skeleton: a division of the skeletal system that includes the main trunk of the body, the skull, the spinal column, the ribs, and the sternum.

axillary: under the arm; the armpit.

axon: an extension of the nerve cell body that conducts impulses away from the body of the nerve cell.

B

bacilli: rod-shaped bacteria.

*bacteria: the plural of bacterium; single-celled microorganisms in the class Schizomycetes.

bacterium: any of the small, single celled microorganisms in the class Schizomycetes.

bag-valve device: a rubber, self-inflating, football shaped device which contains a one-way valve and is used during ventilations of critically ill patients; also referred to as a bag-valve mask.

ball-and-socket joint: a type of joint in which a round end of one bone fits into a cup-like end of another bone, allowing a wide range of movement.

bargaining: the third stage of the dying process as identified by Elisabeth Kubler-Ross in which an individual may try to make a deal with God in an attempt to change the outcome of the situation.

barium enema: the introduction of a barium sulfate solution into the rectum and colon prior to fluoroscopic and radiographic examination of the large intestine.

barium swallow: the fluoroscopic examination of the pharynx and esophagus following the ingestion of barium sulfate.

Bartholin's glands: two small glands located on either side of the vaginal opening.

*basal metabolic rate: the rate at which the body normally burns calories while at rest.

*battery: the unlawful touching of an individual without consent.

bed cradle: a device placed over a part of a patient's body to prevent all linen from coming in contact with the patient's body.

*bedside commode: a portable toilet usually kept by the patient's bedside.

bi-: two.

bi/o: life.

bicuspid valve: the one-way valve located between the left atrium and the left ventricle of the heart; also called the mitral valve.

bile: a secretion of the liver that is stored in the gallbladder and aids in the digestion of fats.

biopsy: the removal of a small piece of living tissue for examination under a microscope.

birth canal: the cervix, vagina, and vulva; the passageway through which the fetus is delivered.

*blood pressure: the pressure of the blood exerted against the arteries.

*body mechanics: the efficient and safe use of the body during activity.

body substance isolation: the use of personal protection equipment to protect against the contraction of a disease through contact with any body secretion.

bone density studies: a method of determining how porous bone is, using radiographic techniques.

bone marrow: the material that fills the medullary canal of bones, and that produces erythrocytes.

bone marrow biopsy: the extraction of a small amount of bone marrow for microscopic examination.

bone scan: a nuclear medicine procedure used to detect fractures, osteoporosis, cancer, and growths, in which a special kind of medication is either ingested or injected directly into a vein. A machine is then scanned over the particular area of the body to detect the amount of radiant energy released from the medication.

bounding pulse: describes a pulse that is unusually strong and may disappear quickly.

Bowman's capsule: a corpuscle at the end of a nephron that contains the glomerulus.

brachi/o: arm.

brachial: pertaining to the arm.

brachy-: short.

brady-: slow.

*bradycardia: a pulse rate below 60 beats per minute.

bradypnea: breathing that is abnormally slow.

brain: the large mass of nervous tissue contained in the cranial cavity that controls the function of the nervous system.

breach of contract: the omission of any of the four components that constitute a contract: duty to act; relevance; compensation; mutual agreement concerning obligations.

*breach of duty to act: the omission of care.

breasts: the mammary glands, made of adipose tissue, that produce milk after the birth of a child.

breathing: the process of taking air into the lungs and releasing it.

bronch/o, **bronchi/o:** bronchial tubes (air tubes in the lungs).

bronchi: the two divisions of the trachea that lead into each lung and that provide a passageway for air.

bronchioles: smaller portions of the bronchi that enter into the alveoli.

bronchitis: inflammation of the bronchial lining.

bronchoscopy: the visual examination of the bronchial tubes and trachea through the introduction of a flexible tube equipped with a light called a bronchoscope.

bucc/o: cheek.

bulimia: a mental illness characterized by overeating binges typically followed by voluntary vomiting, fasting, or induced diarrhea. This disorder is treated with psychiatric intervention and can become life-threatening if left untreated.

burn: a tissue injury caused by exposure to heat, electricity, chemicals, radiation, or gases; may be classified as superficial, partial thickness, or full thickness.

bursa: a sac full of synovial fluid that is located in a joint, and that reduces friction between tendons, bones, and ligaments.

bursitis: inflammation of a bursa in a joint.

C

calcaneus: the heel bone.

calculi: stones usually made up of mineral salts.

*call light: a communication device, located by the patient's bed, that is used by patients to notify the nurses' station of the need for assistance.

*calorie: a unit of heat.

cane: a device used to assist in ambulation by providing support to the patient.

*capillaries: tiny blood vessels in the circulatory system that link arteries and veins.

capitation: a method of payment for healthcare by which the hospital or health group is paid in advance a fixed amount of money for each patient served, regardless of utilization of services.

*carbohydrate: a complex sugar that is a basic source of energy for the body.

carcin/o: cancer.

carcinogen: a substance capable of causing cancer, or that increases the risk of developing cancer.

cardi/o: heart.

cardiac: pertaining to the heart.

*cardiac arrest: asystole; the absence of a heartbeat.

cardiac catheterization: insertion of a catheter through a chamber of the heart or great vessels for the purpose of diagnostic testing.

Cardiac Catheterization Laboratory: a specialized laboratory that performs specific tests to determine diseases of the heart and its vessels.

*cardiac compressions: the controlled and repeated application of pressure to the sternum of a cardiac arrest victim to keep the blood circulating throughout the body.

cardiac enzymes test: a blood test that identifies the probability of the occurrence of an acute myocardial infarction.

cardiac intervention center: a healthcare facility that specializes in treating patients with heart disease.

Cardiac Rehabilitation Services: a department in a hospital that is designed to assist cardiac patients with recovery from cardiac surgery and heart disease.

cardiac sphincter: the two-way valve located between the stomach and the esophagus.

cardiologist: a physician who specializes in the diagnosis and treatment of diseases of the heart and blood vessels.

cardiology: the branch of medicine that deals with the diagnosis, treatment, and prevention of conditions affecting the heart and its blood vessels.

*cardiopulmonary arrest: the sudden absence of a pulse and respirations.

*cardiopulmonary resuscitation (CPR): the basic lifesaving procedure of artificial ventilation and chest compressions that is done in the event of a cardiac arrest.

cardiovascular: of or relating to the heart and blood vessels.

*career: a profession for which one trains and that is undertaken as one's lifelong work.

carotid: the large artery in the neck that carries oxygenated blood to the brain.

carrier: a human or animal who is infected with a pathogen, and who can spread the disease to others, but who does not show any outward signs or symptoms of disease.

cartilage: dense, connective tissue with elastic qualities.

cartilaginous joint: a slightly moveable joint in which there is cartilage attached to the bones, such as the vertebrae in the spine.

cast: a solid mold of a body part, usually made of plaster or fiberglass, that is made to support an unstable body part.

cataract: loss of the transparency of the lens of the eye.

caudal: refers to the lower back or tail.

CDC: the abbreviation for Centers for Disease Control and Prevention.

cecum: the proximal portion of the large intestine, located in the right lower quadrant of the abdomen.

-cele: swelling; tumor; hernia.

*cell: the basic unit of life.

cell membrane: the semipermeable outer surface of a cell.

cellular respiration: the taking of oxygen into cells and the formation of carbon dioxide, resulting in the release of energy.

*Celsius: a temperature scale used in medicine, that uses 100° as the boiling point of water and 0° as the freezing point of water.

*Centers for Disease Control and Prevention (CDC): the government agency responsible for protecting public health through the prevention and control of disease.

*central circulation: refers to the flow of blood to the internal organs.

*central nervous system (CNS): the body system composed of the brain and the spinal cord.

Central Supply Department: the department of the hospital mainly responsible for sterilizing the surgical instruments used in the hospital; also the area designated for the distribution of supplies and equipment.

cephal/o: head.

cerebellum: the part of the brain that is responsible for coordinating body movement.

cerebr/o: cerebrum (part of the brain).

cerebral palsy: a congenital condition that results in a lack of muscle function and coordination due to brain damage.

*cerebrospinal fluid (CSF): the clear, watery fluid that flows through the brain and spinal column, protecting the brain and spinal cord.

cerebrovascular accident (CVA): a stroke; the blockage, hemorrhage, or compression of a blood vessel in the brain.

cerebrum: the largest part of the brain; the part of the brain that is responsible for controlling willful actions as well as coordinating memory, reasoning, and emotions, and interpreting sensory impulses.

certified nursing assistant: an allied healthcare worker who is trained to provide bedside care to patients under the direct supervision of a licensed nurse.

cerumen: ear wax.

cerumen impaction: an abnormal accumulation of cerumen (wax) in the external auditory canal.

cervical: pertaining to the upper portion of the spine; involving the neck; pertaining to the cervix of an organ.

cervix: the neck of the uterus that protrudes into the vagina; the neck or portion of an organ that resembles a neck.

*chain of command: the organizational structure of a given healthcare facility that indicates the person or department responsible for every aspect of the facility's day-to-day operations.

chemical: any substance, such as an acid or alkaline, capable of causing injury either through direct contact on the skin or by the inhalation of the gaseous fumes.

chemical burn: tissue damage caused by caustic chemicals such as hydrochloric acid.

Chemical Dependency Unit: a substance abuse unit.

chemotherapy: the use of drugs or chemicals to treat or control diseases such as cancer.

chest x-ray: a diagnostic test that produces a view of the position, size, and contour of the heart and great vessels, as well as the condition of the lungs, through the use of radiation.

Cheyne-Stokes: a grossly irregular breathing pattern composed of a period of apnea lasting from 10 to 60 seconds, followed by respirations that gradually increase in frequency and depth.

chol/e-, chol/o: bile; gall.

cholecystectomy: the surgical removal of the gall bladder.

cholecystitis: inflammation of the gallbladder.

cholelithiasis: the formation of calculi or stones in the gallbladder or bile duct.

*cholesterol: a waxy, white substance that humans and animals make from fat.

chondr/o: cartilage.

choroid coat: the thin, dark, vascular membrane that covers the white of the eyeball at the back.

chromosome: a structure contained within the nucleus of a cell that contains the genes, which determine the inherited characteristics of a person.

*chronic: slow to develop; persisting for a long time.

*chyme: a semisolid mass found in the stomach, which is formed by the mixture of the gastric secretions and food.

-cid, -cide: kill or destroy.

*cilia: tiny, hairlike structures projecting from the epithelial cells that propel mucus, pus, and dust particles.

circular double frame bed: a special bed that can be used to change a patient's position to prevent pressure sores. Also known as a Stryker frame, it is used for burn patients and those with spinal cord injuries.

circulation: the movement of blood through the blood vessels.

circum-: surrounding; around.

*circumcision: the surgical removal of the prepuce, or foreskin, of the penis.

cirrhosis: a degenerative disease of the liver, which is often caused by chronic alcohol ingestion.

civil law: a statute that provides for the protection of one's private rights and stipulates one's liabilities.

clarification: a communication skill that prompts the sender to explain any part of the message about which the receiver was unclear.

Class A fire extinguisher: a device used to put out fires involving paper, wood, fabric, rubber, and certain plastics.

Class B fire extinguisher: a device used to put out fires involving flammable liquids, oil, paint, fat, and gasoline.

Class C fire extinguisher: a device used to put out fires involving energized electrical equipment such as motors, appliances, and switches.

Class D fire extinguisher: a device used to put out fires involving combustible metals such as sodium, magnesium, potassium, uranium, and powdered aluminum.

*clean technique: the removal or destruction of infected material or organisms; medical asepsis.

clitoris: a small erectile structure that is partially hidden by the labia minora; the structure in the female that corresponds to the penis in the male.

closed-ended question: a type of question that restricts the answer to a simple "yes" or "no".

CO_2: the chemical symbol for carbon dioxide.

cocci: round-shaped bacteria.

cochlea: the cone-shaped tube within the inner ear that contains the organ of Corti.

*Code Blue: the emergency call signal in the hospital for a full arrest situation, which alerts all emergency resuscitation team members to respond to a specific location.

Code of Ethics: statements issued by professional organizations that concern standards and morals that are to be used to govern decisions made by professional healthcare providers.

colitis: inflammation of the colon.

*combining form: a root word plus a combining vowel.

*combining vowel: a vowel that is placed between two word elements to join the two word parts.

communicable: capable of being transmitted from one person to another by direct or indirect contact.

*communication: the verbal or nonverbal exchange of messages, ideas, thoughts, feelings, and information.

communication skills: abilities that facilitate the transmission or exchange of information or thoughts.

community healthcare facility: a healthcare facility that provides care to the general public.

compensate: to adapt or change.

compensation: a type of defense mechanism in which one attempts to make up for physical and/ or mental inferiorities by becoming superior in other areas (eg, a person paralyzed from the waist down may work extra hard on his upper body to build those muscles).

complete blood cell count (CBC): a blood test that determines the number of erythrocytes, leukocytes, and platelets that are present in the patient's blood as well as the hemoglobin and hematocrit.

complex sugar: a sugar that is chemically arranged to form long chains of simple sugars in the form of starches.

computerized tomography (CT) scan: a technique for examining transverse planes of internal structures of the body in which x-rays are used to construct a precise image and show the relationship of structures.

concussion: an injury or loss of function resulting from a blow to the head or a fall.

conduction: a method of heat loss by transference to the surrounding air.

condyloid: a type of joint in which a rounded or oval end of a bone fits into an oval cavity, allowing all types of movement except pivoting.

cones: the flask-shaped cells that receive light in the retina of the eye, making it possible for one to see colors.

congenital: to be born with; from birth.

conization: the excision, or removal, of a cone-shaped piece of tissue.

conjunctiva: a membrane in the eye.

conjunctivitis: an inflammation of the mucous membranes that line the eyelid and coat the anterior part of the eyeball, characterized by redness and a sticky discharge; pink eye.

*connective tissue: tissue that supports and attaches other tissues and parts to each other.

constipation: a condition in which bowel movements are infrequent and the stools are hard and dry.

*constrict: to become smaller.

*contact transmission: direct and indirect transmission of pathogenic microorganisms.

*contagious: capable of being transferred from one person to another, either directly or indirectly.

contamination: the act of making something impure or unclean; infection with pathogens.

contra-: opposite; opposed; against.

*contract: an agreement by all people involved to perform certain obligations.

contracture: abnormalities of connective tissue and shrinkage of scar tissue that prevents normal motion of related joints and tissues.

contraindications: a factor or circumstance that indicates the inappropriate use of a particular treatment or medication.

contusion: a soft tissue injury caused by seepage of blood into tissue; a bruise.

contusion of the brain: bruising of the brain as the result of a blunt force, such as being hit with a baseball bat or hitting one's head on concrete.

convalescent hospital: a facility where patients are admitted following the acute phase of an illness or injury for recovery.

convection: a method of heat loss in which the layer of heated air next to the body is constantly being removed and replaced by cooler air, such as by a fan.

convoluted tubule: a part of a nephron.

cooperation: working together in a harmonious fashion to accomplish a goal.

cooperativeness: the willingness and ability to work with others.

*coping mechanisms: defense mechanisms; the psychological or physical methods by which an individual adjusts or adapts to a challenge or stressful situation.

*core temperature: the internal body temperature.

corium: the true skin, which lies immediately under the epidermis; the dermis.

cornea: the transparent part of the eye; the lens of the eye.

coronal plane: the plane that divides the body into front and back sections.

coronary: pertaining to the heart.

coronary artery disease (CAD): the narrowing of the coronary artery lumen, usually due to arteriosclerosis, which restricts the blood flow to the myocardium.

coronary care nurse: a registered nurse who is specially trained in all areas of critical care including intensive care, cardiac care, and emergency nursing. National certification is possible.

coronary circulation: the flow of blood through the muscular tissue of the heart.

corpus: the middle section of the uterus.

cortex: the outer layer of an organ.

cosmetic and reconstructive surgery: surgical procedures that preserve, restore, or change one's appearance.

cost/o: rib.

counseling centers: healthcare facilities that specialize in the treatment and management of behavioral disorders.

*cover letter: a letter that accompanies a resumé to explain or introduce its contents.

Cowper's glands: two small, tubular glands found on each side of the prostate gland whose ducts end in the wall of the urethra.

CPR: the abbreviation for cardiopulmonary resuscitation; the basic lifesaving procedure of artificial ventilations and chest compressions that is done in the event of a cardiac arrest.

crackles: fine noises caused by air passing through retained moisture in the lungs.

crani/o: skull.

cranial: pertaining to the head.

cranial cavity: the space in the cranium that contains the brain.

cranial nerves: twelve pairs of nerves that originate in the brain, and that control particular body responses.

*crash cart: a portable supply cabinet that contains all of the emergency equipment necessary to treat a full arrest, or Code Blue.

*critical care: the rendering of care to patients with life-threatening conditions.

critical care nurse: a registered nurse who is specially trained in all areas of critical care including intensive care, cardiac care, and emergency nursing. National certification is possible.

Critical Care Unit: a specialized nursing unit that is staffed and equipped to care for the most seriously ill patients.

croup: a viral infection of the respiratory tract that mostly affects children below the age of 3, characterized by a barking cough, hoarseness, fever, and difficult breathing.

crutches: supports used to assist with walking; usually made from aluminum or wood.

cryptorchidism, cryptorchism: a congenital abnormality in which the testes fail to descend into the scrotum.

CT scan: the abbreviation for computerized tomography scan; a technique for examining transverse planes of internal structures of the body in which x-rays are used to construct a precise image and show the relationship of structures.

*culture: a laboratory test for bacterial growth that involves instilling microorganisms in special media and monitoring it for the growth of pathogens; the skills and arts of a given people at a given time.

culture and sensitivity: a laboratory test for bacterial growth that involves instilling microorganisms in special media, monitoring them for the growth of pathogens, and then determining how susceptible the patient's bacterial infection is to certain antibiotics or antibacterial drugs.

Cushing's disease: the excessive secretion of adrenocortical hormones resulting in hypertension, diabetes, obesity, edema, osteoporosis, skin discoloration, loss of protein, and other symptoms.

*custom: a tradition or usual practice of a particular people or social group.

cyan/o: blue.

cyst: a closed sac containing fluid, semifluid, or solid material.

cyst/o: fluid-filled sac; urinary bladder; bag.

cystitis: the inflammation of the urinary bladder.

cystogram: a diagnostic test for the urinary bladder, which involves the use of x-rays taken after the instillation of contrast medium.

cystoscopy: the examination of the urinary bladder using an instrument containing a light and a camera called a cystoscope that is introduced into the bladder through the urethra.

cyt/o, -cyte: cell.

cytoplasm: the protoplasm of a cell that is outside the nucleus.

D

dactyl/o: digits (the fingers or toes).

*damages: a degree of loss that has occurred due to injury to person, property, or reputation.

deafness: the partial or complete inability to hear; may be caused by problems in conducting sound waves or in sensing the sound waves.

*death: the end of life as indicated by the permanent cessation of all vital functions; the absence of brain stem and spinal reflexes, and flat EEGs over at least a 24 hour period.

decreased: below normal; in lung function, refers to very little air movement in the lungs.

decubitus ulcer: a lesion of the skin and surrounding tissue due to prolonged pressure against the skin; a pressure sore.

defamation of character: discussion of a person by another, either in writing or verbally, that damages that person's reputation.

defendant: a person named in a lawsuit; the accused.

*defense mechanisms: coping mechanisms; methods of unconscious behavior that assist people in coping and adapting to life.

defibrillator: an electronic device used to shock the heart into a normal rhythm.

deformity: disfigurement; something out of its natural position.

dehydration: the loss of water from a body or substance; dry.

dendrites: cytoplasmic structures extending from the nerve cell body that transmit impulses to the body of the nerve cell.

denial: the first stage of the dying process as identified by Elisabeth Kubler-Ross in which the patient refuses to believe that which is true or real.

denti-, dent-, dent/o: teeth.

deoxygenated: describes a decreased level of oxygen.

dependability: the degree of reliance or trust that can be placed in a person.

deposition: testimony given under oath concerning the events of a particular incident.

depression: the fourth stage of the dying process as identified by Elisabeth Kubler-Ross in which the patient experiences extreme feelings of sadness or hopelessness.

derm/o, -derma, dermat/o: skin.

dermatitis: the inflammation of the dermis layer of skin, characterized by itching, redness, and skin lesions.

dermatologist: a physician who treats infections, growths, and injuries related to the skin.

dermatology: the branch of medicine concerned with the diagnosis and treatment of disorders and diseases of the skin.

dermis: the layer of skin that contains connective tissue and blood vessels; the true skin.

descending colon: the third part of the large intestine, that is distal to the transverse colon and proximal to the sigmoid colon.

detoxify: to reduce or eliminate toxic or poisonous substances in the body.

development: gradual changes in one's normal growth, leading to maturity.

dextr/o: right side.

dextrose: a simple sugar.

di-: two; twice; double.

dia-: through; complete.

diabetes mellitus: a chronic disorder caused by the failure of the pancreas to produce enough insulin or the failure of cells to accept insulin, causing an increase in blood sugar; commonly referred to as diabetes.

diagnose: to scientifically assess the cause and nature of an individual's illness.

Diagnostic Services: a hospital department that performs diagnostic tests such as EKGs and EEGs.

dialysis: the mechanized diffusion of blood across a semipermeable membrane in order to remove the toxic wastes that have accumulated and disrupted the acid-base balance of the body.

diaphoretic: describes a patient who is perspiring profusely.

*diaphragm: the dome-shaped muscle separating the thoracic cavity from the abdominal cavity; the portion of the stethoscope used for picking up sound.

diaphysis: the shaft of a long bone.

diarrhea: abnormally frequent, watery bowel movements.

*diastolic: the bottom number in a blood pressure reading; refers to the period of time between heart contractions in which the heart relaxes.

Dietary Department: the hospital department responsible for preparing the meals and snacks for both the patients and the hospital staff.

*dilate: to become larger.

dilation and curettage: the surgical dilation of the cervix and scraping of the uterus.

dipl/o: two; twice; double.

diplococci: bacteria that are arranged in pairs.

direct contact: a method of transmitting pathogens through patient care activities that involve close, physical contact between the patient and the healthcare worker.

direct pressure: a method of controlling bleeding in which pressure is applied directly over the wound.

*disaster: an unexpected event that causes great damage and depletes or exhausts currently available resources.

disc: one of the cartilaginous cushions between the vertebrae of the back.

Discharge Planning Department: the hospital department concerned with making appropriate provisions for the patient's care after he or she leaves the hospital.

discretion: showing caution in the way one speaks or acts.

disinfection: the removal of infectious material from an item.

dislocation: the separation of a joint and malposition of an extremity.

displacement: a defense mechanism that involves transferring an emotion (or form of behavior) from the original person or object to another person or object that is less threatening.

distal: farthest from the original reference point on the body.

doctor: one who has earned an advanced degree; a physician.

dorsal: located on the backside.

dorsal cavity: the cavity located along the back of the body, which consists of the cranial and spinal cavities; the posterior cavity.

dors/o, dorsi-: back of body.

drainage bag: a bag connected to an indwelling catheter to collect body fluids such as urine.

*droplet transmission: a method of transmitting pathogens when a susceptible host becomes exposed or infected through the droplets emitted during coughing, sneezing, talking, singing, or while performing ventilations.

duoden/o: duodenum.

duodenum: the first part of the small intestine.

dura mater: the outer membrane of the meninges.

*duty to act: the legal duty to provide care within the scope of practice.

dwarfism: a condition in which one is abnormally small in size; sometimes the result of inadequate production of the pituitary hormones.

-dynia: pain.

dys-: painful; difficult; bad; disordered.

dyspnea: difficult or painful breathing; shortness of breath.

dysuria: difficult or painful urination.

E

early adulthood: a life stage describing people between the ages of 20 and 40 years old; considered to be the most productive life stage.

early childhood: a life stage that describes children between the ages of 1 and 6 years old.

ecchymosis: the black and blue color caused by the seepage of blood into tissue as in a contusion.

ECG: an abbreviation for electrocardiogram.

echocardiography: the use of sound waves to view cardiac structure and function.

-ectasis: dilation; expansion; stretching.

ecto-: external; outside.

-ectomy: surgical removal; excision.

ectopic pregnancy: the growth of a fertilized egg implanted outside the uterus, usually in the fallopian tube.

*edema: swelling due to fluid in the tissues; fluid retention.

edematous: the accumulation of excessive tissue fluid in the tissues, resulting in swelling.

Education Department: the department in a hospital that is devoted to educating the community and staff about a variety of topics related to healthcare and healthy lifestyles.

EEG: the abbreviation for electroencephalogram.

efferent neuron: a nerve cell that originates in the brain or spinal cord and carries impulses to the muscles and glands of the body; motor neuron.

*eggcrate mattress: a special mattress made from foam that is shaped like the bottom of an egg carton, and which is used to prevent skin breakdown.

EKG: an abbreviation for electrocardiogram.

elastic stockings: stockings that provide heavy support to the lower extremities to prevent blood clot formation.

elective surgery: surgery that is scheduled for a specific date and time; surgery that is not done in an emergency.

electric shock: an extreme stimulation of the nerves by the passage of an electric current through the body.

electrocardiogram: EKG or ECG; a diagnostic test for heart disease that measures the electrical activity of the heart.

electrocardiography: the process of recording or tracing the electrical activity of the heart.

electroencephalogram: EEG; a visual picture of the electrical activity of the brain.

*Elisabeth Kubler-Ross: a leading expert in the area of death and dying; the first to identify the five stages of the dying process.

embolus: a circulating clot.

emergency: a medical condition that is life or limb-threatening.

Emergency Department: a specific area of an acute care facility staffed and equipped to handle patients with life-threatening illnesses or injuries; also known as the Emergency Care Unit or ER.

emergency medicine: the branch of medicine that deals with the emergency care of those with life-threatening or limb-threatening illnesses or injuries.

emergency nurse: a registered nurse who is specially trained in the area of emergency nursing; national certification is possible.

emergency surgery: an operation that is performed immediately so as to prevent the loss of a life or limb.

-emesis: vomiting.

*emetic: an agent that induces vomiting.

-emia: blood.

emotional: referring to one's feelings.

emphysema: a chronic lung disease that destroys the alveoli.

encephal/o: brain.

endo-, end/o-: inside, interior, within.

endocardium: the inner-most layer of the heart.

*endocrine: pertaining to a gland that secretes chemicals (hormones) directly into the bloodstream.

endocrine system: the body system that consists of glands that release secretions directly into the bloodstream.

endocrinology: the study of the treatment of disorders affecting the endocrine system.

endometriosis: the presence of endometrial tissue outside of the uterus.

endometrium: the tissue that lines the inner surface of the uterus, and which serves as a nesting place for the fertilized egg.

endoscopy: direct inspection of the lining of a hollow organ through an instrument called an endoscope.

endoscopy nurse: a registered nurse who is specially trained in assisting and preparing for procedures that examine the inside of a patient, usually the gastrointestinal tract. National certification is possible.

endosteum: the lining of the medullary canal of the bone that keeps the yellow marrow intact.

endotracheal tube: a large tube inserted into the trachea through the mouth or nose to assist in administering oxygen.

enter/o: small intestine.

enteritis: inflammation of the intestines which may result in infection.

enzymes: complex proteins, located within the cell mitochondria, that increase the speed of a chemical reaction without changing themselves.

epi-: upon; over; upper.

epicardium: the outermost layer of heart tissue.

epidermis: the outer layer of the skin.

epididymis: the coiled tube next to the testes that stores sperm until they are mature and active.

epidural: refers to the space located outside the outer membrane of the brain and spinal cord.

epiglottis: tissue in the throat that allows air to enter the trachea and food to enter the esophagus.

epiglottitis: inflammation of the epiglottis.

epilepsy: a term that describes a group of nervous system disorders that involve disturbed rhythms of the electrical impulses that fire throughout the cerebrum, resulting in seizure activity or abnormal behavior.

epiphysis: the end of a long bone.

epistaxis: a nosebleed.

***epithelial tissue:** tissue that lines the cavities of the body and the principal tubes and passageways that lead to the exterior of the body.

equilibrium: a person's sense of balance.

erythema: redness of the skin.

erythr/o: red.

erythrocytes: red blood cells.

esophageal airway: a special breathing tube inserted into the esophagus that allows the trachea to be ventilated; also referred to as an airway adjunct.

esophagus: the muscular tube that carries food from the throat to the stomach.

essential hypertension: high blood pressure without an apparent underlying medical cause.

esteem: the fourth level of Maslow's Hierarchy of Needs; refers to one's value, worth, or importance.

-esthesia: sensation; feeling.

***estrogen:** the female sex hormone, produced by the ovaries, which is responsible for the development of secondary sex characteristics and for the cyclic changes in the lining of the uterus.

***ethics:** principles of conduct that establish standards and morals that govern decisions and behavior.

eustachian tube: the internal auditory canal; the tube that joins the nasopharynx and the tympanic cavity.

evaporation: a method of heat loss in which a liquid changes from a liquid to vapor as with perspiration.

ex-: out; outside; away from.

excrete: to remove or expel waste from the body, blood, or organs.

exhalation: the act of breathing out; the second phase of the respiratory cycle.

exo-: out; outside; away from.

***exocrine:** describes glands that transport secretions to another part of the body via ducts.

expiration: to exhale; the act of breathing out.

extended care facility: a long-term care facility.

extension: movement that results in an increased angle between two bones, or the straightening of a body part.

external: near the surface of the body.

external auditory canal: the canal in the ear that leads from the external auditory meatus to the tympanic membrane.

extra-: in addition to; outside of.

extremities: the arms and legs.

F

*Fahrenheit: a temperature scale used in medicine that uses 212° as the boiling point of water and 32° as the freezing point of water.

fallopian tube: the part of the female reproductive system through which the egg travels on the way to the uterus; oviduct.

false imprisonment: restraining a person against his or her will, either physically or with verbal threats.

family practice: the branch of medicine that is concerned with the medical and surgical diagnosis and treatment for all family members.

fascia: the fibrous membrane that covers, supports, and separates muscle.

*fat: a substance made up of lipids or fatty acids that is a source of energy and is vital to growth and development.

felony: a major crime that is punishable by a greater means than a misdemeanor.

femoral: referring to the area in the groin near the femur.

femur: the thigh bone.

-ferous: producing.

fertilization: the union of an ovum and sperm to form a zygote from which an embryo develops.

fetal position: a position in which a patient lies on one side with the arms and legs drawn toward the chest and the head bowed.

fibr/o: threadlike structures; connective tissue.

fibrinogen: a special blood protein responsible for clotting the blood; found in the plasma.

fibrous connective tissue: tissue that supports the joints of the body and helps hold certain structures together.

fibrous joint: an immovable joint such as the cranium.

fimbriae: finger-like projections in the fallopian tubes that receive the mature ovum from the ovary.

*finger sweep: a method of removing a foreign object from a choking patient's mouth.

first aid: the immediate care provided to a person who has sustained an unexpected injury, sudden illness, or other medical emergency.

flat bone: a bone composed of two, essentially parallel plates of compact bone that are separated by spongy bone (eg, the scapula and skull).

flexion: movement that results in a decreased angle between two bones, or the bending of a body part.

fluid overload: excessive fluid within tissue, characterized by tissue swelling.

fluoroscopy: a method of viewing the internal structures while they are in motion through the use of x-rays.

Foley catheter: a tube for draining urine that has a balloon attachment at one end to prevent the catheter from accidentally slipping out of the bladder; an indwelling or retention catheter.

follicle: a small sac or cavity that is secretory in function.

foot board: a board placed at the end of a mattress to keep a patient's feet in proper alignment and to help prevent footdrop.

footdrop: a condition in which a patient is unable to flex the foot backward due to weakness or paralysis of the anterior muscles of the lower leg.

fore-: in front of; before.

-form: resembling; having the form of; shape.

Fowler's position: a position in which the patient is semi-sitting with the head raised 45° to 60°.

fracture: a crack or break in a bone.

fraud and misrepresentation: the intentional witholding of information from a patient to cover up mistakes.

frontal plane: refers to the plane that divides the body into front and back sections; same as coronal plane.

full thickness burn: a burn in which all layers of the skin, and the nerves in it, are destroyed down to the bone; formerly known as a third degree burn.

-fuge: pushing or driving away.

fundus: the main part or base of a hollow organ.

Fungi: the kingdom of organisms that are simple, parasitic plants, including molds and yeasts.

G

gallbladder: the muscular sac located inferior to the liver, from which it receives bile.

*gas exchange: the process of exchanging oxygen for carbon dioxide in the blood during breathing; this process takes place in the alveoli in the lungs.

gaster-, gastr-, gastr/o: stomach.

gastritis: inflammation of the stomach.

gastrocnemius muscle: the calf muscle.

gastroenterology: the area of medicine that studies diseases and disorders of the esophagus, stomach, and intestinal tract.

gastrointestinal nurse: a registered nurse who is specially trained in assisting and preparing for procedures that examine the gastrointestinal tract. National certification is possible.

general hospital: a healthcare facility that does not specialize in a particular type of healthcare.

general surgeon: a medical doctor who is trained to perform non-specialized operations such as an appendectomy or a cholecystectomy.

general surgery: a branch of surgery that is non-specialized in the type of operations performed.

genes: ultramicroscopic structures contained within the chromosomes that determine the physical and mental characteristics of a human being.

gen/o, -genetic, -genic: an originating or producing agent; produced from; pertaining to heredity.

genit/o: genitalia; male and female reproductive organs.

geriatrics: the branch of medicine that deals with the problems of aging; gerontology.

gerontological nurse specialist: a registered nurse who provides care to geriatric patients.

gerontology: the branch of medicine that deals with the problems of aging; geriatrics.

gigantism: a condition in which a person grows to be excessively large in size; sometimes the result of overproduction of the pituitary hormones.

*gland: a structure within the body that secretes a substance used elsewhere in the body.

glans penis: the bulbous structure at the end of the penis.

glaucoma: an eye disorder caused by an increase in intraocular pressure.

glide: a joint in which two facing bone surfaces meet, allowing only gliding movements.

glomerulus: the cluster of capillaries located on the nephron.

gloss/o: tongue.

glottis: the voice apparatus of the larynx consisting of the two vocal cords and the slit between them.

gluc/o: sugar; glucose.

glucose: a simple sugar; used in the human body to produce energy.

glyc/o: sugar; glucose.

glycogen: a carbohydrate made from glucose that is stored in the liver and muscles.

goiter: the abnormal enlargement of the thyroid gland.

gonorrhea: a sexually transmitted disease, characterized by a foul-smelling, white, thick discharge, burning on urination, and abdominal pain.

gout: an accumulation of uric acid crystals in the joint.

-gram: record.

granulocyte: a type of leukocyte that contains granules in its cytoplasm.

-graph: instrument used for recording.

-graphy: process of recording.

gray matter: the term used to specify the portions of the central nervous system that appear gray in color, including the cerebral cortex and nuclei of the brain and the gray columns of the spinal cord.

groin: the area where the abdomen joins the thighs.

growth: refers to changes in the structure or size of a living organism.

gurgling: an abnormal, course sound produced by the movement of air through fluid in cavities; can be heard through a stethoscope.

*gurney: a stretcher with wheels used for transporting patients.

gyne-, gynec/o: woman or female.

gynecological: refers to the healthcare specialty that focuses on diseases and disorders of the female reproductive system.

gynecology: the branch of medicine that focuses on specific problems concerning the uterus, fallopian tubes, ovaries, cervix, vagina, and breasts.

H

hair follicle: a hollow tube in the skin that contains the root of a hair.

hard palate: the roof of the mouth.

*hazard communication label: a label (usually diamond-shaped) with four colored diamonds that each represent a specific aspect of the chemical's hazards.

hazard communication program: a program implemented by healthcare facilities to protect its employees from the dangers of chemicals and medical gases; HazCom.

HCl: the abbreviation for hydrochloric acid.

*head-tilt/chin-lift maneuver: a procedure for opening a blocked airway in which the patient's head is tilted back and the chin is lifted; the most effective method for opening the airway of an unconscious person without a neck or back injury.

*healthcare provider: a professional (such as a physician or advanced practitioner) or institution that provides healthcare.

health clinic: a healthcare facility that is usually formed by several doctors who share a common building.

health maintenance organization: HMO; a type of prepaid group healthcare program that provides health maintenance and treatment services to its members.

*Health Occupations Students of America (HOSA): a professional organization for students of health occupations.

health unit coordinator: unit secretary; ward clerk; a member of the clerical staff who performs reception and clerical functions for the nursing unit and transcribes the physician's orders.

heartburn: a burning sensation in the area of the esophagus and stomach.

*Heimlich maneuver: an obstructed airway maneuver in which a fist is thrust against the abdomen and subdiaphragmatic pressure is applied to remove a foreign body in the airway.

helipad: a landing site, usually designated by an *H*, for helicopters.

hem-, hem/o, hem/a, hemat/o: blood.

hematuria: the presence of blood in urine.

hemi-: half.

hemiplegia: paralysis of half of the body.

hemoglobin: a complex protein that gives erythrocytes their red color.

hemophilia: a congenital condition in which the blood does not clot normally, resulting in excessive bleeding.

hemorrhage: the severe, abnormal internal or external discharge of blood.

hemorrhoids: enlarged veins in the anal area.

hemothorax: blood within the pleural cavity.

heparin: a natural blood-thinner produced by the liver.

hepat/o: liver.

hepatitis: inflammation of the liver.

*hepatitis A: inflammation of the liver that is caused by the hepatitis A virus and spread by the fecal-oral route either from poor handwashing or contaminated food.

*hepatitis B: inflammation of the liver that is caused by the hepatitis B virus and spread through contact with infected blood; the most common form contracted by healthcare workers.

*hepatitis C: inflammation of the liver caused by the hepatitis C virus and spread through contact with infected blood or body fluids.

herpes: a viral infection, a form of which can be a sexually transmitted disease resulting in a chronic viral infection characterized by blister-like vesicles on the genitals.

heter/o: unlike; different; other.

high Fowler's position: a position in which the patient is sitting at a 90° angle with the legs extended.

*high risk: a term used to describe patients who have increased potential for developing life-threatening problems, often without previous warning.

*high-density lipoprotein (HDL): a cholesterol carrier that functions to remove excess cholesterol from the bloodstream and transport it to the liver where it is broken down and excreted.

hinge joint: a type of joint in which the two surfaces are molded closely together, allowing a wide range of flexion and extension along a single plane.

hist/o: tissue.

HIV-positive: refers to a person who is carrying the virus that causes AIDS.

HMO: the abbreviation for health maintenance organization.

Hodgkin's disease: a type of cancer that begins in the lymphoid tissue and, if untreated, will be fatal to the patient by invading or obstructing the vital organs.

Holter monitor: a portable heart monitor worn by a patient to record the patient's EKG. This is usually worn continuously for 24 hours.

hom/o, home/o: alike; the same.

home health agency: an organization that provides extended healthcare to patients in their home.

home/o: alike; the same.

*homeostasis: a state of equilibrium within the body maintained through the adaptation of body systems to changes in either the internal or external environment.

*hospice: a supportive agency offering care and counseling to dying patients and their families; a program consisting of palliative and supportive services.

*hospitalis: a Latin word meaning a house or institution for guests.

humerus: a bone in the upper arm.

hydr/o: water.

hydrochloric acid: a substance that is part of the digestive juice in the stomach.

hyper-: excessive; above; increased.

hypermenorrhea: excessive menstruation.

hyperopia: farsightedness; a condition in which the rays of light entering the eye come to a focus behind the retina, causing objects that are close to appear blurry.

hyperparathyroidism: overactivity of the parathyroid glands resulting in elevated calcium levels in the blood.

hyperpnea: breathing that is faster or deeper than that which is produced during normal activity.

*hypertension (HTN): high blood pressure that has been diagnosed on the basis of several random readings of 140/90 or higher; known as the *silent killer*.

hyperthermia: an unusually high body temperature; a fever.

hyperthyroidism: the excessive production of thyroid hormones resulting in irritability, nervousness, and restlessness.

hyperventilate: to breathe rapidly, increasing the amount of oxygen in the lungs, and resulting in decreased levels of CO_2.

hyperventilation: prolonged, deep, and rapid breathing, resulting in decreased levels of CO_2 in the blood.

hypo-: below, deficient, under.

hypoparathyroism: underproduction of the parathyroid glands, which results in a decreased level of calcium in the blood.

hypotension: an abnormally low blood pressure that impairs functioning.

*hypothalamus: the portion of the brain that controls the temperature of the body.

hypothermia: an unusually low body temperature capable of causing problems with the central nervous system and cardiac arrest.

hypothyroidism: underproduction of thyroid hormones resulting in fatigue and weight gain.

*hypovolemic shock: shock caused by severe blood loss.

hyster/o: uterus; womb.

hysterectomy: the surgical removal of the uterus.

I

-iasis: abnormal condition.

-ic: pertaining to.

idi/o: one's own, or distinct; not known.

ile/o: ileum (last part of small intestine).

ileocecal sphincter: the muscle that separates the ileum from the ascending colon.

ileum: the last section of the small intestine.

ili/o: ilium (part of hip bone).

Imaging Department: another name for the X-ray Department.

immovable: bones that are not able to move (eg, the bones of the skull).

immune system: the body system composed of several different types of blood cells that work together to fight off infections.

incentive spirometer: a hand-held device that encourages a patient to take a deep breath; usually given to patients after surgery to prevent the onset of pneumonia.

incision: a clean, straight, knife-like cut.

incompetent: lacking skills; not mentally able.

incontinence: the loss of bladder or bowel control.

incus: the middle of the three ossicles, or small bones, in the middle ear; also referred to as the anvil.

indirect: a method of fulfilling the hierarchy of needs; this method usually relieves the tension and frustration created by the unmet need, or reduces the particular need.

indirect contact: a method of transmitting pathogens when a susceptible host comes in contact with contaminated, inanimate objects.

industrial accident: an injury that is sustained while working.

industrial illnesses: an illness that is received from an infection contracted at work.

*indwelling catheter: a catheter inserted into a particular area of the body such as the urinary bladder.

infancy: a life stage that describes babies from birth to 1 year of age.

Infection Control Department: the department in a hospital responsible for developing policies and procedures concerned with reducing the risk of transferring communicable diseases to both the staff and patients.

*infection cycle: a pattern that describes the origin and transmission of a disease or illness.

infectious agent: any disease-causing microorganism.

inferior: located below another part.

inferior vena cava: the principle vein that drains deoxygenated blood from the lower body into the right atrium.

infertile: the diminished ability or inability to produce children.

*infertility: a diminished ability or inability to produce children.

informed: made aware.

informed consent: a consent for treatment given by a patient who is fully informed about what will be done, the risks involved, and the options available.

influenza: a highly communicable disease of the upper respiratory tract; the flu.

ingestion: the act of taking something into the gastrointestinal tract through the mouth.

inhaled: breathed into the lungs.

initiative: the drive to first begin an action.

injection: the act of forcing a liquid under the skin or into tissue, a vessel, or a cavity.

in-service: training that takes place while one is fully employed.

inspiration: inhalation or breathing in; the first phase of the respiratory cycle in which the intercostal muscles and diaphragm contract, causing the chest cavity to increase in size.

*insulin: a hormone secreted by the pancreas that causes glucose, or sugar, to leave the bloodstream and enter the cell.

integrity: honesty; undiminished or unimpaired state.

integumentary: relating to the three layers of the skin.

inter-: between.

*intercom system: a communication system between the patient's bedside and the nurses' station.

intermittent positive-pressure breathing machine: a device used by patients who are unable to inhale deeply. It forces oxygen and/or medication into the small tubes of the lungs so the patient can cough up sputum.

intern: a physician in a hospital who has recently graduated, but who is not yet eligible to obtain a license to practice medicine.

internal: within the body.

internal medicine: the area of medicine concerned with the diagnosis and treatment of nonsurgical disorders of adults.

internist: a physician who specializes in the practice of internal medicine.

interstitial fluid: the fluid outside the cell (extracellular fluid), excluding the fluid within the blood and lymph vessels.

intra-: within.

intravenous pyelogram (IVP): a diagnostic test of the kidneys, ureters, and bladder using x-rays following the injection of radiopaque dye.

invasion of privacy: public discussion of private information.

invasive blood pressure: blood pressure measurement that is obtained through the use of special catheters inserted directly into the blood vessel.

involuntary: not under willful control.

IPPB: the abbreviation for intermittent positive-pressure breathing.

iris: the part of the eye that gives the eye its color.

irregular bones: bones of complex shape and structure (eg, facial bones and vertebrae).

*irreversible brain death: a condition in which brain-specific tests show that the patient's brain cells have died, and therefore, the brain is inactive and has no chance for recovery.

islets of Langerhans: clusters of cells in the pancreas that make insulin, glucagon, and pancreatic polypeptide.

isolation: the purposeful act of removing an infectious or contagious patient from the general patient population. An infection-control system developed by most hospitals based on specific Transmission-based Precautions as developed by the CDC. "Precautions" and "isolation" are frequently used interchangeably.

isthmus: a passage or structure that connects two cavities or larger parts together, as in the piece of tissue that connects the two lobes of the thyroid gland.

-itis: inflammation.

IV fluid: a combination of water, dextrose, and other electrolytes such as sodium, potassium, chloride, or lactate, that provides a fast and efficient method of replenishing essential nutrients lost from the body.

*IV infusion pump: a machine that, when attached to IV tubing via an IV pole, allows accurate administration of a solution.

IVP: intravenous pyelogram; a diagnostic test of the kidneys, ureters, and bladder using x-rays following the injection of radiopaque dye.

J

*jaw-thrust maneuver: a method used to open the airway in a neck-injured patient, in which the jaw is lifted up and the neck is not moved.

jejun/o: jejunum.

jejunum: the second section of the small intestine.

*job: a specific duty, role, or function that is performed regularly for compensation.

*joint: a place where two or more bones meet.

judgement: a final decision from a court.

juxta-: near.

K

-kenesis, kinesi/o: movement.

kerat/o: referring to the cornea of the eye.

*kidneys: organs located in the dorsal cavity of the body that are responsible for filtering blood and producing urine.

Kussmaul's breathing: deep, gasping respirations; *air hunger.*

KY jelly: a brand of lubricating jelly.

L

labi/o: lips.

labia majora: the two lips of adipose tissue on either side of the vaginal opening that form the border of the vulva.

labia minora: the two lips of skin between the labia majora and the hymen, if intact, or on both sides of the vaginal opening.

labor: the physiological process of delivering the fetus from the uterus through the birth canal and out of the mother's body.

Labor and Delivery: the department in a hospital where babies are born.

Laboratory: the diagnostic department that obtains and analyzes various specimens such as blood and urine to assist in diagnosing and/or treating a patient.

labored breathing: difficult breathing that uses shoulder muscles, neck muscles, and abdominal muscles (accessory muscles).

laceration: a jagged tear in the flesh.

lacrim/o: tears; lacrimal duct.

lacrimal ducts: ducts that transport tears from the lacrimal lakes to the lacrimal sacs.

lacrimal glands: the glands that produce tears.

lact/o: milk.

lactation: the secretion of milk.

lacteals: lymphatics located on the lining of the intestines that absorb most of the digested fat and transport it into the lymphatic system.

laryngectomy: the surgical removal of the larynx, which leaves a permanent opening in the neck for breathing and causes the loss of speech.

laryngitis: inflammation of the larynx.

laryngopharynx: the third section of the oral cavity, located inferior to the oropharynx, that contains the glottis; also referred to as the hypopharynx.

*larynx: the upper end of the trachea; the voice box.

late adulthood: the life stage that describes individuals over the age of 65 years old.

late childhood: the life stage commonly referred to as preadolescence. It describes children between the ages of 6 and 12 years old.

later/o: side.

lateral: toward the side of the body.

left atrium: the upper chamber on the left side of the heart that receives oxygenated blood from the lungs.

left lower quadrant: LLQ; a section of the abdominal cavity that contains some of the female reproductive organs and intestines.

left upper quadrant: LUQ; a section of the abdominal cavity that contains the spleen, pancreas, stomach, intestines, and left lobe of the liver.

left ventricle: the lower chamber on the left side of the heart that pumps blood through the aorta into the arteries.

lens: the jelly-like substance behind the iris of the eye that refracts light rays to the retina.

leuk/o: white.

leukocytes: white blood cells that are responsible for fighting infection.

licensed practical nurse: a nurse who has completed a practical nursing program and who is licensed by the state; practical nurses are not registered nurses.

licensed vocational nurse: a licensed nurse trained in patient care procedures, treatments, and medication administration who must practice under the supervision of a registered nurse.

licensee: a person who has a license giving him or her the authority to do something.

*life stage: a segment of one's life that spans specific ages, and in which a predictable pattern of growth and development occur.

ligament: a band of white, fibrous, connective tissue, formed from adipose tissue, that helps hold bones together.

lingu/o: tongue.

lingual tonsils: the masses of lymph tissue located near the root of the tongue.

lip/o: fat.

lipase: an enzyme produced in the stomach that helps break down fats.

lipoproteins: cholesterol carriers.

liter: a metric fluid measurement that is equivalent to 1000 milliliters, or approximately 1 quart.

lith/o: stone or calculus.

litigation: a lawsuit.

liver: the largest organ in the body, which functions to secrete bile, neutralize harmful substances, process glucose, etc. Located on the upper right portion of the abdominal cavity, the liver is one of the most complex organs of the body, and performs more than 500 functions.

liver function tests: diagnostic blood tests that evaluate the level of the liver enzymes.

-logist: specialist; one who studies.

*log roll: the method used to turn a patient with a spinal injury, in which the patient is moved to the side in one motion.

-logy: science of; study of.

long bones: bones in which their length is greater than their width (eg, femur or humerus).

long-term care facility: a healthcare facility that provides care to patients with chronic illnesses; also called an extended care facility.

love and affection: one of the levels in Maslow's Hierarchy of needs; includes the need for friendship, social acceptance, and love.

*low-density lipoprotein (LDL): a cholesterol carrier that delivers cholesterol to the cells of the body.

Lubifax: a brand of lubricating jelly.

lumbar: of or relating to the lower back between the thorax and the pelvis.

lumbar puncture: a diagnostic test in which a specimen of cerebrospinal fluid is removed and analyzed for diseases such as meningitis; a spinal tap.

lung: one of the two organs of respiration contained within the thorax.

lung cancer: malignant tumors involving the lung tissue.

lung scan: a test that reveals whether lung tissue is receiving enough blood, in which medication is introduced into the body and a machine measures the amount of radiant energy that is released.

lymph: a colorless fluid that is formed in tissue spaces throughout the body and carried in the lymphatic vessels.

lymphatic capillaries: small tubes that receive the circulating lymph.

lymphatic vessels: thin-walled tubes that carry lymph from the tissues.

lymph nodes: small bodies of lymphatic tissue that filter the lymph of impurities such as pathogens and cancer cells.

lymphocyte: a type of leukocyte found in blood, lymph, and lymphatic tissue that helps fight infection.

-lysis: loosen; dissolve; destruction.

M

macro-: large; long.

macules: flat skin eruptions or discolorations.

magnetic resonance imaging (MRI): a diagnostic procedure in which parts of the body are exposed to an electromagnetic field to produce an image.

major senses: the senses of sight, hearing, taste, smell, and touch.

mal-: abnormal; bad; disordered.

-malacia: softening.

malignant melanoma: a fast-spreading skin cancer that is frequently fatal.

malleus: the largest of the three ossicles of the middle ear.

*malpractice: professional misconduct or lack of professional skill that results in injury to the patient; negligence by a professional, such as a physician or nurse.

*Maslow's Hierarchy of Needs: five categories of needs identified by psychologist Abraham Maslow, including physiological needs, safety and security, love and affection, esteem, and self-actualization.

masticate: to chew.

masto-: breast.

*Material Safety Data Sheet (MSDS): an official required document that identifies all the chemicals that are used in a specific department and that details important information regarding those chemicals.

medial: located near the middle or center.

medical asepsis: the removal or destruction of infected material or organisms; clean technique.

medical assistant: a multi-skilled healthcare worker who is trained to work under the direct supervision of a physician and perform both administrative and clinical duties in physicians' offices, clinics, and outpatient departments of hospitals.

*Medic-Alert: a symbol that indicates important medical information, usually found on a bracelet or pendant provided by the nonprofit organization which bears its name.

medical nurse: a registered nurse who provides nursing care to noncritical and nonsurgical patients.

medical office: a facility in which a physician (or a group of physicians) provides a wide variety of healthcare services to patients, but not overnight healthcare as in a hospital.

medical surgical nurse: a registered nurse who provides nursing care for either medical or surgical patients in the same department; national certification is available.

Medical Surgical Nursing Unit: the nursing unit in an acute care hospital that cares for patients with general medical problems and patients who are recovering from a surgical procedure.

medulla: the inner section of an organ.

medulla oblongata: the lower portion of the brain stem that controls involuntary actions such as respirations, swallowing, blood pressure, and coughing.

medullary canal: the cavity in the diaphysis of a bone that is filled with yellow marrow.

mega-, megal/o, -megaly: enlarged.

***meiosis:** cell reproduction specific to the ovaries and the testes.

melanin: special cells that give color to hair, skin, and the choroid of the eye, and that protect the skin from ultraviolet rays.

men-, men/o: menstruation; monthly.

mening/o: meninges.

***meninges:** the three protective membranes covering the brain and the spinal cord.

meningitis: inflammation of the membranes covering the spinal cord and brain, marked by severe headache, vomiting, fever, and a stiff neck, and usually caused by infection.

meniscus: a curved disc of cartilage filled with synovial fluid.

***menstruation:** the periodic shedding of the endometrial layer of tissue from the uterus.

mental: of or referring to the mind; an aspect of growth and development that includes development of the mind, such as solving problems, judgements, and decision making.

mental health: psychiatry; the branch of medicine that deals with the diagnosis, treatment, and prevention of mental illness.

mental healthcare facility: a healthcare facility staffed with personnel trained to treat patients with emotional and psychological dysfunctions.

Mental Health Department: the Psychiatric Department; the department in an acute care hospital that is devoted to the care and treatment of patients with emotional and psychological dysfunctions.

message: information someone wants to convey to one or more persons.

***metabolism:** the sum of all physical and chemical processes that take place in the body; the conversion of food to energy.

micro-, micr/o: small.

microorganism: an organism that is not visible with the naked eye.

midbrain: the part of the brain responsible for conducting impulses throughout the different areas of the brain.

middle adulthood: the life stage, commonly referred to as *middle age*, that includes individuals between the ages of 40 and 60 years old.

midsaggital plane: the directional plane that divides the body into right and left halves.

***minerals:** inorganic compounds that are essential to body function.

minor: a person who is not of legal age and who, thus, cannot legally consent to medical, surgical, or dental care; the legal age varies from state to state.

misdemeanor: a minor crime; a crime less serious than a felony.

mitochondria: organelles that release energy and are responsible for the chemical reactions that occur within the cell.

***mitosis:** cell reproduction in which a cell divides, forming two daughter cells that are identical to the original cell.

mitral valve: the one-way valve located between the left atrium and left ventricle; also called bicuspid valve.

mixed nerves: a nerve containing a combination of sensory and motor fibers.

molds: a type of fungi.

mon/o, mono-: one; single.

mons veneris: the pad of adipose tissue that covers the lower front bones of the female pelvis.

motor: refers to brain function and muscle stimulation that results in body movement.

*motor neurons: efferent neurons; nerve cells that carry impulses from the brain or spinal cord to the muscles or gland tissue.

mouth: the oral cavity that receives food.

multi-: many.

multitrauma: injuries that affect more than one body system.

*muscle tissue: tissue that is responsible for body movement.

muscle tone: a normal state of balanced and continuous muscle tension.

muscular: pertaining to muscles.

muscular dystrophy: a congenital, progressive disease that results in wasting and atrophy of muscles.

my/o: muscle.

myalgia: muscle pain.

myelogram: an x-ray of the spinal cord and associated nerves after an injection of contrast medium.

*myocardial infarction: a heart attack; a condition caused by the blockage of one or more coronary arteries.

myocardial septum: the division between the right and left halves of the heart.

myocardium: the thick, muscular layer of the heart.

myometrium: the muscular layer of tissue in the wall of the uterus.

myopia: nearsightedness; a condition in which the rays of light entering the eye come to a focus in front of the retina, causing objects that are at a distance to appear blurry.

myositis: inflammation of muscle tissue.

N

nails: flat, horny cell structures, composed of dead epithelial tissue that appear at the ends of fingers or toes.

nares: nostrils.

nasal cannula: special oxygen tubing that is placed just inside each nostril to deliver oxygen.

nasal septum: the cartilage that separates the two nares.

nasopharynx: part of the pharynx located behind the nose, reaching from the back of the nasal opening to just above the soft palate.

National Institute for Occupational Safety and Health: NIOSH; a government agency that investigates requests submitted by employers or employees concerning working conditions and how they relate to illnesses and diseases contracted by employees.

nausea: a sensation leading to the urge to vomit.

nebulizer: a hand-held apparatus that delivers a fine spray or mist of medication.

necr/o: pertaining to death.

necrosis: tissue death due to lack of oxygen to the area.

*need: something (either physical or psychological) that is required by an organism.

*negligence: the failure to give reasonable care or to do what another prudent person with similar experience, knowledge and background would have done under the same or similar circumstances.

neo-: new.

*neonate: an infant from the age of birth up to 1 month old.

neonatology: the branch of medicine concerned with caring for infants from birth to 1 month of age.

neonatology nurse: a registered nurse who is specially trained to provide nursing care for babies from birth up to 1 month old.

neph-, nephr/o: kidney.

nephritis: inflammation of the kidney.

nephrology: the area of medicine concerned with the diagnosis and treatment of diseases and disorders of the kidneys.

*****nephrons:** the functional units of the kidney that act as the basic filtering units of the kidney.

*****nerve:** a combination of nerve fibers located outside the brain or spinal cord, and that connect those structures with various parts of the body.

nerve conduction studies: studies that aid in the discovery of peripheral nerve injuries and diseases by electrically stimulating nerves and measuring the response.

*****nerve tissue:** tissue, made up of neurons, that comprises the nervous system.

nervous system: the body system that includes the brain, spinal cord, and the nerves.

neur/o: nerves or nervous system.

neuralgia: severe pain along the length of a nerve.

neurologist: a physician who specializes in the diagnosis and treatment of diseases and problems affecting the nervous system.

neurology: the branch of medicine that deals with the diagnosis and treatment of diseases and problems affecting the nervous system.

neuron: the primary structural and functional unit of the nervous system; a nerve cell.

nicotine: an extremely addicting poison that is found in all parts of the tobacco plant, especially the leaves.

NIOSH: the accepted abbreviation for National Institute for Occupational Safety and Health.

non-invasive blood pressure: the measurement of the blood pressure using an external sphygmomanometer.

*****nonprofit agency:** an organization that is supported only by contributions.

*****nonverbal:** a form of communication that involves body language, tactile stimulation (touch), and facial expressions.

*****nosocomial infection:** an infection that is acquired during a stay at a hospital.

nuclear medicine: a specialized area of medicine that uses radionuclides for either diagnosis or therapy.

nucleus: the essential body located in the center of the cell that controls vital functions of the cell such as metabolism, reproduction, growth, and the transmission of other characteristics of the cell.

Nursery: the nursing department in a hospital that provides care for the newborn.

Nursing Services: healthcare services that are provided by the nursing staff; includes all of the hospital departments that provide nursing care.

O

O_2: the chemical symbol for oxygen.

OB-GYN nurse specialist: a registered nurse who is specially trained to provide nursing care for women with problems of the reproductive system, throughout pregnancy, and during labor and delivery. Care may be provided for up to 6 weeks after delivery.

objective: that which can be observed.

obstetrics: the branch of medicine that deals with care for the pregnant patient both before and 6 weeks after the delivery of the baby, as well as for the patient who plans to become pregnant.

obstructed airway maneuver: a procedure used to clear a foreign body from the trachea; the Heimlich maneuver.

occult blood: blood, usually found in the stool or gastric contents, that is in such minute quantities that it must be examined microscopically.

*Occupational Safety and Health Administration (OSHA): a government agency that develops safety standards and establishes maximum levels of exposure to many hazardous materials.

ocul/o: eye.

odont/o-: teeth.

olfactory epithelium: the upper part of the nasal cavity.

olfactory nerve: one of two nerves that conduct the sense of smell.

olig/o: few; less than normal; a deficiency.

oliguria: reduced urine production.

-oma: tumor.

onc/o: tumor.

oncology: the area of medicine concerned with the diagnosis and treatment of tumors.

oncology nurse specialist: a registered nurse specially trained to provide nursing care for patients diagnosed with cancer; national certification is available.

Oncology Unit: the nursing department that provides care to patients with cancer.

oophor/o: ovary.

open-ended questions: a question that is phrased in such a way that the answer is not restricted to a "yes" or "no".

operating room: a specific area of the hospital used exclusively for surgical procedures; also called an operating suite or surgical suite.

operating room nurse: a registered nurse who is specially trained to set up for surgical procedures and to assist in the procedures.

ophthalm/o: eye.

ophthalmology: the area of medicine dedicated to the diagnosis and treatment of diseases and disorders of the eye.

ophthalmoscope: an instrument with a light that is used to view the internal structures of the eye, especially the retina and the blood vessels.

opportunistic infections: infections that occur in people with inefficient immune systems.

oral: by way of the mouth.

*organ: a structure within the body made up of tissues that allow it to perform a particular function.

organelles: tiny structures contained within the cytoplasm of a cell that perform specific functions.

organism: any living thing composed of one or more cells.

organ of Corti: the organ in the inner ear that transmits sound waves to the brain via the auditory nerve.

*organ transplant: a surgical procedure in which a vital organ provided from a donor is transferred to a recipient who is suffering from failure of that organ.

oropharynx: the middle section of the pharynx; posterior to the mouth and inferior to the nasopharynx.

orth/o: straight.

orthopedic nurse specialist: a registered nurse who is specially trained to provide nursing care to orthopedic patients.

orthopedic specialist: a physician who specializes in the treatment of disorders affecting the skeleton, its joints, muscles, and other related structures.

orthopedics: the branch of medicine that deals with the treatment of disorders relating to the skeleton, its joints, muscles, and other related structures.

OSHA: the accepted abbreviation for Occupational Safety and Health Administration.

-osis: abnormal condition.

osseous tissue: bone.

ossicles: the three small bones of the inner ear: the malleus, the incus, and the stapes.

ossification: the formation of bone.

oste/o: bone.

osteomyelitis: severe inflammation of bone and bone marrow, resulting from a bacterial infection.

osteoporosis: a condition in which a decreasing calcium level in the bones causes them to become brittle.

ot/o: ear.

otitis externa: inflammation of the external ear canal.

otitis media: inflammation of the middle ear.

otolaryngology: the branch of medicine that studies the diagnosis and treatment of diseases and disorders relating to the ears, nose, and throat.

otoscope: an instrument with a light used to examine the external auditory canal and tympanic membrane.

outpatient: a patient who receives treatment from a healthcare facility without being admitted to a hospital.

outpatient clinic: a facility that allows patients to be treated or have tests completed without being admitted to the facility.

outpatient surgery: an operation performed in a special center or hospital department without the patient being admitted to the hospital; also referred to as ambulatory surgery.

oval window: the oval-shaped structure that, along with the stapes, connects the inner ear to the middle ear.

ovarian cyst: a sac filled with fluid or semi-solid material that develops on the ovary.

ovarian follicle: any of the sacs in the ovaries that each contain one mature egg.

ovaries: the female sex glands.

ovulation: the periodic release of an egg from the ovary.

ovum: a female reproductive cell; an egg.

oxygenated: blood that contains a sufficient level of oxygen necessary for proper functioning of the body systems.

oxygen mask: an oxygen-delivery system that fits over the patient's mouth and nose.

P

palatine tonsils: a mass of lymphoid tissue located on each side of the hard palate (roof of the mouth).

*palliative: care which relieves or eases, but does not heal.

palpate: to examine by feeling with the hands.

*pancreas: the organ in the abdominal cavity that produces insulin and aids in digestion.

pancreatic juice: the secretion produced by the pancreas and made up of water, inorganic salts, protein, and enzymes.

pancreatitis: inflammation of the pancreas.

pap smear: the scraping and examination of cells from the body, especially the cervix and the vaginal walls; used in the detection of cancer; Papanicolaou test.

papules: firm, red areas on the skin.

para-: beside; beyond; apart from; near; abnormal; irregular; opposite; adjacent to.

-para: to bring forth; to bear.

paracentesis: a needle puncture of a cavity followed by the aspiration of fluid for analysis.

parametrium: the outer, serous layer of loose connective tissue of the uterus.

paraplegia: paralysis of the lower part of the body, including both legs.

*parasympathetic nervous system: the part of the autonomic nervous system that acts in specific ways to complement the activities of the sympathetic nervous system.

parathyroid: one of the four small endocrine glands located at the inferior posterior edge of the thyroid gland, that secrete parathormone, a hormone that regulates calcium and phosphorus levels in the blood.

partial thickness burn: an extremely painful burn in which damage extends through the epidermis and into the dermis, but not so seriously that it permanently impairs the regeneration of the epidermis; characterized by blisters and usually accompanied by superficial burns; formerly known as a second degree burn.

-path/o, -pathy: disease.

*pathogen: a disease-causing microorganism.

pathology: the study of the cause and effects of a disease.

*patient advocate: an individual who supports and pleads the cause of the patient.

*patient lift: a piece of equipment used to transfer a bedridden patient out of bed into a chair or bath.

*patient unit: a patient's room, including the bed, overbed table, bedside table, call light, telephone, television, radio, bathroom, and closet.

*Patient's Bill of Rights: a document that identifies the basic rights of all patients.

ped/o: child; foot.

pedal: pertaining to the foot.

pediatric nurse specialist: a registered nurse who is specially trained to provide nursing care for pediatric patients (infants to 18 years old).

pediatrics: the branch of medicine that cares for infants, children, and adolescents to 18 years in age.

pelvic cavity: the lowest section of the anterior cavity that contains the urinary bladder, the last part of the large intestine, and the reproductive organs.

pelvic inflammatory disease (PID): an infection that ascends from the vagina or cervix to the uterus, oviducts, and uterine ligaments.

pelvic ultrasound: the use of sound waves to detect masses or tumors within the pelvic cavity.

-penia: lack of, deficiency.

penis: the male organ of sexual intercourse

pepsin: an enzyme produced by the stomach that speeds the breakdown of proteins.

per-: through.

peri-: surrounding; around.

pericardial fluid: fluid surrounding the heart.

pericardial sac: the pericardium.

pericardium: the fibroserous sac that completely encloses the heart; also referred to as the pericardial sac.

perineum: the part of the body between the inner thighs from the anus in the rear to the vulva in the front of the female, and between the anus and the scrotum in the male.

periosteum: the outer layer of bone.

*peripheral circulation: blood flow to the surface of the skin, extremities, ears, nose, and face.

*peripheral nervous system: the nervous system outside the central nervous system that is responsible for gathering information and carrying the response signals.

*peristalsis: rhythmic, wavelike motion that occurs throughout the digestive tract, and which causes the contents of the alimentary canal to be forced onward.

peritoneal fluid: the clear fluid secreted by the tissue in the peritoneum.

phag/o, -phage: ingest; eat; swallow.

pharmacist: someone who is trained and licensed to prepare and dispense medications.

Pharmacy: the department in a hospital or a store in the community that dispenses medication.

pharyngeal tonsils: lymph tissue located in the back of the throat; commonly called adenoids.

pharynx: the passageway for air and food that extends from the base of the skull to the esophagus; the throat.

phas/o, -phasia: speech.

phimosis: excessive tightness of the prepuce that prevents it from being withdrawn.

phleb/o: vein.

phlebitis: inflammation of a vein.

phob/o: dread; abnormal fear.

physical: relating to the body; an aspect of growth and development that refers to the growth of the body.

physical medicine and rehabilitation: an area of medicine concerned with the treatment of sports and other injuries and the recovery of most, if not all, muscle strength and function and joint range of motion.

physical therapist: a licensed allied healthcare provider who assists patients with physical rehabilitation following an injury, illness, or operation, using heat, cold, electricity, exercise, massage, and/or ultraviolet light.

physical therapy: rehabilitation that is concerned with the restoration of function and prevention of disability following disease, injury, or loss of a body part through the use of heat, cold, electricity, exercise, massage, and/or ultraviolet light.

Physical Therapy Department: the department in a hospital that focuses on providing physical rehabilitation to patients following a disease, injury, or operation.

physiological need: the physical, biological, or basic requirements for life (eg, food, water, sleep, etc.).

*physiology: the study of the function of the body.

pia mater: the innermost layer of the meninges.

pigmentation: coloration of the skin as determined by the amount of melanin that is present in the tissue.

pineal body: the gland-like structure located in the brain that seems to be involved in the function of the sex glands.

pinna: the outer or external ear.

pituitary gland: the endocrine gland at the base of the brain that secretes hormones that regulate body processes such as growth, reproduction, and metabolism.

pivot joint: a type of joint in which a projection fits through a ring made up of bone and ligament, allowing only pivoting motion.

placenta: a structure present in the uterus during pregnancy from which a fetus obtains its nourishment.

plaintiff: the person filing a lawsuit; the injured person in a lawsuit.

plasma: the fluid part of the blood that contains serum, proteins, solids, chemical substances, and gases.

-plasty: surgical repair.

platelets: cells found in the blood that assist in clot formation; thrombocytes.

pleura: the thin layer of tissue that surrounds each lung and extends over the diaphragm and walls of the thorax.

pleural fluid: fluid in and around the lungs.

pleurisy: inflammation of the pleura.

pleur/o: pleura.

pleuro-: referring to the lung, side, or rib.

*PMI: the abbreviation for point of maximal impulse.

-pnea: breathing.

pneum/o: lung.

pneumonia: inflammation of the lungs.

pod/o-: foot.

point of insertion: the end of the muscle where movement occurs.

point of origin: the end of the muscle where movement does not occur.

*Poison Control: an agency for both the general public and professional healthcare providers that provides information and first aid instructions for every poison available.

poliomyelitis: an acute viral disease that inflames parts of the spinal cord and may result in muscular atrophy, deformity, and paralysis.

poly-: many.

polydipsia: excessive thirst; one of the three signs of possible diabetes mellitus.

polyphagia: excessive hunger; one of the three signs of possible diabetes mellitus.

polyuria: excessive urination; one of the three signs of possible diabetes mellitus.

pons: the portion of the brain stem responsible for conducting certain impulses throughout the brain and for some reflex actions such as chewing and producing saliva.

portal of entry: the route by which a pathogen enters the body.

portal of exit: the route by which a pathogen leaves the body.

post-: following; after.

Post Anesthesia Care Unit: a recovery room; an area of a hospital designed to monitor patients immediately following surgery.

posterior: refers to the backside; same as dorsal.

posterior cavity: the body cavity located along the back of the body; contains the cranial and spinal cavities.

Post Partum Unit: a nursing unit that provides care to the mother after delivering her baby.

pre-: in front of; before.

*prefix: a word element placed in front of a root to modify its meaning.

prepuce: the foreskin of the penis.

pressure point: a pulse point on the body, located above an injury, to which pressure can be applied to control bleeding.

*preventive healthcare: healthcare that focuses on patient education that emphasizes the promotion of health and the prevention of disease.

primary care: an approach to nursing in which a registered nurse provides all aspects of patient care, including duties normally assigned to nursing assistants.

*primary survey: an examination of the patient to determine the presence of any life-threatening emergencies; the initial assessment of airway, breathing, and circulation on a patient.

*privileged information: confidential data; all data concerning a patient that is disclosed within the hospital.

pro-: in front of; before; for.

proct/o: rectum.

proctology: the branch of medicine that deals with the treatment of disorders affecting the colon, rectum, and anus.

projection: a type of defense mechanism in which a person attributes undesirable qualities of his or her own to another person, rather than accepting that the problem lies within himself or herself.

prostate gland: the gland that encompasses the neck of the bladder and the urethra in the male, and which secretes a component of seminal fluid.

*protein: any of a class of complex, nitrogenous, organic compounds that function as the primary building blocks of the body.

prothrombin: a protein produced by the liver that helps coagulate the blood.

protocol: a standard treatment procedure approved by an authorized source.

protoplasm: cytoplasm; the contents of a cell outside the nucleus.

protozoa: a pathogenic animal microbe.

proximal: nearest to the point of reference or attachment.

*proximate cause: a legal concept meaning that an aspect of care that was omitted or committed directly caused a patient's injury or death.

pseud/o: false.

psych/o: mind.

Psychiatric Department: the department in a hospital that is set aside for the diagnosis and treatment of patients with mental and emotional problems.

psychiatric nurse specialist: a nurse who is specially trained to provide nursing care for patients with coping and behavioral disturbances. National certification is available.

psychiatrist: a doctor who specializes in the study and treatment of the mind, emotions, and behavior.

psychiatry: the branch of medicine that deals with the study of the mind, emotions, and behavior.

psychology: the study of the mind and behavior patterns.

ptyalin: an enzyme contained in saliva that assists in the breakdown of starches.

puberty: the period of life in which changes occur that enable both the male and female to become functionally capable of reproduction.

pulm/o, pulmon/o: lung.

pulmonary: of or relating to the lungs.

pulmonary angiography: a diagnostic test that allows the physician to view the pulmonary system through the use of radiopaque dye.

pulmonary artery: one of the two vessels that receive low-oxygenated blood from the right ventricle of the heart and pass it into the lungs.

pulmonary edema: the swelling of the lung tissues with fluid.

pulmonary function tests: tests that are used to determine the capacity of the lungs to take in oxygen and release carbon dioxide.

*pulmonary medicine: the branch of medicine concerned with the diagnosis and treatment of disorders and diseases of the lungs.

pulmonary valve: the semilunar valve; the one-way valve located between the right ventricle and the pulmonary artery.

pulmonary vein: one of the two vessels that transport highly oxygenated blood from the lung into the left atrium of the heart.

*pulse: a vital sign; a quantitative measurement of the heartbeat using the fingers to palpate an artery or a stethoscope to listen to the heartbeat.

puncture wound: a soft tissue injury caused by the penetration of a sharp object.

pupil: the opening at the center of the iris in the eye that contracts in light and dilates in darkness.

Purchasing Department: the department in a hospital responsible for purchasing all of the equipment and supplies that are used in the hospital.

pus: fluid, composed of dead leukocytes and other cells that results from infection.

pustules: skin elevations that are filled with a liquid that contains leukocytes and bacteria.

py/o: pus.

pyel/o: pelvis of kidney.

pyelonephritis: inflammation of the kidneys and renal pelvis usually caused by bacteria.

pyloric sphincter: the two-way valve located between the stomach and the duodenum.

Q

quadri-: consisting of four.

quadriplegia: paralysis of the body from the neck down.

R

radial: of or relating to the area of the radius in the wrist.

radial artery: the artery located near the radius in the wrist; one of the places suitable for taking a pulse.

radiation: the release of rays in different directions from a common point; the transfer or loss of heat by or from its source to the surrounding environment in the form of heat waves or rays.

radiation therapy: the use of ionizing radiation to treat cancerous tumors.

radioactive: capable of releasing radiant energy due to the decay of the nucleus of an atom.

radiology: a specific branch of medicine that uses x-rays for diagnosis and therapy.

Radiology Department: the department in a hospital responsible for the diagnosis and treatment of disorders and diseases using x-rays and other radioactive materials.

radiology studies: x-ray films; diagnostic tests that use film and radiation to show most of the body's internal structures.

*range of motion: the extent to which a joint can move.

rash: a general term used to indicate a skin eruption.

rationalization: a defense mechanism in which a reason or explanation is given to explain a particular behavior that makes the behavior seem appropriate.

*receiver: the person or group of people for whom information is intended.

Recovery Room: a Post Anesthesia Care Unit.

rectal: pertaining to the rectum.

red bone marrow: the soft tissue found in spongy bone that produces all types of cells.

reflective statements: statements the receiver makes to indicate to the sender how the message was heard and received.

registered nurse: a nurse who has completed a course of study at a state-approved nursing school and who has passed the state licensing exam for nursing; this nurse is granted the right to practice for hire.

rehabilitation: the restoration of a patient or a part of the body to normal or near normal following an illness or injury.

rehabilitation facility: a specialized facility that assists patients in regaining maximum function and a level of independence following surgery, traumatic injuries, or illness.

ren/o: kidney.

renal basin: the enlarged end of the ureter in the kidney; the renal pelvis.

reoxygenate: to replace or replenish with oxygen.

reproductive system: the body system responsible for procreation.

reservoir host: the individual in which the infectious microorganisms reside.

resident: a physician in training following an internship who is generally a member of the hospital staff.

res ipsa loquitor: a Latin phrase meaning it speaks for itself.

resistance: the ability to fight off a particular force, such as an infection.

*respiration: breathing; the process of bringing oxygen into the body and expelling carbon dioxide from the body.

respirator: a machine that mechanically breathes for a patient who is unable to breathe on his or her own.

respiratory cycle: one inspiration and one expiration.

respiratory therapist: an allied healthcare professional who specializes in performing and providing treatments for patients with respiratory diseases.

Respiratory Therapy Department: a department in a hospital that provides treatments, procedures, and support for patients with respiratory diseases.

respondeat superior: a Latin phrase meaning the employer is responsible for the actions of its employees. Literally, *Let the master answer.*

*resumé: a brief, written account of personal and professional qualifications and experience that is prepared by an applicant for a position.

resuscitate: to revive or bring back to life.

retina: the innermost, nervous tissue membrane of the eye, which receives the light rays from the lens and sends signals to the brain via the optic nerve.

retr/o: located behind; backwards.

*reverse isolation: a method of protecting a patient with a suppressed immune system from pathogens that might be transmitted by the staff, other patients or visitors, or through the air.

-rhage, -rhagia: bursting forth; excessive flow of blood.

-rhaphy: suture or sew up a defect.

-rhea: flow or discharge.

*rheumatology: the branch of medicine concerned with the diagnosis and treatment of disorders and diseases of the joints of the body.

rhin/o: nose.

rhinitis: inflammation of the lining of the nasal cavity.

right atrium: the upper right chamber of the heart, which receives deoxygenated blood from the body and sends it into the right ventricle.

right lower quadrant: RLQ; the section of the abdomen that contains the female reproductive organs, the intestines, and the appendix.

right lymphatic duct: the vessel that receives the lymph from the right side of the head and neck, right side of the chest, and the right upper extremity and carries it into the blood.

*right to die: a controversial issue concerning the right of a terminally ill patient to request that no life-sustaining measures be taken.

right upper quadrant: RUQ; the section of the abdomen that contains the gall bladder, liver, and intestines.

right ventricle: the lower right chamber of the heart, which receives deoxygenated blood from the right atrium and sends it through the pulmonary valve to the pulmonary arteries.

Rinne test: the use of a tuning fork to assess a person's hearing via air conduction and bone conduction of the sound waves.

rods: tiny cylindrical nerve cells on the surface of the retina that respond to dim light.

*rooming-in: keeping the baby in the mother's post partum room instead of in the nursery.

*root word: the main part of a word.

rotation: the process of turning a body part on its axis, resulting in a circular motion.

route of transmission: the method by which a pathogen travels from a reservoir to a new host.

S

saddle joint: a joint in which two surfaces, one convex and the other concave, fit together.

safety: the state of being protected from harm; as the second level of Maslow's Hierarchy of Needs, it includes the desire to feel secure in one's environment and to be free from anxiety and fear.

saliva: a clear fluid secreted by the mouth that moistens and partially digests food.

salping/o: oviduct, uterine tube, or fallopian tube; auditory tube.

scapula: the shoulder blade.

scler/o: hardening; sclera (white of the eye).

sclera: the tough, fibrous membrane that covers the white of the eye, and to which the muscles of the eye are attached.

scoli/o: twisted; curved.

-scope: instrument used to examine or look into a part.

*scope of practice: a legal description of what a specific health professional may and may not do.

-scopy: visual examination.

sebaceous: refers to oil glands contained within the skin layers.

secondary hypertension: high blood pressure that is caused by a medical condition.

*secondary survey: a head-to-toe physical assessment; an additional assessment of a patient to determine the existence of any injuries other than those found in the primary survey.

*seizure: a neurological dysfunction caused by a sudden episode of uncontrolled electrical activity in the brain that may result in involuntary, uncontrolled muscle contractions.

self-actualization: the fifth and last level of Maslow's Hierarchy of Needs, marked by the attainment of an individual's full potential to his or her satisfaction.

sella turcica: a sideways depression crossing the middle of the back of the cranium that houses the pituitary gland.

semen: the thick, white secretion discharged by the male sex organs that carries sperm.

semi-: half.

semicircular canals: three bony, fluid-filled passages that form part of the inner ear.

semi-Fowler's position: a position in which the patient is sitting with the head elevated 45°. The patient's knees may or may not be flexed.

semilunar valve: the one-way valve located between the right ventricle and the pulmonary artery.

seminal vesicles: two sac-like glands near the prostate that secrete a component of semen.

*semipermeable: the ability to permit certain substances to enter and exit through a membrane.

*sender: a person who attempts to transmit information to another person or a group of people.

sensorium: the part of the brain concerned with the senses; the state of a person's level of awareness.

sensory: stimulation through touch, sight, taste, smell, and hearing.

*sensory neurons: afferent neurons; nerve cells that transmit impulses from the sensory organs and the skin to the brain and spinal cord.

sensory system: the body system responsible for the senses of sight, hearing, smell, taste, and touch.

sept/o: poison.

sexuality: the makeup of an individual as related to sexual attitudes and activity.

*sexually transmitted disease: a disease that is acquired during sexual intercourse or other sexually intimate contact with an infected individual.

sharps container: a plastic container, usually red, that is designed for the safe disposal of used sharps.

shock: a condition that occurs when an inadequate amount of blood flows through the body, causing extremely low blood pressure, a lack of urine, and other disorders; a potentially fatal condition.

short bones: bones that are closely joined, and in which there is no relationship between their length and width.

siderails: devices on a bed or gurney that are used to prevent a patient from falling out of bed or off of the gurney.

sigmoid colon: the s-shaped portion of the large intestine through which food passes just before entering the rectum.

sign: an obvious, objective finding, or evidence of an illness or bodily malfunction.

*significant other: a person who is emotionally concerned for or attached to the patient.

*sinoatrial node: the natural pacemaker of the heart, located in the upper part of the right atrium.

-sis: condition or process.

skeletal: refers to the skeleton; a type of muscle tissue that attaches to bone and permits movement.

skilled nursing facility: a type of extended care facility that has skilled nurses available to provide various services requiring the skills of a licensed nurse.

skin scraping: a diagnostic test that involves the scraping of superficial epithelial cells onto a glass slide and examining them.

slit lamp: a microscope used to view the eye under high magnification.

small bowel series: fluoroscopy of the intestines following the ingestion of barium.

small intestine: the coiled portion of the alimentary canal between the stomach and large intestine that is about 20 feet long if uncoiled.

Snellen eye test: a test in which visual acuity is tested by reading the Snellen eye chart from 20 feet away.

sniffing position: the proper position for infant rescue breathing in which the infant's chin is placed in a position that is neither too high nor too low.

social: refers to a person's interactions and relationships with other members of society.

Social Services Department: a department in a hospital that provides assistance to patients with social problems such as child abuse, elder abuse, or food and shelter problems.

soluble: able to be dissolved in water.

somat/o: the body.

somatic: pertaining to the body.

*somatic nervous system: the part of the peripheral nervous system that controls skeletal muscles responsible for voluntary movement.

specialist: someone who has had extensive training and education in a specific area such as cardiology, gerontology, etc.

specialized: focused on a specific area of medicine.

speculum: an instrument, often disposable, used for inspecting canals.

spermatazoa: the mature male sex cells, contained in semen, that fertilize the ova when ejaculated into the female womb.

sphygmomanometer: an instrument for measuring blood pressure.

spinal cavity: the body cavity that contains the spinal cord.

spinal cord: the column of nerve tissue that is attached directly to the medulla oblongata and ends at the level of the second lumbar vertebrae; it conducts impulses and connects the body parts to the brain.

spinal nerves: the 31 pairs of nerves that are attached to the spinal cord; part of the somatic nervous system.

spirilla: spiral-shaped bacteria.

spirochetes: a type of bacteria capable of causing disease.

spleen: the organ in the left upper quadrant behind the stomach that produces lymphocytes and monocytes. It is a reservoir for blood and clears the blood of dead cells and other foreign and toxic substances.

splenomegaly: enlargement of the spleen.

spontaneously: occurring without assistance or apparent cause.

sports medicine: the branch of medicine that deals with the prevention and treatment of athletic injuries.

sprain: an injury to the soft tissues of a joint, characterized by the inability to move, deformity, and pain.

*Standard Precautions: guidelines developed by The Centers for Disease Control and Prevention for protecting healthcare workers from exposure to blood-borne pathogens in body secretions.

stapes: one of the three ossicles in the middle ear; the stirrup.

Staph: the abbreviation for the bacteria staphylococcus.

staphylococci: gram positive, round or oval bacteria that grow in grape-like clusters.

Staphylococcus: singular of staphylococci.

Staphylococcus aureus: a species of bacteria normally found on mucous membranes and the skin.

statute: a law approved by the legislative branch of a government.

statute of limitations: the particular length of time during which a lawsuit can be filed for a certain issue.

sten-, steno-: contracted; narrow.

sterile: aseptic; free from all living microorganisms and their spores.

sterile field: the area considered to be free of contamination during a surgical procedure.

*sterile technique: the procedure used by healthcare workers when performing or assisting with a sterile procedure; surgical asepsis.

*sterilization: the complete destruction of all forms of microbial life.

sternum: the breast bone.

stertorous: labored breathing in which snoring, rattling and/or bubbling sounds are heard.

stethoscope: an instrument used to amplify sounds from within the body; the device used to listen for a pulse, blood pressure, and bowel or lung sounds.

stimulant: an agent that temporarily increases activity.

stomach: an accessory organ of the digestive tract that acts as a churn and a pouch for food and liquid.

-stomy: surgical creation of an opening.

stool: feces.

strabismus: a condition in which the muscles of the eyeballs fail to coordinate movement; cross eyes.

strength testing: diagnostic tests that are done to determine the extent of muscle damage to a patient.

streptococci: bacteria that are arranged in chains.

stress: the result produced when a person perceives that events or circumstances have challenged or exceeded his or her coping mechanisms, and the person's mental, spiritual, and physical state of balance becomes disturbed.

stress test: a diagnostic test that is done to evaluate a patient's cardiovascular fitness. The patient's heart and lungs are carefully monitored while the patient performs a controlled physical activity such as walking on a treadmill.

striated: striped; generally refers to skeletal muscle.

stridor: a high-pitched noise, like a squeak, that occurs from upper airway obstruction, usually laryngeal edema.

Stryker frame: a special bed often used to change a patient's position to relieve constant pressure. Also known as a circular double bed frame, it is used for burn patients and those with spinal cord injuries.

sub-: under; below.

subarachnoid: beneath the arachnoid membrane and above the pia mater of the meninges of the brain or spinal cord.

subcutaneous tissue: the inner-most layer of skin.

subdural: beneath the dura mater and above the arachnoid layer of the meninges.

subjective: that which can be felt or experienced.

subpeona: a document that requires a witness to appear at a trial or other proceeding to provide testimony.

substance abuse: the excessive use of chemicals, drugs, or alcohol in an attempt to cope with daily problems.

Substance Abuse Unit: a specialized unit for patients needing treatment of drug and chemical dependency.

*sudden death: the unexpected and instantaneous cessation of breathing and the pulse, or within 60 minutes of the onset of symptoms in patients without known preexisting heart disease.

sudoriferous: producing or excreting sweat.

*suffix: a word element placed at the end of a root to modify its meaning.

suicide: the voluntary ending of one's life.

super-: over; above.

superficial: near the surface of the body.

superficial burn: a thermal or chemical burn in which only the outer layer of the epidermis is affected; characterized by reddening of the skin; formerly known as a first degree burn.

superior: located near the top; above.

superior vena cava: the principal vein that receives blood from the head and upper part of the body and empties it into the right atrium.

supine: a position in which a patient is lying flat on the back.

Support Services: allied areas of healthcare operations that are not involved with patient care.

supra-: over; above.

surgery: manual and operative procedures that are used to repair injuries, correct deformities and defects, and diagnose certain diseases.

surgical asepsis: the prevention of infection before, during, and after surgery through the use of sterile technique.

surgical nurse: a registered nurse who is specially trained to set up for surgical procedures and to assist in the procedures.

surgical suite: the operating room.

susceptible host: a person capable of being affected or infected by invading microorganisms, depending on the degree of that person's resistance.

sym-: with; together.

*sympathetic nervous system: the part of the autonomic nervous system that controls many involuntary activities of the glands, organs, and other parts of the body.

syn-: with; together.

*syncope: fainting; sudden, brief, and temporary loss of consciousness; passing out.

synovial fluid: the clear fluid surrounding a joint.

*synovial joint: a freely moveable joint such as the elbow, knee, fingers, etc.

syphilis: a chronic, sexually transmitted disease characterized by lesions on an organ or on the skin; may be present without symptoms for years.

syring/o: fistula; tube.

syrup of ipecac: an emetic used to induce vomiting in some cases of poisoning.

*system: a group of organs that work together to perform a common function.

systemic: pertaining to the entire body.

*systolic: the top number in a blood pressure reading; refers to the time between the first and second heart sounds in which the heart contracts.

T

tachy-: fast; rapid; swift.

*tachycardia: a pulse rate above 100 beats per minute.

tachypnea: abnormally rapid breathing.

tars/o: tarsal (ankle bone).

*taste receptors: taste buds; the oval structures located in various areas on the surface of the tongue that transmit the sensation of taste.

-tax/o: order; arrangement; coordination.

team nursing: a method of nursing in which the registered nurse acts as a team leader and supervises other nurses and allied healthcare workers in the provision of direct patient care.

ten/o, tend/o, tendo-: tendon.

tendon: fibrous connective tissue around a joint that connects muscle to bone.

tens/o: stretch; strain.

terminal: describes a disease that has no known cure; fatal.

*testes: the male reproductive glands; responsible for producing testosterone.

testimony: a statement, given under oath in a courtroom, providing details of a particular incident.

*testosterone: the hormone, produced by the testes, which stimulates the growth of secondary sexual characteristics and is essential for normal sexual behavior in males.

therapeutic radiology: a type of therapy usually used in the treatment of cancer patients.

therm/o: heat.

thoracic: pertaining to the area of the body between the base of the neck and the diaphragm.

thoracic cavity: the area in the chest that contains the heart, lungs, and large blood vessels.

thoracic duct: the primary lymphatic duct of the body, which receives purified lymph from all parts of the body except the right side of the head, neck, and thorax, and right upper limb, and empties it into the left subclavian vein.

thoracic surgery: surgery involving the structures within the rib cage.

thready: a weak, fine pulse that can barely be detected.

thromb/o: clot.

thrombocyte: a blood platelet.

thrombus: a blood clot.

thymus gland: the gland located in the center of the chest that produces lymphocytes and antibodies during early life; the thymus atrophies after puberty.

thyroid: the two-lobed endocrine gland at the front of the neck that helps regulate metabolism.

thyroid cartilage: the largest layer of the larynx that forms the "adams apple".

tissue: a collection of similar cells and their intercellular substances that work together to perform a particular function.

-tomy: cutting into; incision.

*tongue-jaw lift: a method of opening the mouth of a choking victim to help ensure that the tongue is not part of the obstruction.

tonometer: an instrument used to measure intraocular pressure of the eye.

tonsillitis: inflammation of the tonsils.

tonsils: small, rounded collections of lymphoid tissue such as those at the back of the throat.

*tort: a private or civil wrong against another person or his property.

tox/o, toxi-: poison.

*toxic: poisonous.

trache/o: trachea (windpipe).

*trachea: the windpipe; a tube of cartilage that extends from the larynx to the bronchial tubes, and which leads air into the lungs.

tracheostomy: a surgical opening into the trachea for the insertion of a breathing tube.

*traction: the process of pulling a part of the body into proper alignment.

trans-: across; through.

Transitional Care Unit: a nursing unit where patients wear mobile heart monitors that allow them to move around while personnel at the desk watch their heart rhythms and rates on the monitors.

*Transmission-based Precautions: guidelines developed by The Centers for Disease Control and Prevention to help prevent transmission of specific infectious and communicable diseases of patients either suspected of having, or confirmed to have, a certain pathogen.

transmit: to transfer.

transverse colon: the portion of the large intestine that passes across the abdomen; lies between the ascending and descending portions of the large intestine.

transverse plane: the directional plane that separates the body by a horizontal line.

trapeze: a triangular piece of equipment that hangs above a bedridden patient to assist with movement.

*trauma: physical or psychological injury caused by an accident, violence, or a poisonous substance.

trauma center: a medical facility or department in a medical facility that is capable of providing care to critically injured patients 24 hours a day.

Trendelenburg position: a position in which the patient lies flat on the back with the feet elevated above the level of the heart to promote the flow of blood to the brain; the position for shock victims and used in abdominal surgery.

tri-: three.

*triage: to sort or prioritize care for a group of patients.

tricuspid valve: the one-way valve located between the right atrium and the right ventricle.

-trophy: nutrition; development; growth.

-tropia: to turn.

trypsin: a pancreatic enzyme that breaks down proteins.

tubal ligation: the surgical tying or partial removal of the fallopian tubes to prevent pregnancy from occurring; a method of sterilization.

tumor: an abnormal growth that may or may not be malignant.

tunica adventitia: the outer layer of a blood vessel.

tunica intima: the inner layer of a blood vessel.

tunica media: the middle layer of a blood vessel.

tympanic: of or relating to the tympanic membrane or eardrum.

U

UGI: the abbreviation for upper gastrointestinal series.

*ulcer: a lesion on the skin or mucous membrane accompanied by sloughing of inflamed, dead skin.

ultra-: excess; beyond.

ultrasound: inaudible sound waves that can be used to create visual images of the internal structures.

uni-: one.

unit secretary: health unit coordinator; ward clerk; a member of the clerical staff who performs reception and clerical functions for the nursing unit and transcribes the physician's orders.

universal adapter: a mechanical device that fits all equipment.

upper GI series: radiography and fluoroscopy of the esophagus, stomach, and small intestine following the ingestion of barium.

upper respiratory infection: URI; a general term used to describe an infectious disease process involving the nasal passages, pharynx, and bronchi.

*ureters: the long, slender, muscular tubes that extend from the kidney basin down through the lower part of the urinary bladder.

urethra: the tube that extends from the bladder to the outside of the body, and which transports urine from the bladder.

urgent care center: a walk-in, free-standing non-emergency care clinic.

URI: an abbreviation for upper respiratory infection; a general term used to describe an infectious disease process involving the nasal passages, pharynx, and bronchi.

-uria: presence in urine.

*urinary bladder: the hollow, muscular sac contained within the pelvic cavity that stores urine until it is excreted from the body.

urinary meatus: the anatomical opening where urine is expelled from the body.

urinary tract infection: UTI; a cluster of symptoms characterized by dysuria, frequent urination, urgency, and white blood cells in the urine.

urine: the liquid waste produced by the body.

uro-: presence in urine.

urology: the branch of medicine that studies and treats dysfunctions of the urinary tract and the male reproductive system.

*uterus: the organ in the female reproductive system responsible for holding the embryo and fetus from conception until birth.

V

vagina: the muscular tube in females that forms the passageway between the cervix and the vulva.

vas/o: duct; vessel; vas deferens.

vascular: pertaining to blood vessels.

vas deferens: the straight extension of the epididymis that acts as a receiving area for the seminal fluid from the epididymis.

vasectomy: the surgical removal of a part of each vas deferens to prevent transportation of seminal fluid through the rest of the reproductive system; a method of sterilization.

vasodilate: to expand a blood vessel.

*vein: a blood vessel that carries low-oxygenated blood to the heart.

ven/o: vein.

venogram: an x-ray of a vein used to confirm the presence of deep vein thrombosis through the injection of iodine into the vein and observation of the progression of the dye.

venography: the process of performing a venogram.

*ventilation: the exchange of air between the lungs and the atmosphere; breathing.

ventilation lung scan: the diagnostic examination of the lungs following the inhalation of a radioactive gas.

ventilator: a machine that mechanically breathes for a patient who is unable to breathe on his or her own; a respirator.

ventr/o: front or belly side of body.

ventral: located on the front; same as anterior.

ventral cavity: the body cavity located along the front part of the body, and which is separated into the thoracic, abdominal, and pelvic cavities.

*ventricle: one of the two pumping chambers of the heart, located inferior to the atria; one of the four cavities of the brain.

venules: microscopic veins that attach directly to capillaries.

*verbal: spoken.

*vermiform appendix: the worm-like tube of tissue directly connected to the cecum.

vertebrae: the individual bone segments of the spine.

vestibule: a small cavity located at the beginning of a canal; as in the middle portion of the inner ear, between the semicircular canals and the cochlea.

villi: finger-like projections found on some membrane surfaces such as those that line the intestines.

*virus: a microscopic, parasitic organism capable of causing an infectious disease.

viscer/o: viscera.

viscera: internal organs.

visceral: pertaining to the internal organs.

visual: pertaining to sight.

vital: essential to life; indispensable.

*vital signs: assessments of temperature, pulse, respirations, and blood pressure; body functions essential to life.

*vitamins: organic substances, other than proteins, carbohydrates, fats, and organic salts that are essential in small quantities for normal body function.

vitreous humor: the clear, jelly-like substance that fills the entire cavity behind the lens of the eye and helps maintain the eye's spherical shape.

*vocal folds: the edges of the lips of the larynx that vibrate to produce a certain pitch of sound.

Vocational Industrial Clubs of America: VICA; a professional organization of health, technical, trade, and industrial courses of study.

vomiting: reverse peristalsis, which results in the expulsion of the stomach contents through the mouth.

*vulva: a collective term referring to the female external genitalia, posterior to the mons pubis.

W

walkers: an ambulation assistance device. Walkers usually are constructed of aluminum and have handles. Some models also have wheels and/or a seat.

ward clerk: health unit coordinator; unit secretary; a member of the clerical staff who performs reception and clerical functions for the nursing unit and transcribes the physician's orders.

warming blanket: a device used for patients who are hypothermic. It is placed directly on the bed's mattress and electrically circulates warm water to warm the patient.

wart: an eruption of the epidermis that resembles a cauliflower in shape; caused by a virus.

*wellness: the state of optimum health.

*wheelchair: a special chair that is equipped with wheels for transporting patients.

wheeze: a high-pitched, whistling sound produced by the flow of air through a narrowed airway.

white matter: white, medullated nerve fibers that compose some of the nervous structures.

withdrawal: a group of symptoms that occurs as a result of the sudden cessation of a psychologically or physically addicting drug or alcohol.

women's hospital: a healthcare facility dedicated to providing healthcare services to female patients.

X

xanth/o: yellow.

xer/o: dryness.

xiphoid process: the bony tip of the sternum.

x-rays: film images, created by the projection of high energy electromagnetic waves through an area of a patient's body onto a photographic plate, which show the bony structures and specific organ outlines in that area of the body.

Y

yeast: a type of fungi, which may cause disease.

*denotes Key Term.

Abbreviations

A

ā: before.

ABC: airway, breathing, and circulation.

abd: abdomen.

ABGs: arterial blood gases.

ABP: arterial blood pressure.

ac: before meals.

Ac: acetest.

Ac and Cl: acetest and clinitest.

ADA: American Diabetic Association; American Dietetic Association; American Dental Association.

ADL: activities of daily living.

ad lib: as desired.

adm: admission.

AF: atrial fibrillation.

AIDS: acquired immune deficiency syndrome.

AM: before noon; morning hours.

AMA: against medical advice; American Medical Association.

AMI: acute myocardial infarction.

amt: amount.

ant: anterior.

Ap: apical.

AP: anteroposterior.

APGAR: a test for newborns based on appearance, pulse, grimace, airway, and reflex.

appy: appendicitis.

AQ or aq: water; aqueous base.

ARDS: adult respiratory distress syndrome.

ARF: acute renal failure; acute respiratory failure.

ARN: authorized radio nurse.

ASHD: arteriosclerotic heart disease.

AT: atrial tachycardia.

B

Bac T: bacteriology.

BBB: bundle branch block.

B and C: biopsy and conization.

BCP: birth control pills.

BE: barium enema; below elbow.

Be: beryllium.

BID or bid: twice daily.

bil: bilateral.

bl: blood.

BLE: both lower extremities.

BM: bowel movement.

BMR: basal metabolic rate.

BP: blood pressure.

BR: bathroom or bedrest.

BRP: bathroom privileges.

BS: blood sugar.

BSC: bedside commode.

BUE: both upper extremities.

BUN: blood urea nitrogen.

Bx: biopsy.

C

C: Centigrade or Celsius.

c̄: with.

CA: cancer.

Ca: calcium.

CABG: coronary artery bypass with graft.

Cal: large Calorie.

cal: small calorie.

cap: capsule.

CAT scan: computerized axial tomography scan.

cath: catheter.

CBC: complete blood count.

CBR: complete bedrest.

cc: cubic centimeter.

CC: chief complaint.

CCU: Coronary Care Unit.

CDA: certified dental assistant.
CE: cardiac enzymes.
CEN: certified emergency nurse.
CHF: congestive heart failure.
CHO: carbohydrate.
cl: clinitest.
Cl: chloride; chlorine.
Cl and Ac: clinitest and acetest.
CL or **Cl liq:** clear liquids.
cm: centimeter.
CNA: certified nursing assistant; Canadian Nurses Association.
CNS: central nervous system.
co or **c/o:** complaining of.
CO$_2$: carbon dioxide.
CODE III: lights and sirens.
comp.: complete.
cont: continue.
COPD: chronic obstructive pulmonary disease.
CP: cerebral palsy or chest pain.
CPK: creatinine phosphokinase.
CPR: cardiopulmonary resuscitation.
CRF: chronic renal failure.
CS: central supply.
C & S: culture and sensitivity.
CSF: cerebrospinal fluid.
CT: computerized tomography.
CTA: clear to auscultation.
CT scan: computerized tomography scan.
CVA: cerebrovascular accident.
CVR: controlled ventricular rate.
Cx: cervix.
CXR: chest x-ray.

D

d: day.
/d: per day.
DAT: diet as tolerated.
DC: doctor of chiropractic; discharge.
dc: discontinue.
D & C: dilatation and curettage.
DCA: Directional Coronary Atherectomy.
DDS: doctor of dental surgery.

dept: department.
diff: differential white blood cell count.
dil: dilute.
DM: diabetes mellitus.
DNR: do not resuscitate.
DO: doctor of osteopathy.
DOA: dead on arrival.
DPM: doctor of podiatry medicine.
Dr: doctor.
dr: drainage; dram.
DTs: delirium tremens.
DW: dextrose in water.
Dx: diagnosis.
Dz: disease.

E

ea: each.
ECG: electrocardiogram.
ECU: Emergency Care Unit.
ED: Emergency Department.
EEG: electroencephalogram.
EENT: eye, ear, nose and throat.
EKG: electrocardiogram.
EMS: Emergency Medical Services.
EMT: emergency medical technician.
ER: Emergency Room.
ERT: emergency room technician.
ESR: erythrocyte sedimentation rate.
ETOH: ethanol.
exc: excision.
exp: exploratory.
ext: extract, extraction, external.

F

F: Fahrenheit.
FB: foreign body.
FBS: fasting blood sugar.
FBW: fasting blood work.
FC: foley catheter.
Fe: iron.
FF or **F Fl:** force fluids.
FH or **FHB:** fetal heart beat.

FHTs: fetal heart tones.
FL or **Full Liq:** full liquids.
Fl or **fl:** fluids.
FUO: fever of undetermined origin.
Fx or **Fr:** fracture.

G

GB: gallbladder.
GC or **Gc:** gonococcus, gonorrhea.
GI: gastrointestinal.
Gm or **gm:** gram.
gr: grain.
Gtt or **gtt:** drops.
GU: genitourinary.
GYN or **gyn:** gynecology.

H

h: hour.
HBV: hepatitis B virus.
Hep B: hepatitis B.
Hct: hematocrit.
Hg: mercury.
HIV: human immunodeficiency virus.
H$_2$O: water.
HOH: hard of hearing.
HS: hour of sleep.
HSV: herpes simplex virus.
ht: height.
HUC: health unit coordinator.
HX: history.
hypo: hypodermic.
hyst: hysterectomy.

I

IABP: intra-aortic balloon pump.
IBP: invasive blood pressure.
ICU: Intensive Care Unit.
I & D: incision and drainage.
IDDM: insulin dependent diabetes mellitus.
IJ: internal jugular.
IM: intramuscular.

inf: infusion or inferior.
ing: inguinal.
inj: injection.
int: internal, interior.
I & O: intake and output.
IUD: intrauterine device.
IV: intravenous.
IVP: intravenous pyelogram.

J

JR: junctional rhythm.
JVD: jugular vein distention.

K

K: potassium.
KCl: potassium chloride.
kg: kilogram.
KO'd: knocked out.
KUB: kidney, ureter, and bladder.

L

L or **l:** liter.
LA: left atrium; left arm.
lab: laboratory.
lap: laparotomy.
lat: lateral.
lb: pound.
LBP: low back pain.
LCTA: lungs clear to auscultation.
L&D: Labor and Delivery.
LFT: left frontotransverse fetal position.
LFTs: liver function tests.
liq: liquid.
LLE: left lower extremity.
LLL: left lower lobe.
LLQ: left lower quadrant.
LOC: level of consciousness; loss of consciousness.
LOM: left otitis media.
LP: lumbar puncture.
LPN: licensed practical nurse.
LR: lactated ringers.

LS: lumbo-sacral.
Lt: left.
LUE: left upper extremity.
LUQ: left upper quadrant.
LV: left ventricle.
LVN: licensed vocational nurse.
LWBS: left without being seen.

M

m: minim or meter.
MA: medical assistant.
MAE: moves all extremities.
MAST: military antishock trousers.
mat: maternity.
MD: medical doctor.
med: medical.
mEq: milliequivalent.
Mg: magnesium.
mg: milligram.
MI: myocardial infarction.
MICN: mobile intensive care nurse.
ml: milliliter.
mm: millimeter.
MOM: milk of magnesia.
MRI: magnetic resonance imaging.
MT or **Med Tech:** medical technologist.
MVA: motor vehicle accident.

N

N: nitrogen.
n: nausea.
Na: sodium.
NA: nursing assistant.
NaCl: sodium chloride.
nc: nasal cannula.
Neur: neurology.
NIBP: non-invasive blood pressure.
NO: Nursing Office.
no: number.
noc: night.
np: nasal prongs.
NPN: nonprotein nitrogen.

NPO: nothing by mouth.
NS: normal saline.
nsy: nursery.
NWB: no weight bearing.

O

O$_2$: oxygen.
OB or **Obs:** Obstetrics.
OD: right eye; overdose.
OP: out-patient.
OR: Operating Room.
ord: orderly.
ORIF: open reduction and internal fixation.
ortho: orthopedics.
OS: left eye.
os: mouth.
OT: occupational therapy.
OTC: over the counter.
OU: each eye.
oz: ounce.

P

p̄: after; post.
P: phosphorous; pulse.
PAC: premature atrial contraction.
PACU: Post Anesthesia Care Unit.
PAST: pneumatic anti-shock trousers.
PAT: paroxysmal atrial tachycardia.
path: pathology.
PBI: protein bound iodine.
pc: after meals.
PCXR: portable chest x-ray.
PDR: Physician's Desk Reference.
peds: pediatrics.
per: by or through.
PERL: pupils equal and react to light.
PERLA: pupils equal and react to light and accommodation.
PET: positron emission tomography.
pharm: pharmacy.
PI: present illness.
PID: pelvic inflammatory disease.

PJC: premature junctional contraction.

PKU: phenylketonuria.

pm: afternoon or evening.

PMD: primary medical doctor.

PMH: past medical history; personal medical history.

po: by mouth.

PO: phone order.

post: posterior; after.

post-op: after the surgery.

PR: paced rhythm.

pre-op: before the surgery.

PRN: whenever necessary or as needed.

psy: psychology, psychiatry.

PT: physical therapy or prothrombin time.

PTCA: percutaneous transluminal coronary angioplasty.

pt: patient.

PTT: partial thromboplastin time.

PVC: premature ventricular contraction.

Q

Q or **q̄:** every.

QD or **qd:** every day; daily.

qh: every hour.

q2h: every 2 hours.

q3h: every 3 hours.

q4h: every 4 hours.

q6h: every 6 hours.

q8h: every 8 hours.

q12h: every 12 hours.

QHS or **qhs:** every night at sleep.

QID or **qid:** four times per day.

QOD or **qod:** every other day.

QS or **qs:** quantity sufficient.

Qt or **qt:** quart.

R

R: rectal; respirations.

RA: right atrium, right arm.

RBC: red blood cell/count.

RLE: right lower extremity.

RLQ: right lower quadrant.

RML: right middle lobe.

RN: registered nurse.

ROM: right otitis media or range of motion.

RR: Recovery Room; respiratory rate.

Rt: right.

RTB: respiratory tract burn.

RUE: right upper extremity.

RUQ: right upper quadrant.

RV: right ventricle.

Rx: prescription; take.

S

S: sacral.

s̄: without.

SAC: short arm cast.

SBO: small bowel obstruction.

SC or **sc:** subcutaneous.

SGOT: serum glutamic-oxaloacetic transaminase (test).

SGPT: serum glutamic pyruvic transaminase (test).

SIDS: sudden infant death syndrome.

Sig: give the following directions.

SL: sublingual.

SOB: short of breath.

Sod: sodium.

sol: solution.

sos: if necessary.

spec: specimen.

Sp Gr or **sp gr:** specific gravity.

SN: student nurse.

s̄s̄: one-half.

SSE or **SS enema:** soap solution, or soap suds, enema.

stat: at once; immediately.

STD: sexually transmitted disease.

sup: superior.

surg: surgical; surgery.

syp: syrup.

T

T or **temp:** temperature.
T & A: tonsillectomy and adenoidectomy.
tab: tablet.
TAH: total abdominal hysterectomy.
Tbs or **tbsp:** tablespoon.
TC: traffic collision.
TEMP: temperature.
TIA: transient ischemic attack.
TIBC: total iron binding capacity.
TIB-FIB: tibia-fibula.
TID or **tid:** three times daily.
TLC: tender loving care.
TO: telephone order.
TPR: temperature, pulse, and respiration.
tr or **tinct:** tincture.
tsp: teaspoon.
TURP: transurethral resection of the prostate.
tx: traction; treatment; transmit.

U

UA: urinalysis.
UCVR: uncontrolled ventricular rate.
ung: ointment.
Ur or **ur:** urine.
URI: upper respiratory infection.
US or **Uz:** ultrasound.
UTI: urinary tract infection.

V

vag: vaginal.
VD: venereal disease.
VDRL: blood test for syphilis; Venereal Disease Research Laboratories.
VO or **vo:** verbal order.
vol: volume.
VS: vital signs.

W

WBC: white blood cell/count.
WC: ward clerk.
w/c: wheelchair.
wt: weight.

X

x: times (3x means 3 times).
XR: x-ray.

Symbols

<   less than.

>   greater than.

@   at.

+   positive.

-   negative.

♀   female.

♂   male.

The Manual Alphabet

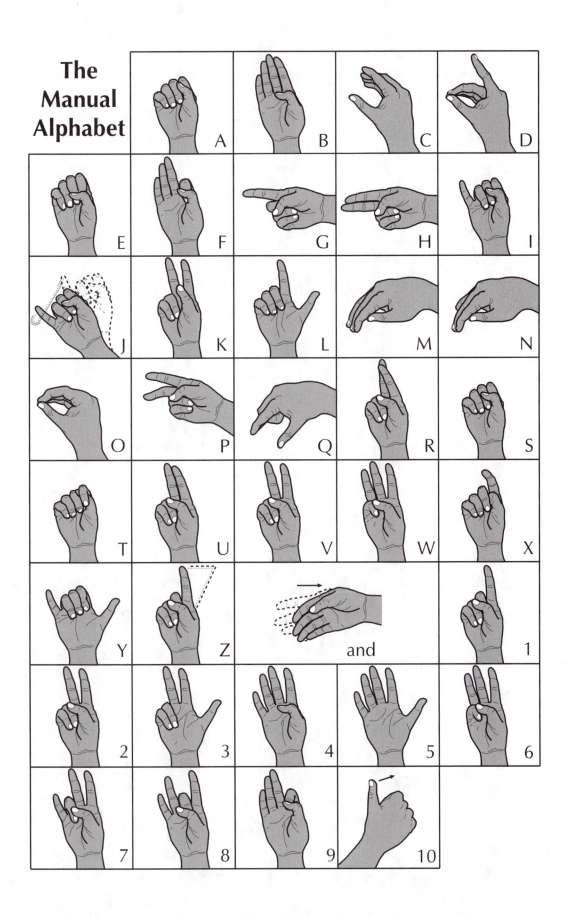

Appendix B-2

Bibliography

Caroline, MD, Nancy. *Emergency Care in the Streets*. Edited by Evan R. Schnittman. Boston: Little Brown, 1995.

Glanze, Walter, ed. *The Mosby Medical Encyclopedia, Revised Edition*. St. Louis: The C.V. Mosby Company, 1992.

Iverson, Cheryl; Dan, MD, Bruce B.; Glitman, Paula; King, MD, Lester S.; Knoll, PhD, Elizabeth; Meyer, MD, Harriet S.; Raithel, Kathryn Simmons; Riesenberg, MD, Don; Young, Roxanne K; *American Medical Association Manual of Style, 8th Edition*. Chicago: American Medical Association, 1989.

O'Toole, Marie T., ed. *Miller-Keane Encyclopedia and Dictionary of Medicine, Nursing, and Allied Health, Sixth Edition*. Philadelphia: W.B. Saunders, 1997.

PHTLS Committee of the National Association of EMTs in cooperation with the American College of Surgeons. *PHTLS Basic & Advanced*. Edited by Claire Merrick. St. Louis: Mosby Lifeline, 1994.

Sanders, Mick J. *Paramedic Textbook*. Edited by Kim McKenna, St. Louis: Mosby Lifeline, Inc., 1994.

Scanlon, Valerie C., and Tina Sanders. *Essentials of Anatomy and Physiology*. Philadelphia: F.A. Davis Company, 1991.

Shaw, Michael, ed. *Illustrated Manual of Practical Nursing*. Springhouse, PA: Springhouse Corporation, 1991.

Thomas, Clayton L., MD, MPH. *Taber's Cyclopedic Medical Dictionary, 18th Edition*. Philadelphia: F.A. Davis Company, 1997.

Yvorra, James G., ed. *Mosby's Emergency Dictionary*. St. Louis: The C.V. Mosby Company, 1989.

Index

A

abandonment   4-8
  defined   4-8
Abbreviations   12-14
abdomen   18-10, 18-11
ABG. *See* arterial blood gas.
Abraham Maslow   6-8
  defined   6-8
  hierarchy of needs   6-8
abrasions   18-17, 18-40
acceptance   5-17
accessory organs   16-13
  diagnostic tests   16-15
acquired immune deficiency syndrome
      2-18, 9-19, 9-21
  defined   9-21
acromegaly   17-12
activities of daily living (ADL), defined   11-13
acute   1-2, 1-4, 2-2
  defined   1-4
acute care hospitals   1-4, 2-1–2-5, 2-9
  in the United States   2-3
  specialized   2-5
  types of   2-3
Addison's disease   17-14
adenitis   15-14
Administration   2-5, 2-6, 2-8
Administrative Services. *See* Administration.
Admissions   2-6
Admitting.   *See* Admissions.
adolescence   5-3, 5-8, 5-9
adrenal gland   17-14
  disorders   17-14
advance directive   4-10
  defined   4-10
aerobic, defined   19-15
AIDS   4-11, 9-2, 9-19, 9-21, 9-23, 9-
      25, 9-27–9-29. *See also* acquired
      immune deficiency syndrome.
  and patient confidentiality   4-11
  defined   9-2, 9-21
air ambulance   2-4
airborne transmission   9-26
  defined   9-26
airway   18-4, 18-12–18-14, 18-16
  anatomical obstruction   18-16
  clearing   18-5

  finger sweep   18-5
  esophageal   18-7
  obstruction   18-5, 18-8, 18-16
    in adults   18-10–18-11
    in children   18-11, 18-15
    in infants   18-15
alcohol   19-5
  abuse   1-3
alignment, defined   7-3
alimentary canal, defined   14-9
allergies   3-12
allergist   3-12
allied healthcare   2-2
  services   2-5
alternating pressure mattress   11-4
alveoli, defined   15-3, 16-4
Alzheimer's disease, defined   5-12
ambulation, defined   11-5
ambulation equipment   11-5
ambulatory surgery   2-12
  centers   1-3, 1-5
amenorrhea   17-19
American Cancer Society   1-6
American Heart Association 1-6, 18-4, 18-8
American Lung Association   1-6
American Red Cross   1-6, 18-8
amniotic fluid, defined   9-28
amputations   18-17
amylase blood test   16-15
anatomy.   *See* Chapters 13, 14, 15, 16 , 17.
  cells   13-2, 13-3
    defined   13-2
  tissues   13-5, 13-6
anemia   15-10
anesthesiologist   3-12
anesthesiology   3-12
anesthetic   1-2
aneurysm   15-10
angina   15-10
angiography   15-11
angioplasty   2-4
anorexia nervosa   5-9
anoxia   16-6
antibiotics   9-8, 9-10
anticoagulants, defined   18-39
antidote, defined   18-34
anuria   16-20
anxiety   10-19, 10-26

apnea 16-6, 18-3
    defined 10-26
appendicitis 16-12
appendicular skeleton 14-4
    defined 14-4
arterial blood gas (ABG) 18-7
    test 15-11, 16-7
arteriosclerosis 15-10
artery 10-19, 15-3, 18-7, 18-17
    carotid 18-8
    defined 10-19, 15-3
arthritis 14-6
arthrogram 14-8
arthroscopy 14-8
asepsis 1-2, 1-3, 9-6, 9-7, 9-10–9-28
    defined 1-2
aseptic, defined 9-10
aseptic technique 9-21
aspiration 14-8
assault 4-8
asthma 16-6
astigmatism 17-5
asymptomatic, defined 9-23
atelectasis 16-6
atherosclerosis 15-10
atrium, defined 15-6
audiometry 17-10
auditory nerve, defined 17-8
autoclave 9-14
autonomic nervous system 15-18
    defined 15-18
avoiding chemical injuries 7-16
avulsions 18-41
axial skeleton 14-4
    defined 14-4
axilla 10-14, 10-16

B

bacilli 9-10
back tips for everyone 7-4–7-6
bacteria 9-8, 9-10, 9-21, 9-28
    controlling 9-8, 9-9
    defined 9-8
    diplococci 9-9
    Gram-staining 9-9
    normal flora 9-8
    shapes 9-9
    Staphylococci 9-9
    streptococci 9-9
bag-valve mask 18-7, 18-12
    pediatric 18-12

bargaining 5-16
barium enema 16-12
barium swallow 16-12
basal metabolic rate 19-15
    defined 19-15
basic first aid 18-1–18-42
basic life support 7-14, 18-1–21
    pediatric 18-11
battery 4-8
    defined 4-8
bed cradle 11-12
beds 11-3
bedside commode 11-9
    defined 11-9
Bill of Rights, patient's 4-4, 4-5
billing 2-6
biopsy 15-14, 16-15, 17-20
bleeding, controlling 18-17, 18-18
blood 9-16, 9-19, 9-29, 10-2, 10-19,
        10-20, 10-25, 15-4, 18-7, 18-8
    analyzing 2-9
    cells 15-4
        types 15-4, 15-5
    exposure 18-2
    flow 10-19
    testing 2-9
    tests 18-7
    transfusions 2-9
    vessels 15-3
blood pressure 2-10, 10-2, 10-31–10-32
    continuous monitoring 10-38–10-40
    auscultating, procedure 10-36, 10-37
    cuff. See sphygmomanometer.
    defined 10-31
    diastolic reading 10-31
    factors affecting 10-31, 10-32
    invasive, defined 10-32
    noninvasive 10-32, 10-45
        defined 10-32
    normal 10-31
    systolic reading 10-31
BMI. See body mass index.
body
    cavities 13-9
    fluids 9-28, 10-2, 18-2
        exposure 9-28, 18-2
    mass index 19-17
    mechanics 2-16, 7-2
        defined 7-2
    planes 13-7, 13-8
    secretions 9-24, 9-28, 9-29

bones 1-3, 14-2, 14-4
  broken 1-5, 2-9
  fracture 2-9
  parts 14-3
  types 14-3
bone marrow biopsy 14-5
bone scan 14-5
bradycardia, defined 10-20
bradypnea, defined 10-26
brain 10-19, 10-25, 10-26, 18-5, 18-9
  tumors 10-18
breach of contract 4-6
breach of duty to act 4-7
  defined 4-7
breasts 2-3
breathing 16-3–16-5, 18-3–18-7, 18-9–
    18-13
  checking for 18-5, 18-15
  rescue 18-5–18-7, 18-9, 18-12, 18-13
    mouth-to-mask 18-6, 18-12
    mouth-to-mouth 18-6, 18-12
    mouth-to-nose 18-6, 18-7
    mouth-to-stoma 18-6, 18-7
bronchitis 16-6
bronchoscopy 9-26, 16-7
bulimia 5-9
burns 18-35
  types of 18-35
bursitis 14-6
Business Office 2-6

C

calculi 16-20
call light 11-13
  defined 11-13
calorie, defined 19-7
cancer 2-10
  treatment of 2-10
canes 11-6
capillaries 15-3, 18-17
  defined 15-3
carbohydrate 19-7, 19-8
  defined 19-7
carbon dioxide 10-25
cardiac 14-9, 18-11
  arrest 18-8, 18-11
    defined 18-8
  diseases 2-4
  function 10-19
Cardiac Catheterization Laboratory 2-4
cardiac compressions 18-6, 18-9, 18-13

  defined 18-6
  procedure for 18-9
  rate for adults 18-9
cardiac enzymes test 15-11
cardiac intervention centers 2-4
Cardiac Rehabilitation Services 2-4
cardiologist 3-12
cardiology 3-7, 3-12
cardiopulmonary arrest, defined 11-11
cardiopulmonary resuscitation (CPR) 7-14,
    9-26, 11-11, 18-8, 18-9, 18-12–18-14
  defined 7-14, 11-11
cardiovascular fitness 2-10
career, defined 20-2
career opportunities 3-2
  employment agencies 20-3
  hospital job opportunity bulletin
    boards 20-4
  job placement counselors 20-3
  networking 20-4
  newspaper advertisements 20-3
career opportunities 2-3
career planning 20-1–20-18
  cover letter 20-12
    sample 20-13
  employee, ideal 20-16, 20-17
  guidelines 20-6
  interview 20-14, 20-15
  planning for success 20-2
  resumé 20-4–20-11
    formatting 20-10, 20-11
    organizing 20-8, 20-9
    sample 20-11
    writing 20-7
  self-assessment 20-7, 20-8
  telephone etiquette 20-5
cataract 17-5
catheter, defined 2-4
CDC 9-2, 9-3, 9-11, 9-25, 9-27–9-29.
    See also Centers for Disease Control
    and Prevention.
cell 13-2
  defined 13-2
  division 13-3
    meiosis 13-3, 13-4
    mitosis 13-3
Celsius 10-4
  defined 10-4
Centers for Disease Control and Prevention
    (CDC) 9-2, 9-3, 9-27. See also CDC.

defined   9-2
central circulation   10-19
    defined   10-19
central nervous system (CNS)   15-16
    defined   15-16
Central Purchasing   2-6
Central Supply Department   2-8, 9-14
cerebral palsy   15-20
cerebrospinal fluid (CSF)
    defined   9-28, 15-16
cerebrovascular accidents (CVA) 10-18,
    10-26, 10-31, 15-20
certified nursing assistant   3-2
chain of command   2-2
    defined   2-2
Chapter Summary   1-7, 2-20, 3-15, 4-15,
    5-18, 6-19, 7-21, 8-10, 10-45, 11-15,
    12-21, 13-10, 14-18, 15-21, 16-21,
    17-23, 18-42, 19-18, 20-18
charting
    blood pressure   10-35, 10-37
    height   10-44
    lung sounds   10-30
    pulse   10-22, 10-24
    respiration   10-28
    temperature   10-9, 10-11, 10-16, 10-18
    weight   10-43
chemical spills   7-16, 18-3
Chemical Dependency Unit   2-18
chemical injuries   7-16–7-18
chemicals   2-9, 7-16–7-18
chemotherapy   2-15, 8-8
chest compressions. See cardiac
    compressions.
    for infants   18-13
chest pain   18-23
chest x-ray (CXR)   15-11, 16-7
Cheyne-Stokes respiration, defined   10-26
cholecystitis   16-14
cholelithiasis   16-14
cholesterol   19-14
    defined   19-14
chronic   1-2, 1-4
    defined   1-4
chyme, defined   16-9
cilia, defined   16-3
circular double frame bed   11-3
circulation   15-6, 18-8, 18-9, 18-12
circulatory path   15-8
circulatory system   15-1, 15-2
    conditions   15-10

diagnostic tests   15-11
circumcision, defined   17-22
cirrhosis   16-13
clean technique   9-10, 9-11. See also
    medical asepsis.
    defined   9-10
Code Blue   11-11
    defined   11-11
Code of Ethics   4-3, 4-4, 4-14
colitis   16-12
Collections   2-6
combining form   12-2, 12-3
    defined   12-2
combining vowel   12-2
    defined   12-2
communication   6-1–6-16, 11-14
    call lights   11-14
    defined   6-2
    devices   6-13
        computers   6-17
        pagers   6-17
        telephones   6-14–6-16
    hearing impaired individuals   6-6
    intercom system   11-14
    learning impaired individuals   6-6
    need for   6-2
    nonverbal   6-3
    receivers   6-2
    senders   6-2
    skills   6-1, 6-2, 6-7
        clarification   6-8
        need for   6-2
        receiving the message   6-5
        reflective statements   6-8
        telephone etiquette   6-14–6-16
        transmitting the intended message   6-4
    verbal   6-3
    visually impaired individuals   6-6
community health clinics   1-3
community healthcare facilities   1-5
    types of   1-5
compensation   6-12
complete blood cell count   15-14
computerized tomography (CT) scan   2-10,
    14-5, 15-11, 15-21, 16-7, 16-12,
    16-15, 16-20, 17-20, 17-23
computers   6-17
concerns, patient   5-13, 5-14
concussion   15-20
conditions. See also diseases.
    ear   17-9

eye 17-5
intestines 16-12
parathyroid glands 17-14
reproductive system
female 17-19
male 17-22
stomach 16-9
urinary system 16-19, 16-20
confidentiality 4-10, 4-11
conization 17-20
conjuctivae 9-26
conjunctivitis 17-5
connective tissue, defined 13-5
consent 4-10
informed 4-10
constipation 16-12
constrict, defined 14-16
contact transmission 9-25
defined 9-25
types of 9-25
contagious, defined 1-2
contamination 9-10, 9-15, 9-19, 9-21, 9-27
accidental 9-16
defined 9-13
self 9-16
continuous monitoring, blood pressure 10-38
contract 4-6
defined 4-6
contusion of the brain 15-20
contusions 18-41
convalescent hospitals 1-4
convection 10-3
coping mechanisms 5-13
defined 5-13
core temperature 10-3, 10-4, 10-18, 10-45
defined 10-3
factors affecting 10-18
coronary artery disease 15-10
coronary vessels 2-4
cosmetic and reconstructive surgery 3-10
cosmetic surgeon 3-12
cosmetic surgery 3-12
counseling centers 3-11
cover letter 20-12, 20-13
defined 20-12
sample 20-13
CPR 18-6, 18-8, 18-9, 18-11–18-14, 18-26. *See also* cardiopulmonary resuscitation (CPR).
adults 18-9
children 18-11, 18-12–18-13
infants 18-11, 18-12–18-13
one-person 18-9
two-person 18-7, 18-9
crash cart 11-11, 18-7
defined 11-11
critical care 2-2, 2-13
defined 2-13
Critical Care Department 18-7
critical care nurses 3-7
Critical Care Unit 2-4, 2-13, 10-32
cross-contamination 9-25
croup 18-16
crutches 11-6
cryptorchidism 17-22
CT scans. *See* computerized tomography scan.
cultural differences 5-14
culture 15-14
defined 5-14
culture and sensitivity 14-18
Cushing's disease 17-14
custom 5-14
defined 5-14
cystitis 16-20
cystoscopy 17-23

D

damages 4-7
defined 4-7
deafness 17-9
death 9-2
and dying 5-15
defined 5-15
defamation of character 4-8
defense mechanisms 6-12
compensation 6-12
defined 6-12
displacement 6-13
projection 6-12
rationalization 6-12
denial 5-16
departments
Chemical Dependency 2-18
Dietary 3-3
Education 2-19
Emergency 3-7
Laboratory 3-3
Medical Records 3-3
Mental Health 2-18, 3-3
Pharmacy 2-11, 3-3
Physical Therapy 2-11, 3-3
Radiology 3-3

Respiratory Therapy   2-11,   3-3
depression   5-17
dermatologist   3-10, 3-12
dermatology   3-10, 3-12
development   5-3–5-7, 5-9
diabetes   10-26, 16-14
   mellitus   17-14
diagnosis   2-6
   defined   2-9
Diagnostic Services   2-5, 2-9–2-10, 2-10
diagnostic tests
   accessory organs   16-15
   alimentary canal   16-12
   circulatory system   15-11
   ear   17-10
   endocrine system   17-15
   eye   17-6
   lymphatic system   15-14
   muscular system   14-13
   nervous system   15-21
   reproductive system
      female   17-20
      male   17-23
   respiratory system   16-7
   skin   14-18
   urinary system   16-20
   diagnostic tests   2-9
diaphragm, defined   10-24, 16-4
diarrhea   16-12
diastolic, defined   10-31
diet   19-7–19-9
   cholesterol   19-14
   nutrient needs   19-9, 19-11–19-13
Dietary Department   2-8
dietetic counseling   2-4
dietician   2-8
digestive juices   16-9
digestive system   16-8–16-12, 16-15
   diagnostic tests   16-12
dilate, defined   14-16
dilation and curettage   17-20
diplococci   9-10
direct contact   9-25
   transmission   9-25
Direct Observation Unit   2-4
direct pressure   18-17
directional terms   13-7,   13-8
disasters   8-1–8-3, 8-10, 9-2
   defined   8-2
   guidelines   8-5
   preparedness   8-4, 8-6

prevention   8-1
   triage   8-2, 8-3
Discharge Planning   2-12, 5-15
diseases 1-3, 1-6, 9-24. *See also* conditions.
   adrenal gland   17-14
   cardiac   2-4
   chronic   1-4
   communicable   9-24, 9-26
   contagious   1-2
      defined   1-2
   flu   1-5
   gallbladder   16-14
   gynecological   2-3
   infectious   9-2, 9-26, 9-28
   kidney   1-5
   liver   16-13
   lung   1-5, 10-26
   muscular   14-13
   pancreas   16-14, 17-14
   pituitary gland   17-12
   prevention and control of   1-6, 9-3
   reproductive system
      female   17-9
      male   17-22
   thyroid gland   17-13
disinfectants, types of   9-13
disinfection   9-6, 9-7, 9-13, 9-29
dislocation   14-6
disorders. *See* conditions and diseases.
displacement   6-13
disposable supplies   9-19
doctors   1-2, 3-5. *See also* physicians.
   education   3-6
donning sterile gloves 9-17, 9-18
drainage bag   11-9
dressings   9-25
   changing   1-5
droplet transmission   9-26
   defined   9-26
drug abuse   1-3
drugs   19-5
duty to act   4-7
   defined   4-7
dwarfism   17-12
dyspnea   10-26, 16-6
   defined   10-26
dysuria   16-20

E

ear 17-7–17-10
  conditions of 17-9
  diagnostic tests 17-10
  equilibrium 17-7
  hearing 17-8, 17-9
early adulthood 5-3, 5-10
early childhood 5-3, 5-5
ECGs. *See* electrocardiograms.
echocardiography 15-11
ectopic pregnancy 17-19, 18-17
edema, defined 13-5
education
  institutions 2-3
  patient 1-6, 2-8
  physician 1-5
  public 1-6
Education Department 2-19
EEGs. *See* electroencephalograms
eggcrate mattress, defined 11-4
EKGs. *See* electrocardiograms.
elastic stockings 11-11
electric shock 7-15
electrocardiogram, defined 2-10
electrocardiography 15-11
electroencephalograms 2-10
electrolytes 19-13
Elisabeth Kubler-Ross, defined 5-15
emergencies 3-12
emergency calls 6-15
Emergency Department 2-4, 2-13, 3-7,
    10-32, 18-7
emergency medicine 3-7
emergency nurses 3-7
emergency physician 3-12
Emergency Room. *See* Emergency Depart-
    ment
emphysema 16-6
employee, ideal 20-16, 20-17
employment agencies 20-3
endocrine 17-12
  defined 17-12
  system 17-2, 17-12–17-14
    diagnostic tests 17-15
endocrinologist 3-12
endocrinology 3-12
endometriosis 17-19
endoscopy 16-12
endoscopy nurse 3-8
endotracheal tube 18-7

enteritis 16-12
Environmental Services Department 9-10
enzymes 16-9
epiglottis 18-10
epiglottitis 18-16
epilepsy 15-20
epistaxis 16-6, 18-39
epithelial tissue, defined 13-5
equilibrium 17-7
equipment 11-1–11-15
  alternating pressure mattress 11-4
  ambulation 11-5
    canes 11-6
    crutches 11-6
    walkers 11-6
    wheelchair 11-5
  and safety 7-14
  bed cradle 11-12
  beds 11-3
  call light 11-13
  circular double frame bed 11-3
  crash cart 11-11
  diagnostic 1-3
  eggcrate mattress 11-4
  elastic stockings 11-11
  excretory 11-9
    bedside commode 11-9
    drainage bag 11-9
    indwelling catheter 11-9
  foot board 11-12
  footdrop 11-12
  gurneys 11-3
  intercom system 11-13
  intravenous therapy 11-8
    IV infusion pump 11-8
  medical 1-6
  operation 11-2
  patient lift 11-10
  respiratory 11-7
    incentive spirometers 11-8
    intermittent positive pressure breathing
      machines 11-7
    nasal cannula 11-7
    nebulizer 11-7
    oxygen mask 11-7
  stryker frame 11-3
  traction
    trapeze 11-5
  warming blanket 11-12
  x-ray 1-3
esteem 6-11

estrogen, defined   17-16
ether   1-2
ethics   4-1, 4-3, 4-4, 4-14
    decisions   4-4
    defined   4-4
    evaporation   10-3
excretion   16-1
excretory equipment   11-9
        bedside commode   11-9
        drainage bag   11-9
        indwelling catheter   11-9
exercise   19-8, 19-15
exhalation   18-5
exocrine   17-12
    defined   17-12
expiration   10-25
extended care facility   1-4
eye   17-3–17-5
    conditions   17-5
    diagnostic tests   17-6
    protection   9-26

F

fahrenheit   10-4
    defined   10-4
fainting   18-25
fallopian tubes   2-3
false imprisonment   4-8
family practice   3-7, 3-12
family practitioner   1-5, 3-12
fat   19-7–19-8
    defined   19-8
FHP   1-6
finger sweep   18-11, 18-15
    defined   18-5
fire   7-18, 7-19, 7-21
    extinguishers   7-19, 7-21
        operation of   7-21
    safety   7-18
first aid   18-1, 18-2
    breathing   18-6
    burns   18-35
    cardiac arrest   18-8
    chest pain   18-23
    defined   18-2
    epistaxis   18-39
    fainting   18-25
    fractures   18-37, 18-38
    guidelines   18-3
    jaw-thrust maneuver   18-4
    log roll   18-26–18-32

    four-person   18-30–18-32
        three-person   18-27–18-29
    nosebleeds   18-39
    poisoning   18-33, 18-34
    primary survey   18-3, 18-8
        defined   18-3
        performing   18-3
    secondary survey   18-19
    seizures   18-22
    shock   18-20
    shortness of breath   18-24
    soft tissue injuries   18-40, 18-41
    sprains   18-37, 18-38
    syncope   18-25
    unconscious patients   18-26
fluoroscopy   16-7
foot board   11-12
footdrop   11-12
Fowler's position   18-24
fractures   18-17, 18-37,   18-38
fraud and misrepresentation   4-8
fundamental skills   10-1–10-45
fungi   9-8, 9-10
    defined   9-8

G

gallbladder, diseases   16-14
gas exchange, defined   15-3
gastritis   16-9
gastroenterologist   3-13
gastroenterology   3-8, 3-13
gastrointestinal tract   9-5
gastrostomy tube feedings   1-5
general hospitals   2-3
general practitioner   1-5
general surgeon   3-8
general surgery   3-13
geriatric nurse specialists   3-9
geriatrics   2-16, 5-2
gerontology   3-9
gigantism   17-12
gland   17-12
    adrenal   17-14
    defined   14-14, 17-12
    parathyroid   17-14
    pituitary   17-12
    sex   17-15
    thymus   17-15
    thyroid   17-13
    types   14-14, 17-12
glaucoma   17-5

gloves 9-15, 9-16, 9-21, 9-25, 9-26, 9-27, 9-29, 10-2, 18-2, 18-5, 18-7
  changing 9-25
goiter 17-13
gonorrhea 17-19, 17-22
gout 14-6
gown 9-26, 9-29
gowns 9-25, 9-26, 9-27
growth and development 5-3–5-9
gurneys 7-8, 7-9, 11-3
  defined 11-3
gynecologist 3-13
gynecology 3-9

H

handwashing 9-11–9-13, 9-26
  guidelines 9-11
  procedure for 9-12, 9-13
hazard communication label, defined 7-17
hazardous waste 9-3
hazards 7-7–7-21, 8-1, 8-6–8-9
head-tilt/chin-lift maneuver 18-4, 18-5, 18-10, 18-12
  defined 18-4
health clinics 1-5
health insurance plans 1-3, 1-6
health maintenance organizations 1-6
  examples 1-6
Health Net 1-6
Health Occupations Students of America (HOSA) 4-14
  defined 4-14
health unit coordinators 3-5
healthcare facilities 1-1–1-7, 2-2, 2-4, 2-5, 2-8
  community healthcare facilities 1-5
  counseling centers 3-11
  health clinics 1-5
  health maintenance organizations 1-6
  history 1-2, 1-3, 1-7
  home health agencies 1-5
  medical offices 1-5
  mental healthcare facilities 1-5
  outpatient clinic 1-5
  policies and procedures 10-20
  skilled nursing facilities 1-5
  types 1-4–1-7, 2-4
  urgent care centers 1-5
healthcare provider 1-6, 1-7
  defined 4-6
  lawsuits 4-2, 4-8, 4-9

healthcare worker 9-10
  obligations 4-2
healthful living 19-1
  alcohol 19-5
  diet 19-7–19-9
    cholesterol 19-14
    nutrient needs 19-9–19-13
  drugs 19-5
  exercise 19-15
  hypertension 19-4
  preventive healthcare 19-2
  smoking 19-3
  stress management 19-6
  weights, suggested 19-16
hearing 17-7–17-9
heart 2-4, 10-19, 15-6, 18-8, 18-9
  anatomy 15-6
  apex 10-20
  conditions 10-19
  function 15-6
  monitor 2-10
  rates 10-20
  relaxation 10-31
  rhythms of 1-3
heart attack 18-11 *See also* myocardial infarction.
heart rate 2-10
heart rhythm 2-4
heart vessels. *See* coronary vessels.
heartburn 16-9
height 10-41, 19-16
Heimlich maneuver 18-10, 18-15, 18-16
  defined 18-10
    procedure for adults 18-10
    procedure for children 18-15
    procedure for infants 18-16
helipad, defined 2-4
hematuria 16-20
hemiplegia 15-20
hemophilia 15-10, 18-17
hemorrhage 18-2, 18-3, 18-17
hemorrhoids 16-12
hemothorax 16-6
hepatitis 2-18, 9-21, 9-25, 9-27, 16-13
  causes 9-21
  defined 9-21
hepatitis A 9-21
  defined 9-21
hepatitis B 9-19, 9-21, 9-27, 9-28
  defined 9-21
hepatitis C 9-21, 9-27

defined   9-21
herpes   17-19
herpes zoster   9-25
high Fowler's position   18-24
high risk, defined   3-9
high-density lipoprotein (HDL), defined 19-14
HIV positive   4-11
HMOs   1-6
   examples of   1-6
Hodgkin's disease   15-14
Holter monitor   2-10
home healthcare   1-2, 1-5
   agencies   1-5
      defined   1-5
      number of   1-5
homeostasis   10-3
   defined   10-3
HOSA   4-14
hospice   5-18
   defined   5-18
hospital(s)   1-2, 1-3, 1-4, 1-5
   as nonprofit agencies   1-6
   children's   1-3
   departments   2-3, 2-5, 2-6
      Admissions   2-6
      Billing   2-6
      Business Office   2-6
      Central Supply   9-14
      Collections   2-6
      Communications   2-8
      Dietary   2-8
      Emergency   1-5
      Engineering and Maintenance   2-8
      Environmental Services   2-8, 9-10
      Grounds Keeping   2-8
      Housekeeping   9-10
      Infection Control   9-3, 9-7
      Laboratory   2-9
      Medical Records   2-8
      Purchasing   2-6
      Radiology   2-10
      Security   2-8
      Transportation   2-6
   employees   3-1–3-15
   environment   2-19
   establishment   1-2
   for the developmentally disabled   1-3
   operation   2-3, 2-5, 2-6
   organizational structure   2-2, 2-3, 2-5
   overcrowding   1-3
   pediatric   2-3

   policies and procedures   9-3, 9-27
   quality of care   1-2
   specialization   1-3
   women's   1-3
hospital job opportunity bulletin boards 20-4
hospitalis   1-2
   defined   1-2
Housekeeping Department   9-10
human needs   6-8
   affection and love   6-8, 6-10
   esteem   6-8, 6-11
   meeting   6-11
   physiological needs   6-8, 6-9
   safety and security   6-8, 6-10
   self-actualization   6-8, 6-11
hypermenorrhea   17-19
hyperopia   17-5
hyperparathyroidism   17-14
hyperpnea, defined   10-26
hyperpyrexia, defined   10-19
hypertension (HTN)   10-31, 15-10, 19-4
   defined   10-31
   symptoms   10-31
hyperthyroidism   17-13
hyperventilation   16-6
hypoparathyroidism   17-14
hypotension   15-10
hypothalamus   10-3, 10-14
   defined   10-3
hypothermia, defined   10-19
hypothyroidism   17-13
hypovolemic shock   18-20
   defined   18-20

I

Imaging Department   2-9
immune system   9-6, 9-21, 9-24
incentive spirometers   11-8
incontinence   16-20
indirect contact   9-25
   transmission   9-25
indirect pressure   18-18
industrial
   accidents   7-2
   illnesses 9-3, 9-11
      defined   9-3
      reducing the risk of   9-11
indwelling catheter   11-9
   defined   11-9
infancy   5-2, 5-4
infection   2-8

control   9-1–9-29
  disposable supplies   9-19
  plan   9-25
cycle   9-4, 9-6, 9-29
  breaking   9-4
  components   9-4–9-6
  defined   9-4
  interrupting   9-6, 9-29
opportunistic   9-23
prevention   1-2
reducing the risk   9-29
Infection Control Department   2-18, 9-3,
    9-7
infectious agent   9-4, 9-6
  defined   9-4
infectious disease   9-25
infertility   3-10
  defined   3-10
influenza   9-26, 16-6
informed consent   4-10
injections   1-5
injuries   1-5, 18-2, 18-4
  spinal   18-4
  traumatic   1-5
inspiration   10-25
instruments   2-8
  surgical   2-8
insulin, defined   16-14
insurance companies   2-6
integumentary system   14-1, 14-14–14-18
Intensive Care Department   18-7
Intensive Care Units   1-3
intercom system, defined   11-13
intermittent positive pressure breathing
    machines   11-7
intern   3-6
internal medicine   3-13
internist   3-13
interviews   20-14, 20-15
intravenous feedings   1-5
intravenous therapy   11-8
invasion of privacy   4-8
irreversible brain death
  defined   3-11
isolation   9-24
  reverse   9-24
IV infusion pump   11-8
  defined   11-8

J

jaw-thrust maneuver   18-4, 18-5, 18-12
  defined   18-4
job, defined   20-2
job fairs   20-4
joints   14-2, 14-6–14-8
  defined   14-6
  diagnostic tests   14-8
  diseases   14-6
  injuries   14-6
  motion groups   14-7
  types   14-6

K

Kaiser Permanente   1-6
kidneys   10-19, 16-16, 16-17
  abnormalities   10-26
  defined   16-16
  function of   16-16
Kussmaul's breathing, defined   10-26

L

Labor and Delivery   2-15
laboratory   2-9, 3-3
laboratory technician   18-7
lacerations   18-17, 18-41
laryngectomy   18-7
laryngitis   16-6
larynx, defined   16-3
late adulthood   5-12
late childhood   5-3, 5-6
law   4-1–4-13
  AIDS   4-11
  confidentiality   4-10
  consent   4-10
  contract   4-6, 4-7
  intentional torts   4-8
  legal terms   4-13
lawsuits   4-9
  malpractice   4-8
  negligence   4-8
legal terms   4-13
licensed practical nurse (LPN)   3-4
licensed vocational nurse (LVN)   3-4
life stages   5-3
  adolescence   5-8, 5-9
  defined   5-3
  early adulthood   5-10
  early childhood   5-5, 5-6

infancy   5-4
  late adulthood   5-12
  late childhood   5-6
  middle adulthood   5-11
listening for lung sounds   10-29, 10-30
liver
  diseases of   16-13
  functions of   16-13
liver function tests   16-15
log roll   18-12, 18-26, 18-32, 18-38
  defined   18-12
  four-person   18-30–18-32
  three-person   18-27–18-29
long-term care facility   1-4
loss of consciousness   18-26
love and affection   6-10
low-density lipoprotein (LDL), defined 19-14
lumbar puncture   15-21
lung(s)   18-9
  cancer   16-6
  diseases   10-26
  scan   16-7
  sounds   10-28
lymphatic system   15-1, 15-12, 15-13
  conditions of   15-14
  diagnostic tests   15-14

M

magnetic resonance imaging 14-5, 15-11,
      15-21, 16-7, 16-12, 16-15, 17-20, 17-23
malpractice   4-8
  defined   4-8
mask(s)   9-26, 9-29, 18-6, 18-7, 18-12
  bag-valve   18-6
  pocket   18-6, 18-7, 18-12
Maslow's Hierarchy of Needs   6-8
  defined   6-8
Material Safety Data Sheet 7-17, 8-8,
      8-10, 9-13
  defined   7-17
measles   9-26
measuring
  apical pulse   10-23, 10-24
  axillary temperature 10-17, 10-18
  height (length)
    adults   10-44
    infants   10-41
  oral temperature
    electronic thermometer 10-5, 10-6
    glass thermometer   10-10, 10-11
  radial pulse   10-21, 10-22

rectal temperature
    electronic thermometer   10-7–10-9
    glass thermometer   10-12, 10-13
  respiration   10-27, 10-28
  tympanic temperature   10-15, 10-16
  weight
    adult   10-42, 10-43
    children   10-41
    infants   10-41
Medic-Alert, defined   18-22
medical
  asepsis   9-10–9-11, 9-11
    defined   9-10
    handwashing   9-11
  assistants   3-2
  nurses   3-9
  specialties   3-7–3-14
  staff   3-1–3-15
  terminology   12-1–12-21
    abbreviations   12-14
    combining form   12-2
    combining vowel   12-2
    prefix   12-2
    root word   12-2
    surgical nurses   3-8, 3-10
    suffix   12-2
    symbols   12-21
Medical Records   3-3
Medical Surgical Nursing Unit   2-14
Medical Surgical Unit   3-8
medication   10-19, 10-41
medicine   2-3
  advances in   1-3
  school of   2-3
meiosis   13-3, 13-4
  defined   13-3
meninges, defined   15-16
meningitis   15-20
menstruation, defined   17-17
mental   5-3
mental health   3-3, 3-11
Mental Health Department   2-18
mental healthcare facilities   1-5
  defined   1-5
metabolism   17-13
  defined   16-14
microorganisms   9-4, 9-8, 9-10, 9-14
  defined   9-8
  infectious   9-4
middle adulthood   5-3
minerals   19-7, 19-11

defined   19-7
minors, treatment   4-7
mitosis   13-3
   defined   13-3
molds   9-8
Mothers Against Drunk Driving   1-6
motor neurons
   defined   15-15
mucous membrane   9-25, 9-26
mumps   9-26
muscle(s)   14-8, 14-10, 14-12
   diseases   14-13
   involuntary   10-25
   movement   14-8
   tissue, defined   13-6
   types   14-9
   voluntary   10-25, 10-26
muscular
   diseases   14-13
   dystrophy   14-13
   system   14-1, 14-8
      diagnostic tests   14-13
myalgia   14-13
myocardial infarction   2-2, 2-4, 15-10
   defined   2-4
myopia   17-5
myositis   14-13

N

National Institute for Occupational Safety
      and Health   8-7
national student health organizations   4-14
   HOSA   4-14
   VICA   4-14
nausea   16-9
nebulizer   11-7
need, defined   6-8
needle sticks   7-7, 9-19, 9-21
needles   1-3
negligence   4-8
   defined   4-8
neonate   2-3
   defined   3-9
neonatology   3-9
neonatology nurse   3-9
Neonatology Unit   2-3
nephrologist   1-5
nephrology   3-8
nephrons   16-17, 16-18
   defined   16-17
nerve, defined   15-16

nerve conduction studies   15-21
nerve tissue, defined   13-5
nervous system   15-1, 15-14, 15-15
   central nervous system   15-16–15-18
   conditions   15-20
   diagnostic tests   15-21
   peripheral nervous system
      autonomic nervous system   15-18
      somatic nervous system   15-18
networking   20-4
neuralgia   15-20
neurologist   3-9, 3-13
neurology   3-9
newspaper advertisements   20-3
NIOSH   8-7
nonprofit agencies   1-6, 1-7
   defined   1-6
   examples   1-6
nonverbal
   communication   6-3, 6-7
   defined   6-3
normal flora   9-8
nose   10-20
nosebleeds   18-39
nosocomial infection   9-3, 9-25
   defined   9-3
   reducing the risk of   9-11, 9-25
nuclear medicine   2-10
nurse(s)   1-5, 3-3, 10-45, 18-7
nursing   2-2, 2-5
   staff   2-6
   units   2-8
Nursing Services   2-5, 2-12
   ambulatory surgery   2-12
   emergency department   2-13
   geriatrics   2-16
   labor and delivery   2-15
   medical surgical nursing   2-14
   oncology   2-15
   orthopedics   2-16
   outpatient surgery   2-12
   pediatrics   2-14

O

OB-GYN nurse specialists   3-9, 3-10
Objectives 1-1, 2-1, 3-1, 5-1, 6-1, 7-1, 8-1,
      9-1, 10-1, 11-1, 12-1, 13-1, 14-1, 15-1,
      16-1, 17-1, 18-1, 19-1, 20-1
obstetrician   3-13
obstetrics   3-9, 3-13
obstructed airway maneuver   18-6

occult blood   16-12
Occupational Safety and Health
    Administration (OSHA)   8-7
    defined   8-7
occupations   3-2
    allergist   3-12
    anesthesiologist   3-12
    cardiologist   3-7, 3-12
    certified nursing assistant   3-2
    cosmetic surgeon   3-12
    critical care nurses   3-7
    dermatologist   3-10, 3-12
    doctor   3-5
    emergency nurses   3-7
    emergency physician   3-12
    endocrinologist   3-12
    endoscopy nurse   3-8
    family practitioner   3-12
    gastroenterologist   3-13
    general surgeon   3-8
    geriatric nurse specialists   3-9
    gynecologist   3-13
    health unit coordinators   3-5
    internist   3-13
    licensed practical nurse (LPN)   3-4
    licensed vocational nurse (LVN)   3-4
    medical assistants   3-2
    medical nurses   3-7, 3-9
    medical surgical nurse   3-10
    medical surgical nurses   3-8
    neonatology nurse   3-9
    neurologist   3-9, 3-13
    OB-GYN nurse specialists   3-9, 3-10
    obstetrician   3-13
    oncologist   3-13
    oncology nurse specialists   3-9
    operating room nurse   3-10
    ophthalmologist   3-13
    orthopedic nurse specialist   3-11
    orthopedic specialist   3-11
    orthopedic surgeon   3-14
    orthopedist   3-14
    otolaryngologist   3-14
    pathologist   3-14
    pediatric nurse specialists   3-10
    pediatrician   3-14
    physiatrist   3-14
    proctologist   3-14
    psychiatric nurse specialists   3-11
    psychiatrist   3-11, 3-14
    radiologist   3-14

    registered nurses   3-3, 3-4
    surgeon   3-13
    surgical nurse   3-10
    thoracic surgeon   3-14
    urologist   3-14
oliguria   16-20
oncologist   3-13
oncology   3-9, 3-13
oncology nurse specialists   3-9
Oncology Unit   2-15
operating room   18-7
operating room nurse   3-10
ophthalmologist   3-13
ophthalmology   3-10, 3-13
ophthalmoscope   17-6
organ, defined   13-6
organ transplant   3-11
    defined   3-11
organism   9-11
    defined   9-8
organs   10-19, 18-9
orthopedic nurse specialist   3-11
orthopedic specialist   3-11
orthopedic surgeon   3-14
orthopedics   2-16, 3-14
orthopedist   3-14
OSHA   8-7
ossicles   17-7
otitis externa   17-9
otitis media   17-9
otolaryngologist   3-14
otolaryngology   3-14
otoscope   17-10
outpatient clinic   1-5
outpatient surgery   2-12
ovarian cyst   17-19
ovaries   2-3, 17-15
oxygen   10-25, 18-6
    consumption   2-10
    equipment   1-3, 11-7, 11-8
    levels in the blood   18-7

P

palliative, defined   5-18
pancreas   17-14
    defined   16-14
    disorders   16-14, 17-14
pancreatitis   16-14, 17-14
pap smear   17-20
paracentesis   16-15
paramedic   18-7

parasympathetic nervous system   15-18
  defined   15-18
parathyroid glands   17-14
  conditions   17-14
pathogens 9-2, 9-4–9-8, 9-10, 9-13,
    9-14, 9-24–9-29
  controlling   9-10, 9-24–9-28
  defined   9-2, 9-8
  types of   9-8
pathologist   3-14
pathology   3-14
patient(s)
  advocate, defined   4-2
  as a person   5-1–5-18
  cardiac   2-4
  care   2-3, 2-5
    advances   1-3
    equipment   11-1
    improvements   1-3
  concerns   5-13, 5-14
  elderly   1-4
  injured   1-2
  lift   11-10
    defined   11-10
  medical records   2-8
  right to die   5-18
  safety   7-7
  stress   5-13, 5-14
  transfers   7-8, 7-9, 7-10
  trust   4-2
  unit   11-13
    defined   11-13
  who smoke   7-13
Patient Care Unit   11-12
Patient Self-Determination Act   4-10
Patient's Bill of Rights   4-4
  defined   4-4
pediatric hospitals   2-3
pediatrician   3-14
pediatrics   2-3, 2-14, 3-14
  defined   2-3
pediculosis   9-25
pelvic inflammatory disease (PID)   17-19
pelvic ultrasound   17-20
pericardial fluid, defined   9-28
peripheral circulation   10-20
  defined   10-20
peripheral nervous system 15-18
  autonomic nervous system   15-18
    parasympathetic nervous system   15-18
    sympathetic nervous system   15-18

defined   15-16
  somatic nervous system   15-18
peristalsis, defined   14-9, 16-8
peritoneal fluid, defined   9-28
personal protection equipment   9-25–9-29
pertussis   9-26
pharmacy   2-11, 3-3
phimosis   17-22
phlebitis   15-10
physiatrist   3-14
physical examinations   1-5, 1-6
physical medicine   3-14
physical therapy   2-6, 3-3
Physical Therapy Department   2-11
physician 1-5, 2-9, 2-10, 9-6, 10-45, 18-7
physiological needs   6-9
physiology   2-14, 13-2
  defined   13-2
pituitary gland   17-12
  disorders   17-12
pleural fluid, defined   9-28
pleurisy   16-6
PMI, defined   10-24
pneumonia   9-26, 16-6
Poison Control   18-34
  defined   18-34
poisoning   18-33, 18-34
poliomyelitis   15-20
polyuria   16-20
portal of entry, defined   9-5
portals of exit   9-5, 9-6
  defined   9-5
portals of entry   9-7
position
  football   18-13
  Fowler's   18-24
  semi-Fowler's   18-24
  supine   18-11, 18-12, 18-13, 18-15
  Trendelenburg   18-21
Post Anesthesia Care Unit   2-17
Post Partum Unit   2-15
prefix   12-2
  defined   12-2
pressure points   18-18
preventing
  falls   7-12
  injuries   7-11
preventive healthcare   19-2
  defined   19-2
primary care   3-4
primary survey, defined   18-3

privileged information, defined   4-11
procedures
   blood pressure
      auscultating   10-36, 10-37
      continuous monitoring   10-39, 10-40
   cardiac compressions   18-9
   CPR
      adults   18-9
      children   18-11, 18-12–18-13
      infants   18-11, 18-12–18-13
   height
      adult   10-44
   Heimlich maneuver   18-10
      adults   18-10
      children   18-15
      infants   18-16
   listening for lung sounds   10-29, 10-30
   pulse
      apical   10-23, 10-24
      radial   10-21, 10-22
   respiration   10-27, 10-28
   temperature
      axillary   10-17, 10-18
      oral
         electronic thermometer 10-5, 10-6
         glass thermometer 10-10, 10-11
      rectal
         electronic thermometer 10-7–10-9
         glass thermometer   10-12, 10-13
      tympanic   10-15, 10-16
   ventilation
      mouth-to-mask   18-6
      mouth-to-mouth   18-6
      mouth-to-stoma   18-7
   weight
      adult   10-42, 10-43
      children   10-41
      infants   10-41
proctologist   3-14
proctology   3-14
professional ethics   4-1
protective devices   18-2
protective eye wear   9-27, 9-29
protein   19-7, 19-8
   defined   19-8
protozoa   9-8
   defined   9-8
proximate cause   4-7
   defined   4-7
Psychiatric Department   2-18
psychiatric nurse specialists   3-11

psychiatrist   3-11, 3-14
psychiatry   3-14
psychology   2-14
Public Health Department   1-5
Public Health Service   9-3
pulmonary angiography   16-7
pulmonary function tests   16-7
pulmonary medicine   3-7
   defined   3-7
pulmonary specialist   1-5
pulse 10-2, 10-19–10-20, 10-25,
      10-45, 18-8, 18-9, 18-13
   apical   10-20
   bounding, defined   10-20
   brachial   18-12
      location   10-20
   carotid   10-19, 18-12
      location   10-19
   defined   10-19
   femoral   10-19
      location   10-19
   pedal, location   10-20
   radial, location   10-20
   sites   10-20
   thready, defined   10-20
puncture wounds   18-40
Purchasing Department 2-6
pyelonephritis   16-20

R

radiation   2-9, 2-10, 10-3
radiologist   3-14
radiology   2-9, 2-10, 3-3, 3-14
Radiology Department   2-10, 8-8
radiology studies   17-23
range of motion, defined   7-4
rationalization   6-12
receiver 6-2, 6-6, 6-7
   defined   6-2
records
   laboratory test results   1-3
   medical   1-3
   pharmacy   1-3
registered nurses   3-3, 3-4
rehabilitation   2-11, 3-14
rehabilitation facilities   1-4
removing contaminated gloves
   procedure for   9-20
reoxygenate   18-7
reproductive system   17-2, 17-16–17-22
   female   17-16 – 17-18

conditions   17-19
diagnostic tests   17-20
male   17-20, 17-21, 17-22
diagnostic tests   17-23
diseases   17-22
reproductive tract   9-5
reservoir   9-5
reservoir host   9-6
defined   9-4
resident   3-6
resistance   9-6
respiration(s)   10-2, 10-26, 16-5, 18-8
defined   10-25
respiratory
arrest   18-8, 18-11
cycle   10-25
devices   11-7
patterns   10-26, 10-28
rate   10-25, 10-26, 10-45
system   16-1, 16-2, 16-4
conditions   16-6
diagnostic tests   16-7
therapist   18-7
therapy   3-3
tract   9-5
Respiratory Therapy Department   2-11
resumé   20-5, 20-7, 20-9
defined   20-4
formatting   20-10
organizing   20-8, 20-9
sample   20-11
writing   20-7
reverse isolation   9-24
defined   9-24
rheumatology   3-9
defined   3-9
rhinitis   16-6
rickettsiae   9-10
defined   9-10
right to die   5-18
defined   5-18
Rinne test   17-10
rooming-in, defined   2-15
root word   12-2
defined   12-2
routes of transmission   9-6
defined   9-5
rubella   9-26

S

safety   6-10, 8-8
accident prevention   8-9
and electric shock   7-15
and equipment   7-14
and hazards   8-6
avoiding chemical injuries   7-16
back tips for everyone   7-4, 7-5, 7-6
body mechanics   7-2
fire   7-18, 7-19
needle sticks   7-7
patient   7-7
patient transfers   7-8, 7-9, 7-10
patients who smoke   7-13
preventing falls   7-12
protecting your spine   7-3
siderails   7-11
workplace   7-1–7-24
saliva   9-28
scabies   9-25
scarlet fever   9-26
scope of practice   4-2, 4-3
defined   4-2
secondary survey   18-19
defined   18-19
secure horizons   1-6
seizure   2-10, 18-22
defined   18-22
self-actualization   6-11
semen   9-28
semi-Fowler's position   18-24
semipermeable
defined   13-2
sender   6-2
defined   6-2
senses
hearing   17-7 – 17-9
vision   17-3, 17-4, 17-5
sensory neurons, defined   15-15
sensory system   17-1, 17-2
ear   17-8–17-10
eye   17-3–17-5
smell   17-11
taste   17-11
touch   17-11, 17-12
sexuality   6-10
sexually transmitted diseases   17-19
defined   17-19
sharps   9-16, 9-19, 9-27
avoiding contamination   9-19–9-21

containers   9-19
guidelines   9-19
shigella   9-25
shock   18-3, 18-17, 18-20
shortness of breath   18-24
siderails   7-11
significant others, defined   6-2
sinoatrial node, defined   15-6
skeletal system   14-2, 14-4
    appendicular   14-4
    axial   14-4
    diagnostic tests   14-5
    disorders   14-5
    functions   14-2
skilled nursing   1-5
    facilities   1-5
skills   10-1–10-45
skin   10-20
    diagnostic tests   14-18
    diseases and disorders   14-17
    functions   14-15, 14-16
    layers   14-14
    parts   14-15
    scrapings   14-18
slit lamp   17-6
small bowel series   16-12
smell   17-11
smoking   2-19, 19-3
Snellen eye test   17-6
sniffing position   18-4
social   5-3
Social Services   5-15
Social Services Department   2-12, 6-6
soft tissue injuries   18-40, 18-41
somatic nervous system, defined   15-18
special systems   17-2
specialties   3-7–3-14
speculum   10-14
sphygmomanometer   10-31, 10-32
spinal injury   18-26, 18-38
spirilla   9-10
splenomegaly   15-14
spores   9-9, 9-14
sports medicine   3-11
sprains   14-6, 18-37, 18-38
sputum   9-28
stages of dying   5-15
    acceptance   5-17
    anger   5-16
    bargaining   5-16
    denial   5-16

depression   5-17
Standard Precautions   9-6, 9-24–9-29
    defined   9-25
Staphylococci   9-8, 9-10, 9-11, 9-25
sterile field   9-15, 9-16
    defined   9-15
    guidelines   9-15
sterile technique   9-10, 9-15–9-16. *See
    also* surgical asepsis.
    defined   9-10
sterilization   2-2, 2-8, 9-6, 9-7, 9-14, 9-19
    defined   2-8
    methods of   9-14
sterilize   9-29
sternum   18-9, 18-13, 18-14
    xiphoid process   18-10, 18-11, 18-15
stethoscope   9-25, 10-20, 10-31
stoma   18-7
strabismus   17-5
streptococcal pharyngitis   9-26
Streptococci   9-10
stress   2-4, 5-13, 19-7
    management   19-6
    patient   5-13
    test   2-10, 15-11
striated   14-10
strokes   10-18, 10-26. *See also*
    cerebrovascular accidents.
Stryker frame   11-3
Student Enrichment Activities 1-9, 2-21,
    3-17, 4-17, 5-19, 6-21, 7-23, 8-11,
    9-31, 10-47, 11-17, 12-23, 13-11,
    14-19, 15-23, 16-23, 17-25, 18-43,
    19-19, 20-19
substance abuse   5-10
Substance Abuse Unit   2-18
suction machine   18-11, 18-15
sudden death, defined   7-14
suffix   12-2
    defined   12-2
suicide   5-10
Support Services   2-5, 2-6, 2-6–2-8, 2-8
surgeon   3-13
surgery   1-2, 1-5, 3-8, 9-10, 10-18, 18-17
    elective   2-17
    emergency   2-17
    open heart   2-4
surgical asepsis   9-10–9-11
    defined   9-10
surgical nurse   3-10
surgical procedures   9-14

surgical suites   2-4
susceptible host   9-7, 9-25, 9-26
   defined   9-6
symbols   12-21
sympathetic nervous system   15-18
   defined   15-18
syncope   18-25
   defined   18-25
synovial fluid, defined   9-28, 14-6
syphilis   17-19, 17-22
syringes   1-3
system, defined   13-6
systolic, defined   10-31
systolic blood pressure   10-33 – 10-35

T

tachycardia, defined   10-20
tachypnea, defined   10-26
taste   17-11
taste receptors, defined   17-11
tastebuds   17-11
team nursing   3-4
telephone etiquette   6-14–6-16, 20-5
temperature   10-2–10-18, 10-19, 10-25
   axillary   10-3, 10-14, 10-16
   environmental   10-18
   oral   10-3
   readings   10-14
   recognizing abnormal   10-18
   rectal   10-3
   scales   10-4
      converting   10-4
   tympanic   10-3, 10-14
terminology, medical   12-2
testes   17-15
   defined   17-20
testosterone, defined   17-20
therapeutic radiology   3-14
Therapeutic Services   2-5, 2-8, 2-11
   cardiac rehabilitation   2-11
   dietary therapy   2-11
   occupational therapy   2-11
   pharmacy   2-11
   physical therapy   2-11
   respiratory therapy   2-11
   speech therapy   2-11
therapy
   exercise   2-4
   radiation   2-10
thermometers   1-3, 10-9, 10-14, 10-16
   digital   10-9

   electronic   10-4, 10-9, 10-14
   glass   10-4, 10-9
      oral   10-9
      rectal   10-9
   tympanic   10-4
thoracic surgeon   3-14
thoracic surgery   3-14
thrombus   15-10
thymus gland   17-15
thyroid cartilage   18-8
thyroid gland   17-13
   disorders   17-13
tissues   1-3, 9-28, 13-5, 13-6
   types of   13-5
tongue-jaw lift   18-11
   defined   18-11
tonometer   17-6
tonsillitis   15-14, 18-16
tort   4-8
   defined   4-8
touch   17-11, 17-12
toxic, defined   18-33
trachea   10-19
   defined   16-3
tracheostomy   18-7
traction, defined   11-5
traction devices   11-5
transfers   7-8–7-10
Transitional Care Unit   2-4, 2-18
Transmission-based Precautions   9-6, 9-
      24, 9-25, 9-26, 9-28, 9-29
   airborne transmission   9-26
   contact transmission   9-25
   defined   9-25
   droplet transmission   9-26
Transportation Department   2-6
trapeze   11-5
trauma   18-5, 18-17
   blunt   18-17
   centers   2-4
   defined   10-26
   facial   18-7
   team   2-4
Trendelenburg position   18-21
triage, defined   8-2
tuberculosis   9-26
   respirator   9-26
tumors   17-22
tympanic membrane   10-14

U

ulcer   16-9, 18-7
    defined   16-9
ultrasound   16-15, 17-23
unconscious patients   18-26
understanding your patient   5-1–5-18
United States Department of Health and
        Human Services   9-3
upper GI (gastrointestinal) series   16-12
upper respiratory infection   16-6
ureters, defined   16-19
urgent care centers   1-5
urinary bladder, defined   16-19
urinary system   16-16–16-20
    conditions of   16-19, 16-20
    diagnostic tests   16-20
urinary tract   9-5
    infection   16-20
urine   9-28
urologist   3-14
urology   3-8, 3-14
uterus, defined   17-17

V

varicella   9-25, 9-26
vein   10-19, 15-3, 18-17
    defined   10-19, 15-3
venography   15-11
ventilation   16-5, 18-6, 18-7, 18-9, 18-12,
        18-14, 18-15
    defined   16-5
    mouth-to-mask procedure   18-6
    mouth-to-mouth procedure   18-6
    mouth-to-nose   18-7
    mouth-to-stoma procedure   18-7
ventilation lung scan   16-7
ventilation to compression ratio 18-13, 18-14
ventilators, defined   18-7
ventricle, defined   15-6, 15-16
venules   15-3
verbal communication   6-3
    defined   6-3
vermiform appendix, defined   16-10
VICA   4-14
viruses   9-8–9-11, 9-14, 9-21, 9-28
    controlling   9-8
    defined   9-8
visceral   14-9

vision   17-3 – 17-5
vital organs   18-9
vital signs   1-3, 10-2, 10-3, 10-19, 10-
        20, 10-31, 10-41, 10-45
    defined   10-2
vitamins   19-7, 19-9, 19-10, 19-12
    defined   19-7
vocal folds, defined   16-3
Vocational Industrial Clubs of America
        (VICA)   4-14
volunteers   1-6
vomiting   16-9
vulva, defined   17-18

W

walkers   11-6
warming blanket   11-12
weight   10-41
    body mass index   19-17
    converting   10-41
    suggested   19-16
    adult   10-42–10-43
    children   10-41
    infants   10-41
wellness   2-2
    defined   2-19
wheelchairs   7-10, 7-11
    defined   11-5
women's hospital   2-3
word elements   12-4
    combining form   12-2
    combining vowel   12-2
    prefix   12-2
    root word   12-2
    suffix   12-2
workplace safety   7-1–7-22

X

x-ray   2-6, 2-9, 2-10, 14-8
    department   2-9
    machine   1-3

Y

yeasts   9-8

Clinical Allied Healthcare Series

*Created by healthcare professionals and experienced educators, this Series brings students the knowledge and training essential for careers in hospitals, medical centers, and physicians' offices. **Career's Clinical Allied Healthcare Series** encourages students to master concepts and skills in its intelligent, reader-friendly text, informative illustrations and graphs, critical thinking exercises, and student enrichment activities. This Series offers administrators the coursework texts that fill classrooms—and students and instructors a text series that is the most versatile and comprehensive in its field.*

Introduction to Clinical Allied Healthcare, 2nd Edition (*Core Text*)

Introduction to Healthcare Facilities • The Acute Care Hospital • Hospital Employees and Medical Staff • The Allied Health Worker, the Law, and Professional Ethics • Understanding the Patient as a Person • Communication Skills • The Safe Workplace • Disasters: Preparedness, Hazards, & Prevention • Infection Control • Fundamental Skills • Fundamental Patient Care Equipment • Introduction to Medical Terminology • Introduction to the Human Body • Support, Movement, & Protection: The Skeletal, Muscular, and Integumentary Systems • Transporting and Transmitting: The Circulatory, Lymphatic, and Nervous Systems • Excretion: The Respiratory, Digestive, and Urinary Systems • The Specialties: The Sensory and Reproductive Systems • Basic First Aid • Healthful Living • Career Planning

ISBN 0-89262-551-1 .... **CALL FOR QUOTE**
***Workbook* ISBN 0-89262-550-3** .... **CALL**
***Instructor's Guide* ISBN 0-89262-552-X**

The Emergency Department Technician

Health Careers in Emergency Care • Introduction to Emergency Medical Services • The Working Environment • Asepsis • Admitting Procedures • Patient Evaluation • Safety In the Emergency Department • Basic Life Support • Emergencies of the Eye, Ear, Nose, and Throat • Medical Emergencies • Abdominal Emergencies • Emergencies of the Reproductive System • Wound Care • Traumatic Emergencies • Bone and Joint Injuries • Moving and Positioning Patients • Environmental Emergencies • Poisoning and Overdose • Emotional and Behavioral Emergencies • Caring for Children • Care of the Elderly

ISBN 0-89262-432-9 .... **CALL FOR QUOTE**
***Instructor's Guide* ISBN 0-89262-440-X**

The Clinical Laboratory Assistant/Phlebotomist

Introduction to the Career of Clinical Laboratory Assistant/Phlebotomist • Departments in the Clinical Laboratory • Medical Terminology for the Clinical Laboratory Assistant/Phlebotomist • Ethical and Legal Considerations for the Clinical Laboratory Assistant/Phlebotomist • Infection Control Practices in the Clinical Laboratory • General Safety Issues in the Healthcare Environment • An Introduction to Blood Drawing: The Circulatory System • Preparing for Blood Collection • Performing the Venipuncture • Performing the Skin Puncture • Special Blood Collection Procedures • Hazards and Complications of Blood Drawing • Obtaining Blood Samples from Animals • Urine Specimen Collection • Collection of Other Non-Blood Specimens • Quality Assurance and the Clinical Laboratory Assistant/Phlebotomist • Transporting, Processing, and Distributing Clinical Specimens • Operating Laboratory Equipment • Measurements and Calculations • Reception and Telephone Technique • The Computer System and Other Office Machines • Health Insurance • Customer Service Skills • Conflict Management in the Clinical Laboratory • Obtaining the Right Job for You • The Excellent Clinical Laboratory Employee • Certification, Regulations, and Continuing Education Requirements

ISBN 0-89262-434-5 .... **CALL FOR QUOTE**
***Instructor's Guide* ISBN 0-89262-442-6**

The Operating Room Aide

Introduction to the Operating Room • Medical Terminology for the Operating Room • Principles of Microbiology & Infection Control • Medical and Surgical Asepsis • Operating Room Design and Surgical Equipment • Safety & Patient Care in the Operating Room • Procedures in the Operating Room • Emergencies in the Operating Room • The Operating Room Aide in the Instrument Room

ISBN 0-89262-433-7 .... **CALL FOR QUOTE**
***Instructor's Guide* ISBN 0-89262-441-8**

The Mental Health Worker: Psychiatric Aide

Mental Health Care: Past and Present • Normal Growth and Development • Anxiety • Trust and Communication • Safety in the Workplace • General Patient Care • Chemical Dependency • Common Psychiatric Disorders • Developmental Disorders Affecting Children and Adults • Alzheimer's Disease and Other Dementias • Mental Retardation and Other Developmental Anomalies • Assaultive and Other Unsafe Behaviors • Documenting Patient Status • Patients' Rights

ISBN 0-89262-437-X .... **CALL FOR QUOTE**
***Instructor's Guide* ISBN 0-89262-445-0**

The Pharmacy Aide

Introduction to the Role of the Pharmacy Aide • The Pharmacy Team The Role and Responsibilities of the Pharmacy Aide • Pharmacology Basics • The Prescription • Inventory Control in the Pharmacy • Staying Healthy as a Pharmacy Aide

ISBN 0-89262-438-8 .... **TBA**
***Instructor's Guide* ISBN 0-89262-446-9**

Introduction to Sports Medicine and Physical Therapy

Introduction • Athletic Training • Personal Fitness Training • Physical Therapy • The Structure of the Human Body — Cells, Skeletal & Muscular Systems, Body Planes & Directional Terms • The Circulatory, Respiratory, & Nervous Systems • Basic Nutrition & Weight Control • Basic Skills — Asepsis, Standard Precautions, Vital Signs, etc. • The First Aid Kits • Emergency Preparedness & Assessment • Treatment of Injuries • Basic Life Support • Prevention of Injuries • Assessment of Physical Fitness • Developing an Individual Training Program • Weight Training • Therapeutic Modalities • Physical Rehabilitation • The Law and Ethics • Resumé and Interview

ISBN 0-89262-436-1 .... **TBA**
***Instructor's Guide* ISBN 0-89262-444-2**

The Electrocardiograph Technician

The ECG Technician • Fundamental Concepts • Cardiac Anatomy & Physiology • ECG Basics—The Heartbeat as a Waveform • The 12 Lead ECG • Recognizing Arrhythmias • Bedside Monitoring & Troubleshooting

ISBN 0-89262-435-3 .... **TBA**
***Instructor's Guide* ISBN 0-89262-443-4**

The Pharmacy Technician

Content to be determined.

ISBN 0-89262-455-8 .... **TBA**
***Instructor's Guide* ISBN 0-89262-446-9**

Phone *Toll Free* — From the U.S./Alaska, Hawaii, Canada & Puerto Rico **1-800-854-4014 (FAX 1-714-532-0180)**

ORDER FORM

Career
PUBLISHING INCORPORATED
VOCATIONAL & APPLIED TECHNOLOGY

910 N. Main Street • Orange, CA 92867-5403
P.O. Box 5486 • Orange, CA 92863-5486

Call our Order Dept. at our
National Toll Free Number
1-800-854-4014
includes Alaska, Hawaii,
Puerto Rico, and Canada

**FAX ORDERS
1-(714)-532-0180
24 HOURS**

Clinical Allied Healthcare Series

PLEASE SEND THE FOLLOWING

QTY.	CODE	TITLE	NET PRICE	TOTAL
	0-89262-551-1	**Intro. to Clinical Allied Healthcare, 2nd Edition** (*Core Text*)		$
	0-89262-550-3	**Introduction to Clinical Allied Healthcare** *Workbook*		$
	0-89262-552-X	**Intro. to Clinical Allied Healthcare, 2nd Ed.** *Instructor's Guide*		$
	0-89262-432-9	**The Emergency Department Technician**	**CALL**	$
	0-89262-440-X	**The Emergency Department Technician** *Instructor's Guide*		$
	0-89262-433-7	**The Operating Room Aide**	**FOR**	$
	0-89262-441-8	**The Operating Room Aide** *Instructor's Guide*		$
	0-89262-437-X	**The Mental Health Worker: Psychiatric Aide**	**QUOTE**	$
	0-89262-445-0	**The Mental Health Worker: Psychiatric Aide** *Instructor's Guide*		$
	0-89262-434-5	**The Clinical Laboratory Assistant/Phlebotomist**		$
	0-89262-442-6	**The Clinical Lab. Assistant/Phlebotomist** *Instructor's Guide*		$
	0-89262-438-8	**The Pharmacy Aide**	TBA	$
	0-89262-446-9	**The Pharmacy Aide** *Instructor's Guide*	TBA	$
	0-89262-436-1	**Introduction to Sports Medicine/Physical Therapy**	TBA	$
	0-89262-444-2	**Intro to Sports Medicine/Physical Therapy** *Instructor's Guide*	TBA	$
	0-89262-435-3	**The Electrocardiograph Technician (EKG)**	TBA	$
	0-89262-443-4	**The Electrocardiograph Technician (EKG)** *Instructor's Guide*	TBA	$
	0-89262-455-8	**The Pharmacy Technician**	TBA	$
	0-89262-446-9	**The Pharmacy Technician** *Instructor's Guide*	TBA	$

Payable in U.S. Funds — F.O.B. Orange CA

Shipping, Handling, & Insurance
A single charge to cover shipping, handling, and insurance will be added as a percentage of the total order as follows:
Orders less than $100.00 .... 13%
Orders $100.00 to $499.99 .... 11%
Orders $500.00 to $999.99 .... 9%
Orders of $1,000.00 and over 7%
There will be a minimum charge of $6.00 per order. These costs may be higher for shipments outside the continental United States.

Subtotal $ _____

*Calif. Orders Add Tax _____

TOTAL AMOUNT $ _____

Shipping, Handling, & Insurance Charges _____

GRAND TOTAL $ _____

*California Sales Tax will be added as applicable without Resale Number on file.
PRICES (INCLUDING SHIPPING) AND PUBLICATION DATES SUBJECT TO CHANGE WITHOUT NOTICE.

School/Company/Individual _____ Date _____

Street _____ Phone (____) _____

City _____ State _____ Country _____ Zip _____

Authorized By _____ Title _____

☐ MasterCard ☐ Visa ☐ American Express Card # _____ Exp. _____
MasterCard   Visa   American Express   16 Digits   Mo/Yr
Signature _____ Exact Name on Card _____

Send me ☐ Order Forms ☐ Catalog ☐ Check enclosed Purchase Order Number (PO) _____

Printed in the U.S.A.